Phenomenology, La

Manfred Spitzer   Friedrich Uehlein
Michael A. Schwartz   Christoph Mundt
Editors

Phenomenology, Language & Schizophrenia

With 41 Illustrations

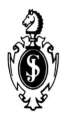

Springer-Verlag

New York Berlin Heidelberg London Paris
Tokyo Hong Kong Barcelona Budapest

Manfred Spitzer, MD, PhD
Christoph Mundt, Prof. Dr. Phil.
Klinikum der Universität Heidelberg
Psychiatrische Klinik
Heidelberg, GERMANY

Friedrich Uehlein, PhD
Philosophische Fakultät II der
Universität Erlangen
Erlangen, GERMANY

Michael A. Schwartz
St. Vincent's Hospital
New York Medical College
New York, NY USA

Library of Congress Cataloging-in-Publication Data
Phenomenology, language, and schizophrenia / [edited by] Manfred
    Spitzer . . .[et al.].
        p. cm.
    Includes bibliographical references and indexes.
    ISBN-13:978-1-4613-9331-3   e-ISBN-13:978-1-4613-9329-0
    DOI: 10.1007/978-1-4613-9329-0
    1. Schizophrenia--Congresses. 2. Phenomenological psychology-
-Congresses. 3. Cognition disorders--Congresses. 4. Delusions-
-Congresses. 5. Schizophrenics--Language--Congresses. I. Spitzer,
Manfred.
    [DNLM: Language--congresses. 2. Philosophy, Medical-
-congresses. 3. Schizophrenia--congresses. WM 203 P5413]
RC54.P48 1993
616.89'92--dc20
DNLM/DLC
for Library of Congress   92-48781

Printed on acid-free paper.

Production managed by Dimitry L. Loseff; manufacturing supervised by Vincent Scelta.
Camera-ready copy prepared by the editors.

9 8 7 6 5 4 3 2 1

ISBN-13:978-1-4613-9331-3

*This volume is
dedicated to the memory of
Hector-Neri Castañeda*

Preface

Phenomenology, Language & Schizophrenia was the title of an international conference, sponsored by the psychiatric University Hospital, Heidelberg. The title of the conference reflects its orientation: "Phenomenology" represents the clinical as well as the philosophical aspect of psychiatric inquiry; "language" not only denotes a subject matter of research, but also a major division within cognitive science, a new interdisciplinary field which bears the prospect of a wealth of new approaches and insights into psychiatric issues. "Schizophrenia" was chosen as the main subject matter and focus of inquiry for this conference for historical and systematic reasons. The Heidelberg University Hospital has a long tradition of influential work in the field of schizophrenia: Many of the people who shaped the concept—Emil Kraepelin, Karl Jaspers, Kurt Schneider, to name but a few—had worked here, and started an influential and fruitful tradition of thought. From a systematic point of view, schizophrenia is one of the most enigmatic, most prevalent, and most devastating disorders, and hence deserves to be one of the major subjects—if not the major subject—of empirical research, clinical study, and conceptual analysis in the field of psychiatry.

The idea of the conference was to bring psychiatrists, psychologists and philosophers together for two days, and have intensive discussions about empirical and conceptual matters in schizophrenia research. The mix of concept-driven and data driven arguments was intended to stimulate fertilization across disciplines, from philosophy to psychiatry, from psychiatry to cognitive science and from cognitive science to philosophy—and back.

The growing interest in the relations between psychiatry and philosophy already was reflected by two previous conferences[1], as well as by the foundation of groups interested in relations between philosophy and psychiatry[2]. Psychology, especially cognitive science, is deeply rooted in philosophy, and societies, journals, and meetings are well established. We are convinced that psychiatry has to offer, and can as well benefit, a lot

---

[1] These conferences took place at the Philosophy Department of the University of Freiburg in 1988, and at the Psychology Department of Harvard University, Cambridge, Mass. in 1989 (cf. Spitzer et al., *Psychopathology and Philosophy*, Heidelberg, Springer, 1988, and Spitzer et al., *Philosophy and Psychopathology*, New York, Springer 1990).

[2] Royal College of Psychiatrys' Philosophy Group, Great Britain; Association for the Advancement of Philosophy and Psychiatry,USA. In Germany, philosophy and psychiatry have always been closer to one another than in the Anglo–American world, and several groups exist.

bridge the gap, to facilitate the dialogue, and to start common projects, we think interdisciplinary work like this conference and book is necessary. Clinical data can be enriched and complemented by data from experimental studies, and both kinds of data can stimulate further analysis of the concepts which were employed to design the experiment and gather the data in the first place. In this way, we will be able to refine our psychopathological concepts, i.e., to enhance their validity and reliability.

This volume is dedicated to the memory of Professor Hector-Neri Castañeda. As a philosopher, he was highly interested in interdisciplinary work of the kind just outlined. In his view, philosophy needs "new data", i.e., has to take into account recent developments in areas of research that produce puzzling findings about man and the various aspects of life. Hence, he was highly interested in the field of psychopathology, which in his view opens up to philosophy thought provoking varieties of human experience. He contributed thoughtful articles to both previous conferences, and would certainly have come to this meeting. Most importantly we missed him as a lively discussant, who—after he seemed to have slept through an entire talk—was able to nail down conceptual difficulties, alternative interpretations, and possible further consequences in an unsurpassed manner. Everybody who had the chance to meet him and talk with him was fascinated by the depth of his philosophical knowledge, his wonderful sense of humor and his brilliant intelligence. He was a person always rewarding to be with.

The symposium was sponsored by the Stiftung Universität Heidelberg, and by the following companies (in alphabetic order): Ciba–Geigy, Desitin, Janssen, Ely-Lilly, Nordmark, Organon, Hoffman LaRoche, Schering, Tropon, and Wander. It was held at the Internationales Wissenschaftsforum, Heidelberg, a site excellently suited to serve the needs of such conferences. We want to express our special thanks to Prof. Ritschl and Dr. T. Reiter for their help with all the "ten thousand little things", as the Chinese would say.

Heidelberg, Erlangen, New York   *Manfred Spitzer*
Spring 1992   *Christoph Mundt*
Friedrich A. Uehlein
Michael A. Schwartz

Contents

Contents

Delusions

Contributors

Winfried Barnett, Dr. med. Dipl. Psych.
Psychiatrische Klinik der Universität
Voss–Str. 4
6900 Heidelberg
FRG

Hinderk Emrich, Prof. Dr. med.
Max–Planck–Institut für Psychiatrie
Kraepelinstr. 10
8000 München 40
FRG

Roselind Fehrenbach, Dr. med.
Psychiatrische Universitätsklinik
Hauptstr. 5
7800 Freiburg
FRG

Jörg Frommer, Dr. med.
Klinik für Psychosomatische Medizin
und Psychotherapie der Universität
Bergische Landstraße 2
4000 Düsseldorf 12
FRG

Mathias Fünfgeld, Dr. phil. Dipl. Psych.
Psychiatrische Universitätsklinik
Hauptstr. 5
7800 Freiburg
FRG

K. William M. Fulford, M.D., Ph.D.
Oxford University
Department of Psychiatry
600 North Wolfe Street
Oxford OX3 7JX
Great Britain

David R. Hemsley, Ph.D.
Department of Psychology
Institute of Psychiatry
De Crespigny Park, Denmark Hill
London, SE5 8AF
Great Britain

Reiner Hess, PD Dr. med.
Abt. Psychiatrie II der Universität Ulm
BKH Günzburg
Ludwig Heilmeyerstr. 2
8870 Günzburg
FRG

Paul Hoff, Dr. med. Dr. phil.
Psychiatrische Klinik der Universität
Nußbaumstr. 7
8000 München 2
FRG

Ralph Hoffman, M.D.
Conneticut Mental Health Center
Clinical Director
34 Park Street
New Haven, CT 06519
USA

Edward Hundert, M.D.
McLean Hospital
Mill Street 115
Belmont, MA 02178
USA

Grant Gillett, M.D.
Department of Surgery, Medical School
University of Otago
Dunedin, New Zealand
New Zealand

Contributors

Theo Manschreck, M.D.
New Hampshire Hospital
Dartmouth Medical School
105 Pleasant Street
Concord, NH 03301-3861
USA

Christoph Mundt, Prof. Dr. med.
Psychiatrische Klinik der Universität
Voss–Str. 4
6900 Heidelberg
FRG

John Z. Sadler, M.D.
Department of Psychiatry
The University of Texas
Southwestern Medical Center
5323 Harry Hines Boulevard
Dallas, Texas 75235
USA

Henning Saß, Prof. Dr. med.
Psychiatrische Klinik der RWTH
Pauwels Str. 30
5100 Aachen
FRG

Louis A. Sass, Ph.D.
Dept. of Clinical Psychology
GSAPP-Busch Campus
Rutgers University
New Brunswick, NJ 08903
USA

Michael A. Schwartz, M.D.
St. Vincent's Hospital
New York Medical College
153 West 11th Street, 3E
New York, N.Y. 10011,
USA

Manfred Spitzer, PD Dr. med. Dr. phil.
Psychiatrische Klinik der Universität
Voss–Str. 4
6900 Heidelberg
FRG

Wolfgang Tress, Prof. Dr. med. Dr. phil.
Klinik für Psychosomatische Medizin
und Psychotherapie der Universität
Bergische Landstraße 2
4000 Düsseldorf 12
FRG

Friedrich A. Uehlein, Prof. Dr. phil.
Philosophische Fakultät II
der Universität Erlangen
Bismarckplatz
8520 Erlangen
FRG

Osborne P. Wiggins, Ph.D.
Department of Philosophy
University of Louisville
Louisville, Kentucky 40292
USA

Introduction

M. Spitzer, F.A. Uehlein
M.A. Schwartz, C. Mundt
(eds.): Phenomenology
Language & Schizophrenia.
Springer-Verlag, New York, 1992

Phenomenology, Language & Schizophrenia: Introduction and Synopsis

Manfred Spitzer, Friedrich A. Uehlein, Michael A. Schwartz

1. The Horizon of Questions: Schizophrenia as Defined in the DSM–III–R

Schizophrenia is one of the most common, most devastating, and most enigmatic of the disorders that plague humankind. About 3 in 1000 people suffer from this disorder at a given time (prevalence: 0.3%), and about 1 in 100 people will be afflicted by the disorder within a year (incidence: 1%). As far as is known, schizophrenia exists in all cultures (with a ten–fold variation of frequency) and has been present throughout history, at least as long as there are records from which some direct or indirect evidence can be derived.

Research on schizophrenia has accelerated over the last two decades. The concept has regained a clear and narrow shape, cases can be reliably identified by explicit criteria, and the biological causes of the disorder are under the scrutiny of more researchers using a more impressive array of research methods than ever. All these efforts promise to bring about a more fruitful understanding of the biological nature of the disorder as well as—the hoped-for ultimate goal—therapeutic advances.

Before we start discussing some recent schizophrenia research issues, we want to clarify what this volume is about. Psychiatrists will be familiar with the concept of schizophrenia as presently employed in research and clinical practice, but some psychologists and most philosophers may not. Hence, we begin this introduction with some lengthy quotes from DSM–III–R, the state–of–the–art manual of psychiatric diagnoses.

"The essential features of this disorder are the presence of characteristic psychotic symptoms during the active phase of the illness and functioning below the highest level previously achieved ... and a duration of at least six months that may include characteristic prodromal or residual symptoms. [...]

Characteristic symptoms involving multiple psychological processes. Invariably there are characteristic disturbances in several of the following areas: content and form of thought, perception, affect, sense of self, volition, relationship to the external world, and psychomotor behavior. It should be noted that no single feature is invariably present or seen in Schizophrenia" (DSM–III–R, pp. 187–188).

As we can see from this preliminary description, there is no "final test" for schizophrenia, no "schizococcus" which can be detected, no X–ray image which can prove the presence or absence of the disorder. All we have, one might say, are basic functions of human beings, such as perception, thought, affect, etc., which are somehow disturbed. The picture is not clear, however, since the disturbances do not seem to show distinct patterns, appear to be unrelated, and, regarding severity, can only be characterized by the criteria of length (6 months) and global "functioning". Even these two criteria are debatable. The International Classification of Diseases, 10th edition (ICD–10), the other major classificatory system, has a different criterion of length (1 month) and of severity (functioning need not necessarily be below the highest level previously achieved, i.e., total recovery is thought to be possible).

It must be emphasized at the outset that when we discuss schizophrenia we discuss the mind and its functions, and hence, that we are engaged in a psychological and also a philosophical enterprise. For the philosopher, phenomenology becomes important when we want to study these mental functions and their disturbances in detail. The psychologist will add that most of the thought processes mentioned are mediated (to say the least) by language, and therefore, that it is necessary to study language and its disorders in schizophrenia.

"*Content of thought.* The major disturbance in the content of thought involves delusions that are often multiple, fragmented, or bizarre (i.e., involving a phenomenon that in the person's culture would be regarded as totally implausible, e.g., thought broadcasting, or being controlled by a dead person). Simple persecutory delusions involving the belief that others are spying on, spreading false rumors about, or planning to harm the person are common. Delusions of reference, in which events, objects, or other people are given particular and unusual significance, usually of a negative or pejorative nature, are also common. For example, the person may be convinced that a television commentator is mocking him.

Certain delusions are observed far more frequently in Schizophrenia than in other psychotic disorders. These include, for instance, the belief or experience that one's thoughts, as they occur, are broadcast from one's head to the external world so that others can hear them (thought broadcasting); that thoughts that are not one's own are inserted into one's mind (thought insertion); that thoughts have been removed from one's head (thought withdrawal); or that one's feelings, impulses, thoughts, or actions are not one's own, but are imposed by some external force (delusions of being controlled). Less commonly, somatic, grandiose, religious, and nihilistic delusions are observed" (DSM–III–R, p. 188).

Delusions are far from being understood, as can be seen from the many theories about their origin and the almost complete lack of literature regarding appropriate treatment approaches. In this book, an entire section is devoted to delusions and several articles in other sections deal with delusions in some way.

Form of thought. A disturbance in the form of thought is often present. This has been referred to as "formal thought disorder,' and is different from a disorder in the content of thought. The most common example of this is loosening of associations, in which ideas shift from one subject to another, completely unrelated or only obliquely related subject, without the speaker's displaying any awareness that the topics are unconnected. Statements that lack a meaningful relationship may be juxtaposed, or the person may shift idiosyncratically from one frame of reference to another. When loosening of associations is severe, the person may become incoherent, that is, his or her speech may become incomprehensible.

There may be poverty of content of speech, in which speech is adequate in amount, but conveys little information because it is vague, overly abstract, or overly concrete, repetitive, or stereotyped. The listener can recognize this disturbance by noting that little if any information has been conveyed although the person has spoken at some length. Less common disturbances include neologisms, perseveration, clanging, and blocking" (DSM–III–R, p. 188).

Disorders of the form of thought are noticed as disturbances of the patient's utterances. Topics may shift in consecutive sentences, several sentences may lack meaningful relatedness, or the speech may become totally incomprehensible. Single words may be affected, i.e., the patient may produce new words (neologisms), repeat the same word, sometimes over and over (perseveration), use words because they rhyme without conveying any meaning (clanging), or merely stop talking before the idea is finished (blocking).

Cognitive science has contributed a lot to our understanding of normal language processes, and therefore, experimental studies heavily influence by cognitive science represent the majority of the papers in the section on language and cognition.

Other aspects of the symptomatology of schizophrenia, for example affect, volition, and psychomotor behavior, are as important as the ones already mentioned and are not covered in special sections in this book. As these areas are the subject of discussion in some of the papers, we will further quote from the DSM–III–R description in order to provide an overview of these clinical phenomena:

"*Perception.* The major disturbances in perception are various forms of hallucinations. Although these occur in all modalities, the most common are auditory hallucinations, which frequently involve many voices the person perceives as coming from outside his or her head. The voices may be familiar, and often make insulting remarks; they may be single or multiple. Voices speaking directly to the person or commenting on his or her ongoing behavior are particularly characteristic. Command hallucinations may be obeyed, which sometimes creates danger for the person or others. Occasionally, the auditory hallucinations are sounds rather than voices.

Tactile hallucinations may be present, and typically involve electrical, tingling, or burning sensations. Somatic hallucinations, such as the sensation of snakes crawling inside the abdomen, are occasionally experienced. Visual, gustatory, and olfactory hallucinations also occur, but with less frequency, and, in the absence of auditory hallucinations, always raise the possibility of an Organic Mental Disorder. Other perceptual abnormalities include sensations of bodily change; hypersensitivity to sound, sight, and smell; illusions; and synesthesias.

Affect. The disturbance often involves flat or inappropriate affect. In flat affect, there are virtually no signs of affective expression; the voice is usually monotonous and the face immobile. The person may complain that he or she no longer responds with normal emotional intensity or, in extreme cases, no longer has feelings. In inappropriate affect, the affect is clearly discordant with the content of the person's speech or ideation. For example, while discussing being tortured by electrical shocks, a person with Schizophrenia, Disorganized Type, may laugh or smile. Sudden and unpredictable changes in affect involving inexplicable outbursts of anger may occur.

Although these affective disturbances are almost invariably part of the clinical picture, their presence is often difficult to detect except when they are in an extreme form. Furthermore, antipsychotic drugs have effects that may appear similar to the affective flattening seen in Schizophrenia.

Sense of self. The sense of self that gives the normal person a feeling of individuality, uniqueness, and self-direction is frequently disturbed in Schizophrenia. This is sometimes referred to as a loss of ego boundaries, and frequently is evidenced by extreme perplexity about one's own identity and the meaning of existence, or by some of the specific delusions described above, particularly those involving control by an outside force.

Impaired interpersonal functioning and relationship to the external world. Difficulty in interpersonal relationships is almost invariably present. Often this takes the form of social withdrawal and emotional detachment. When the person is severely preoccupied with egocentric and illogical ideas and fantasies and distorts or excludes the external world, the condition has been referred to as "autism". Some with the disorder, during a phase of the illness, cling to other people, intrude upon strangers, and fail to recognize the excessive closeness makes other people uncomfortable and likely to pull away" (DSM–III–R, pp. 188–189).

Apart from references to onset, course, outcome, and differential diagnoses, these descriptions define what it is that psychiatrists are so used to calling "schizophrenia". Notice that schizophrenia is thereby defined using features of a peculiar nature: These features are neither observable in the same manner as a wound, a fever, or other *signs* of an illness, nor do many of them seem to reside on the same level as ordinary *symptoms*, such as the experience of pain or of feeling hot. It seems as if many of the subjective features of schizophrenia do not resemble the experience of the disorder of a particular function as much as they resemble disordered experience itself, i.e., *modifications of the experiences of the patient as conveyed through language.*

How can we be sure that our descriptions of such phenomena are adequate? Which field of inquiry deals with problems of this kind?

2. Phenomenology & Language

The word "phenomenology" has various meanings. For most clinicians it merely means *signs and symptoms.* For many psychiatrists, it means *psychopathology in the Jaspersian tradition,* and for philosophers it means *philosophy in the Husserlian tradition.* As we will see, these facets of phenomenology can illuminate aspects of some of the problems stated above. They lead to fruitful conceptual analyses as well as to questions that can be empirically answered.

Phenomenology provides a rich conceptual framework for the description of states of mind. In this sense, it is concerned with "signs and symptoms", but in a much more detailed sense than is usually implied. This is also the Jaspersian meaning of phenomenology, and part of the Husserlian meaning as well. Husserl developed the concepts of *intentionality*, of *passive synthesis*, and of the *flow of inner time* (see Uehlein, this volume). These concepts can be highly useful for any understanding of the way in which patients experience their disorder (see, for example, Wiggins et al. 1990). Phenomenology thus sheds light upon the realm of psychopathology.

From the point of view of the philosophy of science, phenomenology provides *tools* for description, i.e., provides a method for arriving at general concepts which all descriptive work must use. Husserl has shown how we form truly general concepts by means of *eidetic variation*, a process which clarifies the boundaries of concepts of all kind (Uehlein, this volume).

Husserl's phenomenology dealt with the broader problem of how we form general concepts and with the more specific problem of how we describe mental life as we—i.e., I for myself, and you for yourself—know it. In comparison, the main problem for Jaspers and his phenomenology was that of how we understand another person. Needless to say, this problem lies at the heart of psychiatric theory and practice (see Spitzer & Uehlein, as well as Wiggins et al., this volume).

Just as the study of phenomenology leads to insights on different levels of generality, the study of language bears upon the understanding of schizophrenia on several levels. Language processes can be studied on the interactional and the social level, where complex meaning structures, e.g., situations and stories, are involved; on the level of sentences, where more simple meaning–structures are at issue; on the level of single words; and even on the level of phonemes, morphemes and semes, i.e., on the level of minimal distinctive phonetic, structural and semantic features.

From a more practical point of view, yet another distinction between levels of inquiry is important: In psychiatry, symptoms are often much more important than signs. Symptoms are, however, *subjective experiences as reported by the patients*, i.e., symptoms are *necessarily mediated by language*. Patients must use language in order to report changes in their experiences to clinicians. Therefore, the way in which patients use language to describe their symptoms deserves close scrutiny.

When it comes to the symptoms of schizophrenia, language is not only the medium in which pathology is reported, but language is itself subjected to pathological deformation. These pathologies of the processes involved in the production of language and thought are indeed at the very center of schizophrenia (see the above quotes from DSM-III-R).

3. Overview of this Volume & Discussion

This introduction is followed by a brief history of the Heidelberg psychiatric tradition, in particular, of the figures who have played an important role in the process of conceptualizing modern psychopathology. As Mundt illustrates with pictures and words, the Heidelberg Psychiatric University Hospital was the environment in which many of the psychiatric concepts that we now take for granted came into existence.

3.1 Phenomenology

The section on phenomenology starts out with a discussion of the various meanings of phenomenology (Spitzer & Uehlein), followed by a critique of a view on phenomenology which is widely held, but in our opinion nonetheless wrong; Using a recent paper of G.E. Berrios as their target—a target which has the virtues of being short, to the point, well written, and representative—Wiggins et al. point to the limitations of this view.

The methodological contribution of phenomenology to the description of mental life and to the clarification of general concepts is the subject of two contributions by Uehlein.

Sadler endeavors to show the importance of the method of free fantasy variation for psychiatric practice. It remains an open question, however, whether there are enough empirical clinical data to support any conceptual analysis of psychiatric symptomatology which can be claimed to be the final one.

Given the importance of Emil Kraepelin for present day psychiatry, it is appropriate to critically re-evaluate Kraepelin's nosological positions and to highlight the philosophical implications of his work. As Hoff points out, these philosophical overtones are often quite well hidden in Kraepelin's writings but nonetheless demonstrate how closely and necessarily philosophy and psychiatry are linked. Hoff uses Kraepelin as an example of his more general point that mutual disadvantages are the consequence of mutual ignorance between philosophy and psychiatry.

Following Kraepelin's original contributions to psychiatric nosology, successors attempted to extend his conclusions with results that have often been forgotten but which are of interest today. For example, around 1920, Heinrich Körtke tried to improve Kraepelin's classification by proposing the simultaneous usage of two different diagnostic systems for each patient: One for the somatic level of illness and one for the psychopathological level. Hoff recalls Ernst Kretschmer's criticism of this work as terminologically dualistic, strange, artificial, and impractical. Ironically, conceptual dualism is precisely what we find today in DSM-III and DSM-III-R, with its Axis I lists of psychopathological disorders and Axis III lists of physical disorders. In recent decades, innovations of this magnitude have been introduced in the absence of conceptual reflection, yet they have profound consequences for psychiatric practice.

L. Sass attempts to view some basic features of the schizophrenic syndrome as disturbances of experience itself, rather than as disturbances of what is experienced. In his view, the normal interpretation of schizophrenia is modeled on an understanding of what is acceptable as "real" in everyday life. As a result, schizophrenic patients are said to suffer from delusions, poor reality-testing and a poverty of the content of speech. According to L. Sass, the application of Heidegger's ontological difference between Being and beings may open up a more genuine understanding of the lived-world of schizophrenic patients. He proposes that these patients might especially be in touch with, or have a heightened awareness of, Being and the ontological difference. L. Sass believes that Heidegger himself suggested such an application, since his major example of writing that captures the oblivion of the ontological difference and the revelation of Being "is the late work of Friedrich Hölderlin, a poet who was manifestly schizophrenic at the time of producing most of the poetry in question." This link between Heidegger's ontological difference and the schizophrenic experience, however, proves to be rather brittle. It is true that the importance of Hölderlin's poetry for Heidegger can hardly be overestimated. As late as 1963, in an interview in the magazine *Der Spiegel* (9/23/1963), Heidegger confessed: "My own thought stands in an uneliminable relationship to the poetry of Hölderlin"[1] The *Oden, Elegien* and *Vaterländische Gesänge,* which Heidegger quotes and interprets in his own way to form the grand testimonia of the withdrawal and the advent of Being were written between 1799 and 1803: *Gesang des Deutschen* and *Wie wenn am Feiertage* (1799); *Der Gang aufs Land* (1800); *Brod und Wein; Heimkunft; Versöhnender der du nimmergeglaubt; Die Wanderung; Der Rhein; Germanien* (all 1801); *Friedensfeier* (1802); *Patmos; Andenken; Der Ister; Mnemosyne* (all 1803); *In lieblicher Bläue* (of uncertain date, presumably written after 1803). Hölderlin's schizophrenic disorder, however, became evident only in 1804, i.e., when he developed clear signs of formal thought disorder, after he had already suffered from two depressive episodes in 1802 and 1803 (cf. Peters 1981). Therefore, on purely historical grounds, it remains questionable whether those poems of Hölderlin which were the major source for Heidegger already contained signs of, or were already influenced by, schizophrenic symptoms.

From a systematic point of view, it must be asked whether Heideggerian philosophy can in fact serve as an adequate conceptual framework for the analysis of the changes of mental life which happen to schizophrenic patients. Heidegger explicitly dismissed the idea of a subject which construes experience as an active agent. Therefore, it is unlikely in our view that a Heideggerian framework could serve the conceptual needs of psychiatrists interested in schizophrenic psychopathology. L. Sass's chapter may serve as an interesting example of an attempt of elucidating the nature of human experience by general philosophical theories (cf., for

---

1 "Mein Denken steht in einem unumgänglichen Bezug zur Dichtung Hölderlins." The interview appeared after Heidegger's death: Der Spiegel, vol. 30, 1976, nr. 23, p. 193-219

other such attempts Binswanger 1957, 1960, 1965, Blankenburg 1971, Spitzer 1985, Hundert 1989, Wiggins et al. 1990).

3.2 Language and Cognition

The historical roots of one important aspect of the field of language and cognitive psychology are the subject of Spitzer's chapter on word associations in experimental psychiatry. Spitzer shows that experimental "cognitive" approaches played a major role in the very beginnings of academic psychiatry, not only in research but also in the formation of concepts for clinical practice. Kraepelin, Jung, and Bleuler, to name merely the most influential psychiatrists, all believed that association psychology was the way to come to grips with the otherwise confusing symptomatology of schizophrenia. However, for several reasons they failed, and research on word-associations almost ended in the 1920s—only to be revived recently by the emerging field of cognitive science.

H. Sass examines the historical roots of the concept of Zerfahrenheit (any translation of this word has its problems, hence we follow Sass in not translating it at all) which are used to account for thought disorder up to the present day. In the paper, two arguments are presented, one regarding phenomenology as a method and the other regarding a knowledge claim. With respect to the first argument, Sass points out that the phenomenological notion of understanding is helpful in the diagnosis of formal thought disorder. In particular, he claims that the idea that mental events are related in understandable ways is helpful in a proper account of formal thought disorder. While such an approach is certainly "more inferential" than the approach favored by Andreasen, it may come closer to the actual experience of the patient, and hence, closer to one of the most prominent and important subjective psychological aspects of schizophrenic symptomatology. The knowledge claim made by Sass upon such phenomenological grounds, i.e., that "Zerfahrenheit" can be distinguished from "Verschrobenheit" (eccentricity), has to await empirical testing.

Many of the bizarre symptoms of schizophrenia correspond to alterations in the experience of the will. The DSM–III–R gives the following description:

"*Volition.* The characteristic disturbances in volition are most readily observed in the residual phase. There is nearly always some disturbance in self-initiated, goal-directed activity, which may grossly impair work or other role functioning. This may take the form of inadequate interest, drive, or ability to follow a course of action to its logical conclusion. Marked ambivalence regarding alternative courses of action can lead to near-cessation of goal-directed activity" (DSM–III–R p. 189).

Hoffman provides an phenomenological analysis of involuntary actions. Schizophrenic patients often report ideation experienced as deriving from an alien, nonself force. According to Hoffman, such ideation reflects internally coherent cognitive plans which unfold independently of, and are in conflict with, the conscious goals and actions of the individual. The author exemplifies his hypothesis by examining the speech disturbances of schizophrenic patients. At the syntactic and the discourse level of speech production, different planning structures simultaneously compete for expression. These plans may be further elaborated but may nonetheless remain more or less out of consciousness. According to Hoffman, such preconscious language plans form the mental nucleus of experiences of both alien thoughts and auditory hallucinations.

Texts of schizophrenic patients show significantly more incoherence than those of patients with other syndromes and normals. Frommer and Tress define incoherence as a disorder in the implicit dialog structure of text, and claim that it is based on deficits in the capacity of taking the role of the other person. Patients are unable to see themselves in a stable and consistent way as both an object and a subject. It remains an open question whether disturbances in the process of role–taking in social interaction are caused by fundamental disturbances in the self–awareness and self–consciousness of schizophrenic patients. Empirical studies by Frommer and Tress are presented to support their theoretical approach.

In his chapter on cognitive abnormalities and the symptoms of schizophrenia, Hemsley gives an information processing account of schizophrenic psychopathology. He argues that schizophrenia, and in particular delusion formation, is characterized by a weakening of the influence of the regularities of previous input on current perception. Hemsley summarizes recent experimental work relevant to his model. His paper exemplifies how paradigms derived from animal learning theory can influence biological models of schizophrenia.

The psychopathological nature of negative schizophrenia is investigated by Barnett and Mundt. Contrary to widely held opinions and to what was expected, the results of their study suggest that affective rather than cognitive dysfunction plays the primary role in the development of negative symptoms. However, it must be taken into account that their sample consisted of young inpatients who were recently recovering from a major psychotic episode.

Abnormalities of motor behavior are an essential part of schizophrenic symptomatology.

"*Psychomotor behavior.* Various disturbances in psychomotor behavior are observed, particularly in the chronically severe and acutely florid forms of the disorder. There may be a marked decrease in reactivity to the environment, with a reduction in spontaneous movements and activity. In extreme cases the person appears unaware of the naute of the environment (as in catatonic stupor); may maintain a rigid posture and resist efforts to be moved (as in catatonic rigidity); may make apparently purposeless and stereotyped, excited motor movements not influenced by external stimuli (as in catatonic excitement); may voluntarily assume inappropriate or bizarre postures (as in catatonic posturing); or may resist and actively counteract instructions or attempts to be moved (as in catatonic negativism). In addition, odd mannerisms, grimacing, or waxy flexibility may be present" (DSM-III-R, pp. 189-190).

The importance of understanding these abnormalities of motor behavior and of relating them to other aspects of schizophrenic pathology is
highlighted by Manschreck. Results from several empirical studies are
presented which demonstrate the frequent occurrence of motor abnormalities and their association with a variety of psychopathological features.
The evidence indicates that motor anomalies constitute a core disturbance
in schizophrenia.

Fünfgeld et al. present a study on laterality in schizophrenic and
depressed patients. They use a divided visual field paradigm with either
words or faces which are to be distinguished from non-words and non-
faces. In addition, they investigate the effect of emotional stimulation.
Their results are largely in line with the findings of other investigators of a
bilateral hemispheric deficit in schizophrenia and of major right hemispheric involvement in depression. From a methodological perspective, the
finding that accuracy and speed may vary independently in opposite
directions requires further study. This finding reveals difficulties in
assessment strategies of laterality that use reaction times and error rates as
dependent variables.

Hess et al. report preliminary data on a comparative study of attention
in schizophrenic patients and normal control subjects. The results of the
two paradigms indicate a poorer performance by schizophrenic patients
and additionally point to a previously unrecognized attentional deficit.
These experiments are interesting from a systematic as well as a
methodological point of view: If schizophrenic patients are given enough
time to perform a required task, there remains surprisingly little difference
in the number and type of errors reported as compared to controls.
Therefore, it is possible that the only attentional deficit in schizophrenic
patients consists of a need for more time to process information.

3.3 Delusions

In their clinically oriented chapter, Schwartz and Wiggins advance the
hypothesis that schizophrenic patients may believe and disbelieve their
delusions at the same time. What appears to the clinician as delusional
certainty may in fact be more accurately accounted for as a striving for
certainty. From a methodological perspective, this hypothesis is motivated
by anecdotal evidence only. However, it has empirically testable consequences and therapeutic potential. As the authors rightly point out, these
findings have to be settled empirically; for example, how frequently the
phenomenon of a double orientation really occurs, in what kind of patients
it is found, and in what manner it is related to other features of delusional
syndromes. The effectiveness of the proposed therapeutic strategy could
even be tested by means of an experimental design. In our view, such
clinically oriented studies are of value and have been neglected in the
recent history of our field: Without accurate clinical work to generate

hypotheses such as the one proposed in the paper, clinical research cannot progress to new insights.

Gillett develops an interpersonal or intersubjective view in his analysis of the kind of rationality which allows us to distinguish between rational behavior and delusions. According to Gillett, mental content is based on doing things and relating to others rather than on receiving and connecting data from a purely objective world; i.e., the construction of mental life does not proceed via purely formal or causal, truth–preserving operations. Instead, rationality and truth are linked to rule–governed techniques of articulating one's activity with the world. Beliefs, rationality, and values combine to form an interconnected cognitive repertoire which is holistic and instrumental, explains behavior, aims at truth, and arises in discourse. Psychotic patients suffer from a disruption of their integrity as human agents; they are split from the sensus communis as well as from the vita communis. Several features of delusions, such as their tendency to have personal content, their tendency to be relative to a culture, and the specific relation of delusions and insight are discussed within this framework.

The nature of the relation between emotions and delusions is discussed in Spitzer's chapter. In order to do so, the concept of affect (emotion) is analyzed from a systematic and historical perspective. Then, views about the role of affect on the formation of delusions are presented: Hagen, Specht and Bleuler favored the idea that affective changes, even if we do not notice them, are among the main causes of delusions. In contrast, Jaspers, Gruhle and Schneider proposed the opposite view, i.e., that real (primary, proper) delusions are not caused by affects. The issue has not yet been resolved. Examples are provided to demonstrate that present day psychiatry seems to fail to handle the problem of affect and delusion in a scientifically sound way. It is argued that conceptual and empirical questions have to be disentangled in order to ask the right questions and to answer them in a non–prejudiced manner.

Hundert emphasizes the adaptive role that some delusions may have. As he correctly states, it is nearly always possible to ask if a psychotic symptom represents primary brain pathology or a reparative effort of the healthier part of the individual's mental apparatus to find a way to continue living with that pathology. In the case of delusions, most theorists, including Hundert, favor the latter "adaptive" view: Delusions are viewed not a disorder but rather as the healthy reaction of a person to some kind of disorder. Hundert then goes on to investigate the dilemma that the truth–value of many statements is either never defined or is context dependent (as Hegel emphasized with his famous example "it is raining now"). Clinicians can in fact distinguish between delusions and other statements, but they do so not by determining the truth value of these statements, but rather by determining how the statements in question are justified in a dialogue. Hundert goes on to correctly emphasize the meaning of delusions for therapeutic interventions. Before we treat patients with delusions, we should know whether their delusions serve any function or purpose. If so, we still may want to treat them, but we will do more justice to the patient's needs if we assess what their function or purpose is.

Starting with the Wittgensteinian assumption that the use of a concept is a better guide to its meaning than a definition, Fulford examines the notion of insight in psychiatry. He points out that difficulties in defining psychotic loss of insight are due to the adoption of the disease paradigm of mental disorder. Fulford contrasts this standard view with his approach towards insight in the general framework of an illness paradigm of mental disorder. Psychotic loss of insight is relatively transparent in meaning if the notion is derived from certain general features of the patient's actual experience of illness. The analysis of the differential diagnoses of certain psychotic symptoms—thought insertion, hallucination and delusion—serves to illustrate this point.

Emrich analyses delusions in terms of a theory of subjectivity which employs concepts from modern Western philosophy as well as from systems theory. Based on a model of how human beings actively perceive the outside world, Emrich discusses a possible mechanism of delusion formation which involves the misconstrual of sense data caused by a failure to correct for certain errors.

4. Conclusion: Synthesizing Conceptual & Empirical Analyses

This volume is based on a conference of the same title which took place in Heidelberg on the 12th to 14th of September in 1991. It was our goal to bring together psychiatrists and psychologists who work on empirical questions using experimental approaches on the one hand, and on the other hand psychiatrists, psychologists and philosophers who engage in conceptual analyses of the presuppositions and concepts that underlie our field and drive the research. Our aim was to provide a basis for discussions which would be empirically grounded as well as conceptually rich, detailed and deep. In this way, we anticipate the advancement of knowledge in clinical work and in research.

In our view, it is unfortunate that philosophically minded psychiatrists are sometimes regarded as "merely soft" as opposed to "hard–nosed" biologically minded psychiatrists; that the discussions seem to reflect more polemics than an interest in real solutions; that there even seems to be competition between two approaches, etc.

On the contrary, we are convinced that real progress will only be made through a integration of approaches as different as the fine–grained analyses of subjective phenomena *and* the collection of detailed biological parameters. Such a synthesis of empirical approaches together with conceptual ones enlarges the foundations of a genuinely comprehensive psychiatry.

References

American Psychiatric Association: Diagnostic and Statistical Manual of Mental Disorders, third edition, revised (DSM–III–R). Washington, DC, American Psychiatric Association, 1987

Berrios GE: What Is Phenomenology? A Review. Journal of the Royal Society of Medicine 82: 425-428, 1989

Binswanger L: Schizophrenie. Pfulingen, Neske, 1957

Binswanger L: Melancholie und Manie. Pfulingen, Neske, 1960

Binswanger L: Wahn. Pfulingen, Neske, 1965

Blankenburg W: Der Verlust der natürlichen Selbstverständlichkeit. Stuttgart, Enke, 1971

Hundert EM: Philosophy, Psychiatry, and Neuroscience: Three Approaches to the Mind. Oxford University Press, 1989

Peters UH: Hölderlin: Dichter, Kranker – Simulant? Nervenarzt 51: 261–268, 1981

Spitzer M: Allgemeine Subjektivität und Psychopathologie. Frankfurt, Haag und Herchen, 1985

Spitzer M: Why Philosophy? In: Spitzer M, Maher BA (eds) Philosophy and Psychopathology, pp. 3–18, Springer, New York, Heidelberg, Berlin, London Paris, Tokyo, Hong Kong, 1990

Wiggins OP, Schwartz MA, Northoff G: Toward a Husserlian Phenomenology of the Initial Stages of Schizophrenia. In: Spitzer M, Maher BA (eds) Philosophy and Psychopathology, pp. 21–34, Springer, New York, Heidelberg, Berlin, London Paris, Tokyo, Hong Kong, 1990

M. Spitzer, F.A. Uehlein
M.A. Schwartz, C. Mundt
(eds.): Phenomenology
Language & Schizophrenia.
Springer-Verlag, New York, 1992

The History of Psychiatry in Heidelberg

Christoph Mundt

The beginning of academic psychiatry in Heidelberg in 1878 was preceded by a long struggle between the medical faculty and non-academic care-takers for the mentally ill. In 1827, the Ministry of the Interior of the State of Baden appointed a young and ambitious physician, Karl Friedrich Roller, to give lectures and work out plans for a modern psychiatric hospital (Middelhoff 1979). The medical faculty, however, refused to permit Roller to lecture because he had not yet written a thesis and there-fore did not possess a medical degree. Perhaps because of this personal insult, or possibly for more sincere reasons, after an educational tour of the European madhouses of his time, Roller developed a philosophy for hospital-based care of the mentally ill which was totally opposed to the needs of academic psychiatry. He recommended to the Ministry of the Interior that mentally ill patients should be isolated in rural areas and separated from their families and their usual social surroundings in order to calm down their emotions. Furthermore, Roller proclaimed that the tasks of hospital director and academic professor were so demanding that they were incompatible and should not be taken over by the same person (a view which may be not so wrong after all). The ministry followed his recommendations and, as a result, instead of a psychiatric university hospital, the mental hospital Illenau was built to the southwest of Heidelberg and opened in 1842. Over the following two decades, this hospital gained a very high reputation and even outshined academic psychiatry at the university. Its directors, von Gudden (later chairman in Munich), Krafft-Ebing (later chairman in Vienna), and Schüle (who declined several academic appointments), made the Illenau internationally well known. At the same time, psychiatric lectures in Heidelberg were provided by internists and neurologists. This early clash between academic and non-academic psychiatry at Illenau and Heidelberg unfortunately characterized the relationship between the two institutions for many decades. Indeed, only in the present era have the two hospitals finally reconciled through a day hospital joint venture. One practical consequence of Roller's victory over Heidelberg was the prominent development at

Illenau of services for acute and chronic patients. On the other hand, the Psychiatric University Hospital in Heidelberg was often criticized for its lack of therapeutic accomplishments and engagement, even in its best period in the 1920s.

In 1878, the year of Roller's death, the university psychiatric hospital finally overcame all obstacles and was opened. Figures 1 and 2 show the old construction plans of the front building (Figure 1) and the rear buildings (Figure 2), in both cases viewed from both sides. Despite several renovations, these buildings are essentially unchanged today. Friedreich, a neurologist and dean at Heidelberg, recruited the neuropathologist Fürstner to be the university's first psychiatry chairman (Table 1). Fürstner's neuropathological work was not very influential. In 1890, he went to Straßburg and took his assistant Hoche along with him. Later on, as chairman in Freiburg, Hoche played an unfortunate role in German psychiatry as a promotor of euthanasia. In 1920, together with the lawyer Karl Binding, he published the book: *The Abolition of Life Unworthy of Living*. The book promoted euthanasia for chronically ill patients, especially psychiatric patients, with Hoche lending his full academic authority to these suggestions. This publication may have facilitated the actions that the Nazis took in the 1940s, although Hoche himself did oppose the Nazis (Schimmelpfenning 1990).

Fürstner's successor Kraepelin (Figure 3) was called from Dorpat (a town in Estonia which is now called Tartu) in 1891. Kraepelin's first text-book had been published in 1883, and the second edition in 1887. The decisive sixth edition of his textbook, in which he worked out his dichotomy of the endogenous psychoses, was prepared and published in Heidelberg in 1899. Kraepelin left for Munich in 1903, unwilling and disappointed, since his main wish, to relieve the hospital from mandatory admissions from its catchment area, had not been fulfilled (Kraepelin 1983).

During his chairmanship, Kraepelin attracted many co-workers who were to become famous psychiatrists. The best known internationally is Alois Alzheimer, who followed Kraepelin to Munich after only about one year at the Heidelberg Hospital. Another important neuropathologist, Nissl, who described the neuropathology of paralysis, remained at the hospital and later on became its director. Among co-workers who are internationally less well known, Robert Gaupp should be mentioned. Later chairman in Tübingen, he wrote an extensive case report (1920) on a spectacular forensic case of paranoia, a man who slaughtered several persons. Gaupp explained the biographical and inner world development of this patient in detail and concluded that the logic of a person's psychological development can be a constituting factor for psychosis. This idea was adopted and further developed by Ernst Kretschmer, one of Gaupp's successors to the Tübingen chair, in a monograph on the sensitive delusion of reference (1927). Kretschmer's work in this monograph as well as his studies on temperament, character and psychosis (1931) led him to postulate that transitions occur between personality variants and psychosis. However, transitions and psychological interpretations of the psychotic process were strictly rejected by Kraepelin, and later by Jaspers (1913) and Kurt Schneider (1946, 1976). This controversy between the Tübingen and Heidelberg schools provoked many papers in the following decades. Jaspers approached this question by differentiating between the psychological process of "understanding," which is relevant to psychological developments in psychic life, and the process of "explaining," which pinpoints causal connections applicable to physical and somatic events in "process" psychoses. Here, according to Jaspers, the biographical net of meanings and purposes is torn asunder. Kurt Schneider, in his *Clinical Psychopathology*, again referred to this question with a somewhat overexact differentiation between an understandable paranoid reaction which arises out of the emotional background of a patients' actual biographical situation, and delusional perception, wherein this emotional background is missing—an absolute border, as Kurt Schneider put it, between a psychosis and a non-psychotic paranoid reaction. Fortunately for psychiatry, the rivalry between Tübingen and Heidelberg schools, although rather academic, did lead to sharp differentiations in psychopathological terms which remain valuable for the present day operationalizing of diagnoses.

In 1928, on the occasion of the 50th anniversary of the hospital's foundation, a symposium was held which celebrated the hospital's accomplishments. Most emphasized, of course, was Kraepelin's revolutionary simplification of the diagnostic system, with clear-cut triadic categories (organic psychiatric diseases; endogenous psychoses; and abnormal personalities, reactions and developments) and the dichotomy of the endogenous psychoses. By the time of this conference, Kraepelin's views had long since succeeded Griesinger's concept of unitary psychosis and were also outweighing opposing tendencies towards more differentiation of the psychoses proposed by Wernicke and later, by K. Leonhard. These views of Wernicke and Leonhardt would begin to be appreciated again in years to come, when difficulties with the Kraepelinian system came up in the form of the schizoaffective psychoses. It is of interest that the only critical remarks regarding contributions to this symposium came from Mayer-Gross (1929), who stated his view that Kraepelin lacked regard for the historical dimension of life histories and the inner logic of developments in the psychic life of his patients.

Kraepelin's successor, Karl Bonhoeffer, the author of the concept of exogenous reaction types and later chairman of psychiatry in Berlin, stayed for only two months. Janzarik (1978) reported a nice anecdote on the encounter of Kraepelin and Bonhoeffer. Bonhoeffer, carelessly enough, addressed the topic of alcoholism. Instantly, he was trapped in a twelve hour sermon by Kraepelin on alcohol pathology and the advantages of U-boat warfare. Bonhoeffer eventually withdrew with a severe attack of migraine.

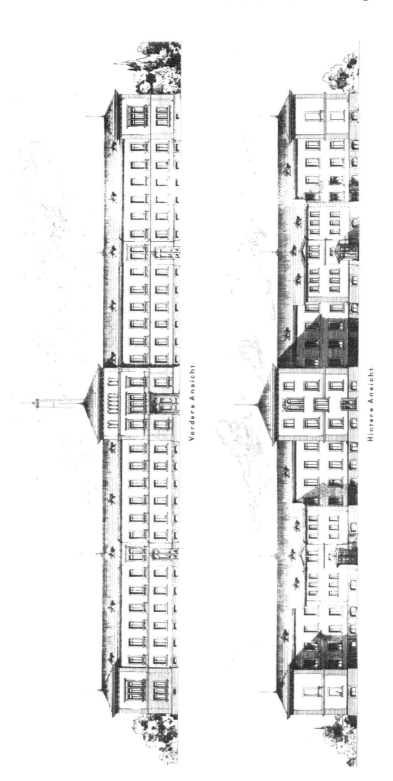

Figure 1: Construction plan of the front building of the Psychiatric University Hospital

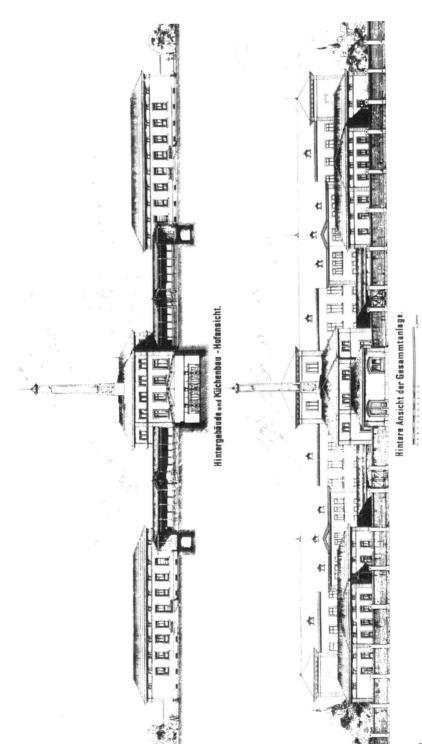

Figure 2: Construction plan of the rear building of the Psychiatric University Hospital

Although Bonhoeffer's successor Nissl's (Figure 4) main interest was neuropathology, under his chairmanship the hospital gained new renown because of the prominence of its psychopathologists. Nissl managed to foster a creative atmosphere with controversial, often critical discussions and yet at the same time with a feeling of belonging and working together in an important stage of the development of clinical psychiatry. Jaspers wrote that without this atmosphere and without prominent co-workers gathered together in the hospital during the Nissl era his book would never have been written. Jaspers especially viewed Gruhle as indispensable, and in a unpublished letter Janzarik quotes Jaspers as praising Gruhle for his "daily critical thrashing". Jaspers (Figure 5), freed from every day clinical work as a result of bronchiectasis, published his *General Psychopathology* in 1913. His main intention, he declared, was to develop a methodological approach to clinical psychopathology which would rely on philosophical categories and clinical empirism. If methodological distinctions were not carefully reflected upon, cloudy concepts would arise. As a consequence of his approach, Jaspers strictly rejected the intermingling of psychopathological and existential or transcendental issues. He did not appreciate the philosophical turn in Heidelberg psychopathology in the 1950s and 1960s which was based on the work of Husserl and Heidegger. Therefore, concerning Jaspers work, the term phenomenology may be misleading. One should speak of descriptive phenomenology as compared to anthropological phenomenology in the sense of Husserl's use of this term as a psychology of the transcendental organization of the mind.

Mayer-Gross (Figure 6), another one of Nissl's co-workers, needs hardly any introduction for Anglo-Saxon readers. In the German literature, his work on oneiroid states is probably better known than the textbook that he wrote together with Eliot Slater and Sir Martin Roth. Mayer-Gross' psychopathological descriptions of the short term course of schizophrenia and of patients' different attitudes towards their illness (1920) are still worth reading. In the Anglo-American literature, McGlashan has taken up these ideas with his descriptions of modes of integration and sealing over in delusional patients. In 1928, Mayer-Gross together with Beringer founded the journal *Der Nervenarzt*, which today is the most influential and best selling German-speaking psychiatric journal.

Beringer became famous for studies on experimental psychoses with mescaline and other substances which he administered to volunteers from among his colleagues in the hospital (1927). Subjects in these experiments invariably underwent characteristic stages of drug effect: 1) autonomic (vegetative) dysregulation 2) decline of attention, and 3) affective derailment. Therefore, for Beringer, perception, state of consciousness, and affective experience belong together as areas of disturbance in experimental psychoses.

Gruhle (Figure 7) played a predominant role in the Nissl-Wilmanns era in the hospital, although the publications of others' became better known. His monograph on the psychology of schizophrenia in 1929

(Berze and Gruhle) is considered the most comprehensive and mature of his publications. However, the substantial influence that Gruhle exerted on the hospital was based on his wit and criticism, which was met with admiration as well as apprehension. One of his sayings was: "Comments in discussion have to be short and insulting".

Table 1: Directors of the Psychiatric University Hospital Heidelberg

Director	Chair	Later famous co-workers
C. Fürstner	1878-1890	(A. Hoche)
E. Kraepelin	1891-1903	A. Alzheimer, G. Aschaffenburg, R. Gaupp, F. Nissl, E. Rüdin, E. Trömner, K. Wilmanns
K. Bonhoeffer	1904	
F. Nissl	1904-1918	H.W. Gruhle, A. Homburger, K. Jaspers, A. Kronfeld, W. Mayer-Gross, O. Ranke
K. Wilmanns	1918-1933	W. v. Baeyer, H. Bürger-Prinz, K. Beringer, H. Prinzhorn, H. Ruffin
C. Schneider	1933-1945	
K. Schneider	1945-1955	W. de Boor, G. Huber, W. Janzarik, K.P.Kisker, H. Leferenz, H.H. Wieck
W. v. Baeyer	1955-1972	W. Blankenburg, W. Böker, W. Bräutigam, H. Häfner, H. Tellenbach, D.v. Zerssen
W. Janzarik	1973-1988	

Nissl's succession by Wilmanns (Figure 8) can be considered as a continuity until the Nazis took over. Wilmanns' daughter, the American psychoanalyst Ruth Lidz, married to Teodore Lidz, has told stories about the destitute persons Wilmanns studied (1906). Some of them turned up in his private home, borrowed money from him and, to his daughter's amazement, repaid their debt months later. Wilmanns was forced by the Nazis to give up his chair, probably due to his comment on Hitler's hysterical blindness.

Hans Prinzhorn spent only two years at the hospital, 1919 to 1921. He enlarged the collection of paintings, drawings, sculptures and other objects made spontaneously by patients before the era of psychopharmacology. Figure 9 shows wooden sculptures of arthropods made by Brendel, which resemble African art. Figure 10 shows the phenomenon of contamination of two objects which is often found in the drawings of schizophrenic patients. Prinzhorn's monograph describing similarities between the art of psychiatric patients and modern art, especially Art Brute, has become a classic (1922). The landmark publication for prewar psychopathology investigations in Heidelberg is the schizophrenia volume in Bumke's textbook, published in 1932, to which most of these authors contributed.

Carl Schneider marks a dark period in the history of the hospital. Although he was said to be an engaged therapist who introduced elements of work therapy to the hospital, he nonetheless participated in euthanasia programs. In 1940, he became the top assessing judge in Germany on euthanasia for chronic patients, a direct appointment by T 4, the central authority for this action, so named because of its address Tiergartenstraße 4 in Berlin. At this time, Schneider also received a grant of 31 million marks for his research programs.

It is not yet clear if patients from the Heidelberg university hospital were deported to special euthanasia hospitals and camps; it is certain, however, that schizophrenic patients were sterilized against their will.

Six staff members were expelled in 1933, with the exception of Willmanns, all of them because of their Jewish origins. Carl Schneider committed suicide shortly after his imprisonment in 1945.

After the war, the Heidelberg faculty recruited Kurt Schneider (Figure 11) as chairman from the Psychiatric Research Institute in Munich. Schneider managed to revive the traditions and spirit of the hospital. The international regard for his work stems mainly from his first rank symptoms of schizophrenia, a non-theoretical hierarchy of symptoms set up for mere diagnostic reasons. In contrast, Bleuler's primary and secondary symptoms imply a functional hierarchy. Another important part of Schneider's work is his clinical description of psychopathy-types (1923). Quite unlike the Tübingen school, Schneider regarded these diagnoses as variants of normality, a view which was quite controversial because of its consequences for forensic psychiatry.

With Walter von Baeyer (Figure 12), Heidelberg psychopathology moved in the anthropological direction, as represented by monographs by Kisker (1960), now chairman in Hannover, the early Häfner (1961), Tellenbach (1961), and Blankenburg (1971), now chairman in Marburg (Table 2). Janzarik's work (1959, 1988), while difficult to categorize, belongs to this group because of its extensive interpretative element. Tellenbach's book, *Melancholia* (1961), on the premorbid personality of melancholic patients, has by now been translated into five languages. As is the case with Kurt Schneider's *Clinical Psychopathology* (1976), which has been translated into seven languages, Tellenbach's clinical descriptions have been operationalized and proven valid, although not as generally applicable as Tellenbach believed. It is of interest that Tellenbach's work as well as the work of his disciple Alfred Kraus (1977) have been much better received in Japan and in the Latin world, Spain, France, Italy, South America, than in English speaking countries. The translation of Tellenbach's *Melancholia* into English was the last of the five foreign language translations.

Table 2: Outstanding publications in psychopathology by members of the "Heidelberg School"

E. Kraepelin	Psychiatrie, 6th ed., 1899
K. Jaspers	Allgemeine Psychopathologie, 1913
H. Prinzhorn	Die Bildnerei der Geisteskranken, 1922
W. Mayer-Gross	Selbstschilderungen der Verwirrtheit (Die oneiroide Erlebnisform), 1924
K. Beringer	Der Meskalinrausch, 1927
H.W. Gruhle	Die Psychologie der Schizophrenie, 1929
K. Schneider	Klinische Psychopathologie, 1946
W. Janzarik	Dynamische Grundkonstellationen in endogenen Psychosen, 1959
K.P. Kisker	Erlebniswandel der Schizophrenen, 1960
H. Häfner	Psychopathen, 1961
H. Tellenbach	Melancholie, 1961
W.v.Baeyer, H. Häfner, K.P. Kisker	Psychiatrie der Verfolgten, 1964
W. Blankenburg	Verlust der natürlichen Selbstverständlichkeit, 1971

Von Baeyer himself was greatly concerned with the psychiatry of the persecuted. He assessed a large number of Jewish patients who survived concentration camps and developed psychiatric syndromes afterwards. On the basis of this work, Von Baeyer broke with the notion of a strict endogenous-reactive dichotomy, asserting instead that psychotic developments can emerge from what he called "annihilation" in adolescence or early adulthood as long as bridging symptoms are present between events of persecution and the onset of illness. Von Baeyer's ample experience with such patients was published in a monograph that he wrote with Häfner and Kisker (1964).

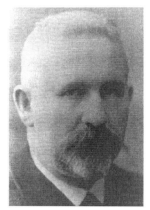

Figure 3: Emil Kraepelin

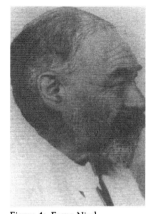

Figure 4: Franz Nissl

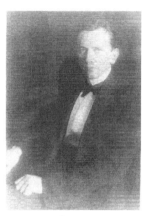

Figure 5: Karl Jaspers

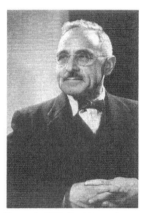

Figure 6: Wilhelm Mayer-Gross

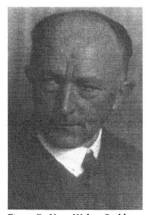

Figure 7: Hans-Walter Gruhle

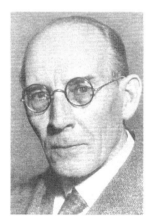

Figure 8: Karl Willmanns

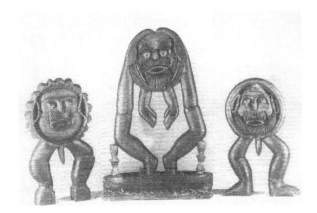

Figure 9:
Wooden Sculptures
by Brendel
(Prinzhorn
collection)

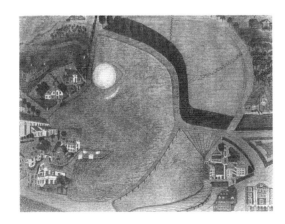

Figure 10:
Example of contamination
of two objects in the
drawing of a schizophrenic
patient
(Prinzhorn collection)

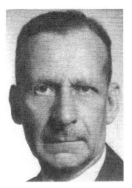 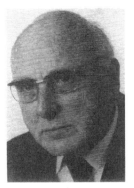 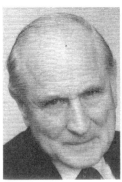

Figure 11: Kurt Schneider   Figure 12: Walter von Bayer   Figure 13: Werner Janzarik

At the end of von Baeyer's chairmanship, the left wing students' movement hit the hospital and continued on for a while in the time of his successor Janzarik (figure 13). A former co-worker in the hospital later blended into the terrorist underground and took a few patients with him. After Janzarik took over, ideology gradually subsided and scientific thinking and clinical work was re-established. Janzarik developed a very systematic approach to endogenous psychoses in his work on the interplay between the "dynamism" of the personality and its "structure" (cf. Janzarik 1959, 1988). These terms were taken from over from psychology, especially from the Gestalt psychology of Krüger and Wellek, and were then applied to the endogenous psychoses. Janzarik's model not only explains many heterogeneous clinical phenomena of endogenous psychoses, but also reaches beyond as a general psychology of personality development.

With respect to the subject of this volume, a note should be interjected on the Heidelberg School's work on thought and language disturbances. Gruhle's chapters on this topic in his and Berze's monograph (Berze & Gruhle 1929) and in the schizophrenia volume in Bumke's textbook (cf. Bumke 1932) belong to the best of what he has written. Gruhle differentiated "formal intelligence" from "higher intelligence" and maintained that higher intelligence alone is disturbed in schizophrenics. According to him, the schizophenic's comprehension of symbols is inconclusive. Patients suffer from the predicament of having no adequate language available for their abnormal feelings and experiences. Gruhle strictly objected to Kleist's assumption that neologisms are paraphasias. Instead, Gruhle regarded schizophrenic talk as an immediate play of feelings without terms, similar to a poem or a song (German Lied). Beringer's (1926) "reduced intentional span" turned up again in Gruhle's writings as a "lack of teleological discipline". Carl Schneider (1930) later used the metaphor of little ships (naviculae) which were severed from their tows at shore and taken by the stream of associations without control and rule. The merit of the work of these classical authors is in their clinical descriptions whereas the nature of the underlying processes is approached in a merely metaphorical way.

Anthropological psychiatry dominated the hospital after the war. In the 1960s, Kisker emphasized the problem of self-presentation in language. He suggested that distorted language should be taken seriously and that the therapist should listen to the pre-predicative meaning of the patients' desultory speech. This approach has some similarity to interpretations of delusions as pseudo-predicative or concretistic phenomena. Wit, and even deep truth, which some authors find in schizophrenic talk, e.g. Bertaux in his interpretation of Hölderlin in his later years, are considered unintentional by most psychopathologists. Avenarius (1991) described case histories of schizophrenic patients who need self-elation and an intent to present themselves in order to go on talking. Blankenburg (1971) proposed that reduced transcendental organization of the patient's ego is the basis for unobtrusive thought disorders in simple and hebephrenic schizophrenics, an approach much agreed about by Japanese psychopathologists who wrote about a psychopathology of the human in-between (cf. Kimura 1980) or about common sense psychopathology. In the 1980s, younger authors[1], influenced by Goldstein's concept of concretism and Cameron's concept of overinclusion, continued these lines of investigation with experimental studies. Tress and Pfaffenberger (1991) operationalized cohesion and coherence in the narrative talks of schizophrenics and control groups and demonstrated specific schizo-phrenic deficiencies. In a similar manner, Holm-Hadulla (1991) operationalized the intermingling, substitution and transfer of meaning from one sentence to the next. They also investigated the interpretation of proverbs by acutely disturbed schizophrenic patients and non-schizo-phrenic controls and found marked differences (Frommer & Tress 1991). As a whole, these authors delineated different aspects of language in psychopathology, for example: language as a message, as two-way communication, as self-presentation and as preformed symbol patterns of reality.

The hospital is currently in the midst of a stage of reorientation. Research activity will continue to emphasize psychopathology, but the methods and the guiding questions must shift. Research methods will involve more empirical work such as psychopathometry and experimental psychopathology. Nonetheless, the tradition of working on holistic psychopathological disease models will not be interrupted. An active group of biological psychiatrists will provide the necessary counterbalance of methods and contents to prevent autistic undisciplined thinking by psychopathologists.

Although Kisker (1979) summed up severe criticism of the Heidelberg School, including therapeutic disengagement, arrogance, and hostility towards psychoanalysis, and although he considered the work of Zurich's Burghölzli and Munich's Psychiatric Research Institute to be superior, the Heidelberg School has done innovative and important work in psychopathology for many decades , right up to the present time.

What made the old authors so successful?

Looking back to publications which exerted influence and are still read and quoted today (Table 2), it seems that two features have made them so prominent:

(1) Sober clinical observation, combined with relentless criticism towards one's own prejudices, which prevents these authors from overly speculative or shallow theoretical constructions.

(2) Conceptual thinking which keeps in mind the fundamental questions of our science: How access is possible to the psychopathological phenomena of a subjective world of feelings and experiences and, the problems of nosology in psychiatry given its body-mind-problem. Both of these questions are linked to each other.

---

1 For examples of these works and further references, see Kraus and Mundt (1991).

As Jaspers predicted, both empirical particulars as well as speculative amplifications of theories did not gain lasting interest but fell into oblivion, as for example experimental-psychopathological studies of Kraepelin or the enormous work of Arthur Kronfeld. Instead, in those great old days in the hospital, work on what today is called the "molar level" was rewarded with extremely useful and practical knowledge for scientific psychiatry. To some of us today, however, this molar level of symptom inventories and fundamental conceptions seems to be more or less exhausted. Some time ago, Kurt Schneider commented that the harvest of psychopathology was already brought in. Instead, the old ideas are now pursued with new technologies and methods on the molecular level. If new concepts arise, they will come out of this broad stream of molecular level findings. For example, important and abundant results reported from neuroimaging studies on schizophrenics not only produce new factual knowledge but also generate new models of pathogenesis (even if the earliest concepts for these findings go back to the 19th century and, in more detail, to Berze at the beginning of this century; cf. Berze 1914). Other examples may be drawn from psychosocial research, such as expressed emotion, social support and social network research. The mere method of clinical observation, which served Kurt Schneider so well in his evaluation of symptom ranking, is by itself hardly acceptable today as a sufficient research tool. Still, even the most sophisticated experimental study must be interpreted on the basis of clinical experience. In my view, the ultimate framework within which empirical results and theoretical constructs can be evaluated remains the personal encounter with the patient over time. We have no safer grounds. And that is it what we can learn from the old boys.

Summary

The first attempt to found a Psychiatric University Hospital in Heidelberg ended with a clash between non-academic care for psychiatric patients and the academic bodies responsible for the tuititon of students in Heidelberg. After this setback for psychiatry in Heidelberg, which lasted about 50 years, the refounded hospital gained importance at the end of last century. In the following two decades, the hospital made very substantial contributions to the development of terms and concepts of general psychopathology as well as to the specific disease entities which build up today's nosological order. After the dismal period of the 1930s and the war years this tradition was resumed. It was followed in the 1950s by a period of phenomenological–anthropological approaches to psychopathology based upon the application of philosophical tools. Furture tasks can be seen in bridging the gap between this tradition and biological psychiatry and in connecting psychopathology with therapy–oriented research.

References

Avenarius R: Emil Kraepelin, seine Persönlichkeit und seine Konzeption. In: W
    Janzarik W (ed): Psychopathologie als Grundlagenwissenschaft, pp. 62-73.
    Stuttgart, Enke, 1979
Avenarius R: (1991). Über Größenwahn und Sprachverwirrtheit. In: Kraus A, Mundt
    Ch (eds): Schizophrenie und Sprache, pp. 105-116. Stuttgart, Thieme, 1991
Baeyer W v, Häfner H, Kisker KP: Psychiatrie der Verfolgten. Berlin Göttingen
    Heidelberg, Springer, 1964
Beringer K: Denkstörungen und Sprache bei Schizophrenen. Z ges Neurol Psychiat
    103: 185-197, 1926
Beringer K: Der Meskalinrausch, seine Geschichte und Erscheinungsweise. Berlin
    Göttingen Heidelberg, Springer, 1927
Berze J: Die primäre Insuffizienz der psychischen Aktivität. Ihr Wesen, ihre
    Erscheinung und ihre Bedeutung als Grundstörung der Dementia praecox und
    der Hypophrenien überhaupt. Leipzig Wien, Deuticke, 1914
Berze J, Gruhle HW: Psychologie der Schizophrenie. Berlin Göttingen Heidelberg,
    Springer, 1929
Binding K, Hoche AE: Die Freigabe der Vernichtung lebensunwerten Lebens. Ihr Maß
    und ihre Form. Leipzig, Barth, 1920
Blankenburg W: Der Verlust der natürlichen Selbstverständlichkeit. Ein Beitrag zur
    Psychopathologie symptomarmer Schizophrenien. Stuttgart, Enke, 1971
Bumke O (ed): Handbuch der Geisteskrankheiten. Vol. 9, V. Schizophrenie. Berlin
    Göttingen Heidelberg, Springer, 1932
Frommer J: Sprachauffälligkeiten Schizophrener: Historische Wurzeln moderner
    Forschungsperspektiven. In: Kraus A, Mundt Ch (eds): Schizophrenie und
    Sprache, pp. 117–139. Stuttgart, Thieme, 1991
Gaupp R: Der Fall Wagner. Z ges Neurol Psychiat 60, 312, 1920
Häfner H: Psychopathen. Daseinsanalytische Untersuchungen zur Struktur und
    Verlaufsgestalt von Psychopathien. Berlin Göttingen Heidelberg, Springer, 1961
Hoche AE: Die Fürstner'sche Ära. Arch Psychiatr Nervenkr 87: 24-29, 1920
Holm-Hadulla R: Zur Struktur schizophrenen Denkens und Sprechens—eine mittels
    Sprichwortinterpretation empirisch fundierte psychopathologische Perspektive.
    In: Kraus A, Mundt Ch (eds): Schizophrenie und Sprache, pp. 61–70. Stuttgart,
    Thieme, 1991
Janzarik W: Dynamische Grundkonstellationen in endogenen Psychosen. Berlin
    Göttingen Heidelberg, Springer, 1959
Janzarik W: 100 Jahre Heidelberger Psychiatrie. Heidelberger Jahrbücher XXII, pp.
    93-113, Berlin Heidelberg New York: Springer, 1978
Janzarik W: Strukturdynamische Grundlagen der Psychiatrie. Stuttgart, Enke, 1988
Jaspers K: Allgemeine Psychopathologie (1st ed). Berlin Heidelberg New York,
    Springer, 1913
Kimura B: Phänomenologie des Zwischen—zum Problem der Grundstörung der
    Schizophrenie. Z G klin Psychol Psychother 28: 34-38, 1980
Kisker K: Der Erlebniswandel der Schizophrenen. Ein psychopathologischer Beitrag
    zur Psychonomie schizophrener Grundsituationen. Berlin Göttingen Heidelberg,
    Springer, 1960
Kisker K: Die Heidelberger Psychopathologie in der Kritik. In: Janzarik W (ed):
    Psychopathologie als Grundlagenwissenschaft, pp. 122-136, Stuttgar, Enke,
    1979
Kraepelin E: Psychiatrie. Ein Lehrbuch für Studierende und Ärzte (7th ed). Leipzig,
    Ambrosius Barth, 1903
Kraepelin E: Lebenserinnerungen (eds: Hippius H, Peters G, Ploog D). Berlin
    Heidelberg, Springer, 1983
Kraus A: Sozialverhalten und Psychose Manisch-Depressiver. Eine existenz- und

rollenanalytische Untersuchung. Stuttgart, Enke, 1977

Kraus A, Mundt Ch (eds): Schizophrenie und Sprache. Stuttgart, New York, Thieme, 1991

Kretschmer E: Der sensitive Beziehungswahn. Ein Beitrag zur Paranoiafrage und zur psychiatrischen Charakterlehre (2nd ed). Berlin Göttingen Heidelberg, Springer, 1927

Kretschmer E: Körperbau und Charakter. Untersuchungen zum Konstitutions-problem und zur Lehre von den Temperamenten. Berlin Göttingen Heidelberg, Springer, 1931

Mayer-Gross W: Über die Stellungnahme zur abgelaufenen akuten Psychose. Zschr ges Neurol Psychiatr 60: 160-212, 1920

Mayer-Gross W: Selbstschilderungen der Verwirrtheit. Die oneiroide Erlebnisform. Berlin Göttingen Heidelberg, Springer, 1924

Mayer-Gross W: Die Entwicklung der klinischen Anschauungen Kraepelins. Arch Psychiatr 87: 30-42, 1929

Middelhoff HD: C.F.W. Roller und die Vorgeschichte der Heidelberger psychia-trischen Klinik. In: Janzarik W (ed): Psychopathologie als Grundlagen-wissenschaft, pp. 33-50, Stuttgart, Enke, 1979

Prinzhorn H: Bildnerei der Geisteskranken. Ein Beitrag zur Psychologie und Psychopathologie der Gestaltung. Berlin Göttingen Heidelberg, Springer, 1922

Schimmelpenning GW: Alfred Erich Hoche. Das wissenschaftliche Werk: "Mittel-mäßigkeit?" Joachim Jungius-Gesellschaft der Wissenschaften 8/3, pp. 3-39, Göttingen, Vandenhoeck & Ruprecht, 1990

Schmitt W: Karl Jaspers und die Methodenfrage in der Psychiatrie. In: Janzarik W (ed), Psychopathologie als Grundlagenwissenschaft, pp. 74-82, Stuttgart, Enke, 1979

Schneider C: Die Psychologie der Schizophrenen. Leipzig, Thieme, 1930

Schneider K: Die psychopathischen Persönlichkeiten. Leipzig, Thieme, 1923

Schneider K: Klinische Psyachopathologie (1st ed 1946). 11th ed, Stuttgart, Thieme, 1976

Tellenbach H: Melancholie. Problemgeschichte, Endogenität, Typologie, Pathogenese, Klinik. Berlin Heidelberg, Springer, 1961

Tress W, Pfaffenberger U: Die sprachliche Verwendung des Begriffs "schizophren"— eine sprachphilosophische und linguistische Untersuchung. In: Kraus A, Mundt Ch (eds): Schizophrenie und Sprache, pp.38–52. Stuttgart, Thieme, 1991

Wilmanns K: Zur Psychopathologie des Landstreichers. Leipzig, J.A. Barth, 1906

Phenomenology

M. Spitzer, F.A. Uehlein
M.A. Schwartz, C. Mundt
(eds.): Phenomenology
Language & Schizophrenia.
Springer-Verlag, New York, 1992

Phenomenology and Psychiatry

Manfred Spitzer & Friedrich A. Uehlein

The term "phenomenology" is frequently mentioned in present day medicine and psychiatry. As this term is used by different authors to denote various topics, its meaning may sometimes be obscure. Hence, it is the aim of this article, to clarify the diverse facets of the term, and then, to focus upon the ways in which phenomenology has been used by investigators in psychiatric studies and monographs.

1. Facets of "Phenomenology"

Phenomenology is taken by many authors to denote the description of patient's signs and symptoms. Even here, however, distinctions can be made. Rotov (1991), for example, contrasts what he calls the Husserl–Jaspers–Binswanger school of phenomenology with an alternative approach involving the application by psychiatrists of statistical methods to symptoms and syndromes. Obviously, Rotov sees a major difference in the study of *individuals* on the one hand and *groups* on the other. This distinction within empirical phenomenological research—the detailed study of individuals in contrast to the (supposedly not so detailed) study of groups—may be viewed as a fundamental dichotomy within the domain of "phenomenological" approaches to signs and symptoms. According to this view, both the group statistical and the individualistic case study approach to signs and symptoms belong to the general class of phenomenological research.

In contrast to the view just stated, other psychiatrists claim that only the study of *individuals* can justify the label "phenomenology". In any event, both kinds of phenomenology, individual or statistical, use *empirical* methods. "Phenomenology" in either case plainly means "the study of signs and symptoms". Furthermore, when descriptions of signs and symptoms are called "phenomenological", it often but not always means that the descriptions are more detailed than usual. Examples of such views of the meaning of "phenomenology" can be found in many articles and textbooks in present day psychiatry (Andreasen 1991, Kaplan & Sadock 1988, p. 148, Shepherd 1983, pp. 1–3, to give just three examples).

If a phenomenological account of a state of affairs is meant to be purely descriptive, *no inferences* about possible causes are made. No explanatory theory is given, and the situation is merely described. In this sense, diagnostic manuals with an emphasis on clinical description, such as the Diagnostic and Statistical Manual of Mental Disorders, DSM–III, can be said to exemplify a phenomenological approach.

When it comes to the diagnosis of psychotic and neurotic disorders, the experiences of patients as reported to the psychiatrist is still the most important source of information for diagnosis. Behavioral aspects play a minor role. Possibly because of this, the emphasis in "phenomenological" is on *subjective* (i.e., *first–person*) reports of mental activity, rather than on objectively observable behavior. Therefore, the term is more closely linked to (subjective) symptoms than to (objective) signs.

Detailed descriptions of single patients are more likely to include *idiosyncratic* features than descriptive sums and averages of groups of people. Hence, for many psychiatrists, "phenomenological" means "emphasis on idiosyncrasies rather than on generalities."

Additionally, a phenomenological account of a patient can be contrasted to a psychodynamic account. According to psychoanalysis, symptoms (i.e., the experiences of the patients) are produced by an interplay of hypothetical intrapsychic entities. The existence of these entities is inferred from psychoanalytic theory which in turn is based on analogies and inferences. Hence, interpretations which psychoanalysts give go far beyond the actual experiences of patients and are opposed to the spirit of phenomenology. This *anti–inferential* sense of phenomenology was already pointed out in detail by Karl Jaspers in his writings on psychopathology (cf. Jaspers 1913/1963).

In addition to and as an elaboration of its meaning "descriptive in detail", the term "phenomenological" has become linked with the notion of *anti–reductionism*. The connection is one of presupposition and attitude: Psychiatrists who overwhelmingly concern themselves with the brain and the body ("only matter really matters") will have little interest in the detailed description of hallucinations, delusions, disturbed emotions, etc. These psychiatrists will only to a small extent be interested in phenomenology. He or she may simply not engage in the enterprise at all. In contrast, psychiatrists who believe that there is much more to mental illness than merely neuronal or brain dysfunction are likely to be extremely interested in the details of the experience of the patient.

To sum up, the term "phenomenology" and the derived adjective "phenomenological" have a special meaning in the context of psychiatry, which can be grasped through an appreciation of the following characteristic features: "Phenomenology" in psychiatry means a *descriptive* account of the *signs and symptoms* of a patient, which is

(1) *empirical* (as opposed to speculative)
(2) *detailed* (with emphasis on the idiosyncratic features of a particular person)

(3) *individualistic* (as opposed to statistical)
(4) *subjective* (i.e., heavily or entirely dependent on a first–person account)
(5) *anti–inferential*
(6) *atheoretical* with respect to etiology
(7) *anti–reductionistic.*

2. The Art of Description

A chronic paranoid schizophrenic patient "distinguished voices that talked directly from the outside, through walls and pipes, from those voices bought by a current which his persecutors used to force him sometimes to hear inwardly. These inward voices were neither localized outside not were they physical; he distinguished them from 'made thoughts' unaccompanied by any inner hearing and directly conducted into his head..." (Jaspers 1963, p. 74).

Compare this description of a hallucinating patient with the description which is most widely used at present (i.e., the hallucinations–item on the *Brief Psychiatric Rating Scale, BPRS,* cf. Overall & Gorham 1976):

hallucinations

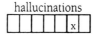

"A patient noticed the waiter in the coffee–house; he skipped past him so quickly and uncannily. He noticed odd behavior in an acquaintance which made him feel strange; everything in the street was so different, something was bound to be happening: A passer–by gave such a penetrating glance, he could be a detective. Then there was a dog who seemed hypnotized, a kind of mechanical dog made of rubber. There were such a lot of people walking about, something must surely be starting up against the patient. All the umbrellas were rattling as if some apparatus was hidden inside them" (Jaspers 1963, p. 100).

This description of a patient with delusions may be compared, again, with the standard description given to such experiences in most research papers:

delusions

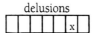

Of course, we do not deny the necessity of "compressing" data for the sake of the computability of sums and means, and we additionally do not claim that the narrative account of a patient's symptoms is best suited for all purposes. However, we intentionally contrasted the two approaches in order to demonstrate how much gets lost in the process of compression and in the "reduction" of data.[1]

Standard symptom checklists such as the *BPRS* not only highly compress or reduce psychiatric data but additionally omit some forms of

---

[1] The reader should keep in mind, of course, that *both* kinds of descriptions may be found in sections on "signs and symptoms", "psychopathology", and "phenomenology" in research papers.

experience altogether. For example, the following descriptions of disorders of the experience of space and time do not have any equivalent in most rating scales:

"I was suddenly caught up in a peculiar state; my arms and legs seemed to swell. A frightful pain shot through my head and time stood still. At the same time it was forced on me in an almost superhuman way how vitally important this moment was. Then time resumed to its previous course, but the time which stood still stayed there like a gate" (Jaspers 1963, p. 84).

"I still saw the room. Space seemed to stretch and go on into infinity, completely empty. I felt lost, abandoned to the infinities of space, which in spite of my insignificance somehow threatened me. It seemed the complement of my own emptiness ... the old physical space seemed to be apart from this other space, like a phantom" (Jaspers 1963, p. 81).

It is easier and faster to check off a mark on a scale than to write a descriptive paragraph. Furthermore, everyone who attempts to write narrative accounts of patient's mental states will find him– or herself having great difficulty saying even the most simple things about mental processes. The detailed description of mental phenomena is to some extent an art, which has to be developed by the psychiatrist if he or she wants to provide appropriate accounts of the experiences of patients. However, the accurate rendering of such experiences is not merely an art. Two problems appear which can be, and have been, approached scientifically: (1) How can we know what is going on in other minds; and (2) how are mental phenomena constituted, both in our own mind as well as the minds of others. Both problems have been solved by thoughtful arguments labeled "phenomenology", the first by Karl Jaspers, and the second by Edmund Husserl.

3. The Empirical Science of Other Minds: Phenomenology in Karl Jaspers' Sense

At the turn of the century, the distinction between *understandable* mental phenomena (e.g., someone has lost a friend and for this *reason* is sad) and those mental phenomena which can only be *explained* in causal terms (e.g., someone has a brain tumor in his left parietal lobe which *causes* sadness in this person) was already in the air. In the latter case, something goes wrong, and a material process must be invoked. The following quote on "aberrations of thought", from William James' *Psychology (Briefer Course)*, first published in 1892, may serve as an example of this view:

"It is a suggestive fact that Locke, and many more recent Continental psychologists, have found themselves obliged to invoke a mechanical process to account for the *aberrations* of thought, the obstructive prepossessions, the frustrations of reason" (James 1892/1984, p. 225).

Karl Jaspers was the first to explicitly realize the psychiatric significance and implications of the dichotomy of "understanding" and "causal explanation".

Several causes for mental dysfunctioning, such as tumor, infection, and obstruction of or bleeding from the brain's blood vessels, were already known. Moreover, the cause of syphilis, a deadly veneral disease with a plethora of neurological and psychiatric manifestations, had just been discovered: A small spiral-like bacterium, the spirochete, was found to cause a variety of mental disorders, ranging from megalomania to depression, and from delusions of persecution to dementia. As syphilis is a chronic disease, such symptoms sometimes took decades to develop, and long years of mental changes could now be appreciated as the result of a disease process.

It was only reasonable to suppose that other mental disorders with known chronic courses—and most importantly, the disorder which had just been described by Kraepelin and Bleuler—were similarly caused by disease processes. However, in the case of dementia praecox or schizophrenia, nothing had yet been found by investigations using the microscope or other objective techniques. However, invoking syphilis as a model and referring to the idea of a disease-entity developed by Kahlbaum and Kraepelin, Jaspers reasoned that it might be possible to infer the disease process from the course by using a derivation rule as follows: If in the course of a persons life mental changes occur which cannot be *understood* in terms of *reasons* for such changes, then a disease *process* has to be assumed to *cause* them. Therefore, in cases where the microscope does not provide the answer, the burden of proof rests on the psychiatrist, who attempts to understand the patient and his life course, and fails. Given this state of affairs, and given Jaspers' life-long interest in methodological issues, the question of understanding in psychiatry necessarily occupied an important place at the very center of his studies.

The contrast of understanding versus explanation, between issues that can be understood and issues that have to be explained, was introduced as a psychiatric diagnostic framework by Jaspers. It was "in the air" not only in psychology, but also in philosophy. Wilhelm Dilthey had emphasized the distinction between explanation as the method and aim of the natural sciences on the one hand, and understanding as the aim and method of the *Geisteswissenschaften*.[2] "Nature is what we explain, mental life is what we understand", as Dilthey (1894/1982, p. 144) put it in a famous phrase. Jaspers was the first to consequently apply this to psychiatry: He saw that psychiatrists could not be content with being "pure" natural scientists

---

2 The term Geisteswissenschaft cannot be translated directly. The term "Humanities" denotes a number of subjects and branches of activity at universities which partly overlap with "Geisteswissenschaft". However, Geisteswissenschaft contains the term "science" and hence, bears connotations different from "Humanities". The distinction between *idiographic* and *nomothetic* science is sometimes employed to denote the difference between Geistes- and Naturwissenschaft, although this distinction, too, is not fully congruent with the one in question. Lastly, the social sciences are also not equivalent to the Geisteswissenschaften.

(Naturwissenschaftler), as they were constantly engaged in activities of understanding and interpretation, i.e., activities thought to constitute what the *Geisteswissenschaftler* does.

Jaspers was able to draw on Dilthey to make basic distinctions. In Dilthey's works (Dilthey 1926/1979, pp. 205-227), there is a detailed account on the understanding of other people. Here, Dilthey describes the various ways in which we understand others by what they say, by their behavior and by their expressions. Moreover, we can interpret other peoples utterances, actions and expressions, and thereby gain a complicated picture of other minds.

In his *General Psychopathology*, Jaspers set out to bring to psychopathology these and other aspects of Geisteswissenschaft as developed by Dilthey. We have already seen that the difference between understanding and explanation was used by Jaspers as a tool to discover disease processes that were undetectable by other means. He clarified the notion of understanding in psychiatry by introducing two major concepts of understanding: *genetic* and *static* understanding.

By means of genetic understanding the psychiatrist finds out how mental events are related to one another. In Jaspers' own words,

"In some cases ... we understand directly how one psychic event emerges from another" (Jaspers 1963, p. 27). "Psychic events 'emerge' out of each other in a way which we understand... The way in which such an emergence takes place is understood by us, *our understanding is genetic*" (Jaspers 1963, p. 302, his italics).

As can be seen from the quote, genetic understanding is the means by which the psychiatrist clarifies whether a particular mental condition (sadness, for example) can be understood in terms of other mental conditions (as opposed to being explained by a causal/material/bodily/disease process). In conclusion, genetic understanding is a major diagnostic tool which enables the psychiatrist to detect disease processes indirectly, i.e., without direct objective evidence.

Not all that is meant by the word "understanding"—in its ordinary language sense—is captured in the notion of genetic understanding. If somebody says that he is in pain, for example, we might say that we "understand" what that means. That is to say, we know what he means because we have experienced pain ourselves. Note that this kind of understanding is different from genetic understanding. When we "understand" someone feeling pain, we do so because we *know what it is like* to feel pain, to be in the state of pain, as some philosophers might say. Jaspers saw that this kind of understanding is important for psychiatrists, who simply have to *know what it is like* to be in a large variety of mental states in order to correctly appreciate their nature. He appropriately called such understanding *static understanding*.

Static understanding includes more than the mere recall of sensual qualities, and in the broadest sense, includes all of the contents of consciousness as experienced by us. Only the psychiatrist with detailed knowledge about the varieties of conscious experience, will be able to fully appreciate these experiences in other people as well as the broader array of experiences due to pathology. For this reason, Jaspers turned to the early philosophy of Edmund Husserl, as this philosopher had already set out to do exactly what is needed: To give a detailed and veridical description of the content of mental life (conscious experience in the widest sense of the term). In other words, Husserl's phenomenology was adopted by Jaspers and then modified to some extent to solve the general problem of the description of mental phenomena as such.

This problem and Husserl's solution deserve a closer look.

4. Descriptive Dimensions of Consciousness: The Relevance of Husserlian Phenomenology for Psychopathological Reasoning

Psychopathology as a clinical practice has developed general schemes for organizing subjective data. Although these schemes differ slightly in various cultures, countries, and even hospitals, they all utilize similar basic concepts, such as hallucinations, delusions, disturbances of formal thought, disturbances of affect, descriptions of motor phenomena, and so forth. It is easy to see that these descriptive concepts rest upon mental concepts such as perception, the flow and coherence of thought, consciousness and its modifications, affective states, etc. How, we may ask, have we developed our descriptive concepts? We certainly need them in order to describe! Can we give a more satisfying answer to this question than the obvious response that they have somehow evolved in clinical practice?

Our general problem seems to be that we are asking where the tools for description (the descriptive concepts) come from, while our answer so far is that they came from clinical practice, i.e., from descriptions of patients. So we need descriptions in order to be able to describe!—Is there a way out of this circle?

The situation is not very different from that seen in craftsmanship. In order to be a good craftsman, good tools are needed. Where do good tools come from? The answer is simple: Good craftsman make good tools! How?—With other tools!

In practice, of course, there is no infinite regress making good crafts-manship impossible, and there is also no infinite regress making good descriptions in psychiatry impossible. However, just as good craftsmen and the best tools are required to improve the tools themselves, it takes experienced clinicians and skilled, rigid conceptual reasoning to improve descriptive terminology, the tools of psychopathology.

With this in mind, the question of the description of consciousness in all its varieties, the central issue of Edmund Husserl's phenomenology, becomes critically relevant to general psychopathology.

As much as possible, we must avoid starting descriptions of mental life with prejudices of whatever kind. Therefore, phenomenological descrip-

tions of what is called the life-world are the starting point of attempts to
obtain unbiased knowledge of our mental life. Such descriptions attempt
to depict only what is really present in actual, conscious experience. As
experiencing subjects, we always experience something, i.e., in experience
there is always something which is experienced. This fundamental nature
of experience—somebody experiences something—was elaborated by
Husserl, who used the term *intentionality* to refer to it. Husserl called single
acts of experience intentional acts; and he called the objects experienced
intentional objects. Such objects need not necessarily be perceived. On the
contrary, one reason for requiring the concept of intentionality is the need
to account for "objects" which only exist in the mental life of an experiencing subject (e.g., subjective perspectives of something; imagined
objects; goals). The notion of the *intentional object* serves the purpose of
denoting whatever is experienced in mental life. In other words, an
"intentional object" is an "object" in the broadest, and at the same time, in
the most subjective sense. A cat perceived is an intentional object, but so is
a hallucinated cat. A delusional system of connected meanings, fears and
desires is an intentional object. Intentional objects can be described and
we can refer to them.

How does a uniform synthetic experience of something come into
being? We know from cognitive psychology that experience is the final
result of complicated processes. However, information processing accounts
of experience start with "data" rather than with experience itself. As we
have already pointed out, the phenomenologist's ultimate bedrock is
experience. Unlike the cognitive psychologist, the phenomenologist does
not even attempt to explain experience in non-experiential terms.
However, phenomenologists can go further than merely asserting (and
describing in detail) that experience is synthetic and unified. As Husserl
pointed out, this feature of experience is the result of synthetic processes in
which we are not actively engaged (as in deliberately thinking of
something; or as in purposely watching something), but which we
passively perform. We might even say that such passive synthetic processes
are performed for us, but if we do so, we run the risk of losing the agent of
these processes, which, for the phenomenologist, is the experiencing
subject: Passive synthetic processes are performed by *us*; they are not
performed by some component of our cognitive-perceptual apparatus. By
passing the experiencing subject and invoking a cognitive-perceptual
mechanism has all of the virtues of cognitive psychological hypotheses (for
example, such a mechanism can be linked to physiological and computational theories of certain features of experience). At the same time,
however, such bypassing suffers from the crucial drawback of all non-
phenomenological accounts of experience, i.e., the loss the subject of
experience as well as the *phenomenal* characteristics of experience.[3]

---

3 This statement does not imply any oppositional view of the relation between phenomenology and
cognitive science. On the one hand, cognitive science needs a phenomenological interpretation of its
physiological and computational hypotheses. Otherwise it would not be clear what these hypotheses

Without going into details at this point, such phenomenal characteristics are the "qualia" of experience (phenomenological qualities in a narrow sense, i.e., the experience of red, of the sound of a violin, of a bitter taste), the synthetic unity of experience (we do not see pixels, but objects, we do not hear single frequencies, but tones with a certain color and timbre, etc.), the intentionality of experience (which always consists of the two closely related poles of the subject and the intended object), and the temporality of experience.

We conclude this section with a brief comment on temporality. We are aware of its constant flux. Things and events pass in alteration, duration and succession, there is always now, no more and not yet. As Husserl pointed out in detail, the constitution of temporal objectivity is grounded in the internal temporality of the self. Temporality is constituted by us; by our synthetic ability to experience a durational presence, and to bring successive events together in consciousness, along with transitions and differentiations of these events in experiential life. In short: we do not experience time in the same way that we experience clouds and trees; instead, time is a characteristic feature of all our experience, a product of the synthetic unifying activity of the experiencing subject.

5. Eidetic Variation and the Boundaries of General Concepts: Husserl's later Phenomenology

One focus of Husserl's interest is the problem of the formation of general concepts. This is an issue for all sciences which aim at general knowledge and hence at general concepts. However, this problem deserves specific scrutiny by psychiatrists, because (a) psychopathology must contend with critics who claim that it is not a science, and (b) psychiatric concepts are particularly troubled by vagueness and inconsistency.

Eidetic variation is a way of reasoning which is in constant implicit use in all scientific work. When we form a general concept, we do not simply add data: we would not know which datum to add and which to leave out if there were no "guidelines" which tell us how to do so. However, the presupposed guidelines must be general if they are to be of any value, i.e., they must represent exactly what we set out to look for: general concepts. In other words: Whenever we collect data and form a general concept, the general concept formed has already somehow been "at work". In order to describe a mentally ill patient, for example, we may use some concept of perception and some concept of thought, for example, to distinguish hallucinations from delusions. We may use such concepts of perception and thought without ever having subjected them to reflective scrutiny. If we do so, to pursue our example a bit further, we may ask how close a thought can come to a perception before it reaches the point where we

are about. On the other hand, phenomenology, as a theory of embodied persons, implicates physiology and cognitive science as a theory of the bodily foundation of experience, and therefore as a necessary complement of mental phenomena.

would be justified in regarding it as a perception. In this way, we might think about patients with passively experienced thoughts, audible thoughts, and auditory hallucinations. Of course, we have to know many patients very well in order to partake in any informed reasoning about these matters. However, even the detailed knowledge of a large number of patients (if this were possible without already using a variety of concepts) does not, in itself, provide us with any general descriptive concept. In order to form a truly general descriptive concept, we have to engage in reflective thought about what is already at work when we describe any patient in the first place. The concepts we use become subject to various "observations" of the following kind: We engage in the variation of one specific aspect of the concept (the passivity of perception, for example), holding the other features fixed. In contrast to empirical data which are always discrete, in our minds we can continuously change a feature, i.e., we can put it at variation. In this manner, with good knowledge of all the relevant empirical data (and only with such knowledge), we may be able to clarify the concept of perception with respect to the feature of passivity.

The point here is not that all of this has been worked out for psychiatric purposes, and needs only to be learned and then applied. On the contrary, the point here is that the use of general concepts in an informed manner requires us to engage in this kind of reasoning: What, for example, would we say about whether this particular object belongs to the class of objects denoted by this particular concept, if this particular feature of the concept were changed just a bit, and what if we changed it even a little bit more...

Thinking about concepts in this way rather than merely using them (as they appear within our minds in one or another disguise with a meaning guaranteed by common usage) is an inevitable part of scientific reasoning. Husserl went to great length to illuminate this process and to demonstrate its validity. Eidetic variation is by no means identical with "limitless" speculation. Instead, it is informed, reflective reasoning.

Summary

Various facets of the term "phenomenology" are discussed, starting with connotations of the adjective "phenomenological" in the field of psychiatry, such as "empirical", "detailed", "individualistic", "idiosyncratic", "subjective", "anti–inferential", "atheoretical", and "anti–reductionistic". For many psychiatrists, "phenomenology" refers to the "signs and symptoms" of a patient, i.e., the clinical picture as described as accurately as possible. Jaspers contributed to phenomenological psychiatry by his account of "understanding" patients. Husserl's phenomenology is relevant, providing both a conceptual framework for the description of conscious phenomena as well as a method, free eidetic variation, through which general concepts can be sharpened.

References

American Psychiatric Association: Diagnostic and Statistical Manual of Mental Disorders, Third Edition, Revised (DSM-III-R). American Psychiatric Association, Washington, DC, 1987

Andreasen NC: Reply to "Phenomenology or Physicalism?". Schizophrenia Bulletin 17/2, pp. 187–189, 1991

Dilthey W: Ideen über eine beschreibende und zergliedernde Psychologie (1894). In: Gesammelte Schriften V (7th ed), pp. 139-240. Stuttgart, Göttingen, Teubner, Vandenhoeck & Ruprecht, 1982

Dilthey W: Der Aufbau der geschichtlichen Welt in den Geisteswissenschaften (1926). In: Gesammelte Schriften VII (7th ed), pp. 205-227. Stuttgart, Göttingen, Teubner, Vandenhoeck & Ruprecht, 1979

James W: Psychology (Briefer Course), first published in 1892

Jaspers K: Allgemeine Psychopathologie (1913). (General Psychopathology, transl. Hoenig J, Hamilton MW). Chicago, The University of Chicago Press, 1963

Kaplan HI, Sadock BJ: Synopsis of Psychiatry, 5th ed. Baltimore, London, Williams & Wilkins, 1988

Overall JE, Gorham DR: Brief Psychiatric Rating Scale. In: Guy W: ECDEU Assessment Manual for Psychopharmacology, Rev. ed., Rockville, Maryland, pp. 157–169, 1976

Rotov M: Phenomenology or Physicalism?. Schizophrenia Bulletin 17/2, pp. 183–186, 1991

Shepherd M: Introduction: The sciences and general psychopathology. In: Shepherd M, Zangwill OL (eds): Handbook of Psychiatry, vol. 1, General Psychopathology, pp. 1-8. Cambridge University Press, 1983

Spitzer M: Why Philosophy? In: Spitzer M, Maher BA (eds): Philosophy and Psychopathology, pp. 3–18. New York: Springer 1990

M. Spitzer, F.A. Uehlein
M.A. Schwartz, C. Mundt
(eds.): Phenomenology
Language & Schizophrenia.
Springer-Verlag, New York, 1992

Phenomenological/Descriptive Psychiatry: The Methods of Edmund Husserl and Karl Jaspers

Osborne P. Wiggins, Michael Alan Schwartz, & Manfred Spitzer

1. Introduction: Psychiatry and Philosophy

While there can be no doubt that philosophy and psychiatry are different fields of inquiry, there can also exist little doubt that there is a growing interest in philosophical issues in psychiatry.[1] How are these two fields related? How are we to appreciate both their differences and their common ground? What can psychiatry expect from philosophy, and vice versa? In this paper we will focus on phenomenology, which for several reasons remains at the heart of the questions just posed. We will do so by addressing the similarities and differences of the meaning of the term "phenomenology" as used in psychiatry and philosophy. Our focus on phenomenology should not obscure, however, our firm conviction that psychiatry must employ a variety of methods, concepts, and theories in order to illuminate and treat mental disorders.

2. Phenomenology in Psychiatry—Present and Past

A discussion contained in two recent papers published in the *Schizophrenia Bulletin* indicates some of the problems lingering behind any account of phenomenology in the context of present day psychiatry (cf. Rotov 1991, Andreasen 1991). The term has various meanings and is associated with a number of authors who espouse divergent views. An example of one such view is provided in the following quote from Andreasen:

> "The word 'phenomenon' has been expanded in contemporary medical usage beyond its original meaning of 'appearance,' and it is now roughly equivalent to reported or observed experiences of patients (or 'signs and symptoms' in

---

1 By sheer coincidence, in 1989, unbeknownst to each other, the Royal College of Psychiatry's interest group in philosophy and the Group (now: Association) for the Advancement of Philosophy and Psychiatry had their inaugural meetings in Great Britain and in the United States in the very same month.

psychopathology). It is also used more generally in ordinary language or in psychology to refer to the experience and behaviors of normal individuals. The study of all of these kinds of phenomena is referred to as 'phenomenology.' This type of study focuses on human experience at a fine-grained and detailed level and does not make inferences about specific disease states" (Andreasen 1991, pp. 187-188)

This conception of phenomenology as the descriptive study of signs and symptoms is commonly accepted in psychiatry today. Furthermore, according to the commonly accepted view, a phenomenological account in psychiatry does not make inferences about any possible causes. The "phenomenology of schizophrenia," for example, does include descriptions of hallucinations and delusions but does not include references to dopamine receptors, the limbic system, brain ventricles, the regressed superego, latent homosexuality, or whatever may be assumed to be causally involved in the genesis of the disorder. In other words, "phenomenology" signifies an *atheoretical spirit with respect to etiology*. In the standard view, the classification system of *DSM-III-R* is phenomenological in two crucial respects: (1) it emphasizes the importance of the description of signs and symptoms of the patient, and (2) it deemphasizes speculation about the possible etiology of such signs and symptoms. According to *DSM-III-R*, for example:

"The major justification for the generally atheoretical approach taken in *DSM-III* and *DSM-III-R* with regard to etiology is that the inclusion of etiological theories would be an obstacle to use of the manual by clinicians of various theoretical orientations, since it would not be possible to present all reasonable etiological theories for each disorder. For example, Phobic Disorders are believed by many to represent a displacement of anxiety resulting from the breakdown of defense mechanisms that keep internal conflicts out of consciousness. Others explain phobias on the basis of learned avoidance responses to conditioned anxiety. Still others believe that certain phobias result from a dysregulation of basic biological systems mediating separation anxiety. In any case, clinicians and researchers can agree on the identification of mental disorders on the basis of their clinical manifestations without agreeing on how the disturbances come about" (American Psychiatric Association 1987, p. xxiii.)

As can be seen from this passage, there exists a prevailing consensus about the nature of phenomenology. Within this consensus, however, phenomenology as originally imported into psychiatry by Karl Jaspers is obscured or misconstrued. G.E. Berrios, a forceful advocate for descriptive psychiatry, has pointed this out. Regarding the way in which phenomenology is used nowadays, Berrios has written:

"This usage is conceptually uninteresting, a consequence of self-inflicted confusion, and, to a certain extent, parasitical upon ... the idiosyncratic usage started by Karl Jaspers...." (Berrios 1989, p. 425).

Berrios here dismisses the term "phenomenology," as it is used in psychiatry today, as "conceptually uninteresting." Moreover, he thinks Jaspers' usage—the historical source of the present-day meaning—is "idiosyncratic." Berrios' position entails that Jaspers was at least misleading when he asserted that he was employing phenomenology in a manner like

Edmund Husserl. We shall maintain in this paper that, although differences exist, Jaspers' notion of phenomenology significantly resembles Husserl's. For Jaspers chose to apply phenomenology to psychopathology, and Husserl had limited it to philosophy and psychology. The resemblances, however, clearly indicate that Jaspers did derive his notion of phenomenology from Husserl while modifying it to fit his own professional experience as a practicing psychiatrist. This Jaspersian notion of a phenomenological psychopathology, we shall argue, should be revived and employed again in psychiatry today. Only this method can furnish detailed and precise descriptions of the psychopathological experiences of patients. The currently accepted notion of "phenomenology" as a description of the signs and symptoms of a disorder, on the other hand, leaves the patient's psychopathological experiences ill-defined. What is needed in present-day psychiatry are the detailed and exact descriptions of psychopathological events that a Jaspersian phenomenology can provide. And, following Jaspers and Husserl, these detailed descriptions can be obtained while remaining strictly neutral with regard to etiology.

Recent articles by G. E. Berrios and C. Walker will serve as examples of the view of Jaspers' phenomenology that seems to be held by many psychiatrists today. In this paper, we shall first address the claims of Berrios and Walker. Secondly, we shall explicate some of the main concepts in Husserl's phenomenology. Thirdly, we shall discuss Jaspers' version of phenomenology, with particular regard to Husserl's influence on it. Fourthly and briefly toward the end of our essay, we shall indicate how present-day psychiatry may benefit from the refined view of phenomenology that we propose. In our judgment the phenomenologies of Husserl and Jaspers offer important methodological insights for researchers and for clinical psychiatrists.

2. Berrios on Phenomenology

In a recent article entitled, *What Is Phenomenology? A Review*, G.E. Berrios addresses the topic of the relationship of phenomenology to psychiatry (Berrios 1989). Berrios' concern with this relationship is commendable because it demonstrates the need to re-examine the influence that movements of thought outside of psychiatry actually have had in the past or potentially could have in the future on psychiatry. In this article, however, Berrios' findings are almost entirely negative. He concludes that phenomenologists, despite their claims to devise and utilize a purely descriptive approach to mental entities, have in all likelihood failed to do so (Berrios 1989, p. 427).

We contend that matters are not as dire as Berrios asserts. Through a critical examination of Berrios' review, we shall maintain that his depiction of phenomenology remains far too limited for him to appreciate adequately (1) the influence that Husserl's early phenomenology had on Karl Jaspers in the *General Psychopathology,* or (2) the relevance of Jaspers' phenomenology for present-day psychiatry.

Berrios begins his article by claiming that,

> "The term 'phenomenology' refers to a set of philosophical doctrines loosely sharing: (a) assumptions as to what the world is like (metaphysical) and how it can be known (epistemological), and more importantly, (b) strategies for the descriptive management of the mental entities relating to such a world" (Berrios 1989, p. 425).

Phenomenologists, however, do not share, even "loosely," "assumptions as to what the world is like (metaphysical)." Husserl, for example, endorses a "transcendental" phenomenology precisely in order to "bracket" or "set aside" all metaphysical assumptions regarding the world. Husserl's philosophy remains metaphysically neutral (Husserl 1973a, 1982). On the other hand, later phenomenologists, like Heidegger and Sartre, are ontologists who are indeed concerned with the *being* of the world and of the human beings who exist in this world (Sartre 1956, Heidegger 1962). Furthermore, contrary to what Berrios writes, phenomenologists do not share "assumptions" as to "how (the world) can be known (epistemological)." Husserl and other early phenomenologists, like Alexander Pfänder, devoted their efforts to an epistemology of logic, mathematics, and science (Husserl 1969, 1970a, Pfänder 1963). For these thinkers, the world can be known through empirical science and through a philosophy that is itself a "rigorous science" (Husserl 1965). Heidegger, on the other hand, dismissed the "calculative reckoning" involved in logic, mathematics, and science and sought to replace it with a "poetic dwelling" that made the poet and not the scientist the intimate of Being (Heidegger 1966, 1971). More recently, phenomenological discussions of epistemology center around the "hermeneutic interpretation" of action, language, and symbols (Ricoeur 1974, Gadamer 1975).

Berrios comes closer to the mark when he writes that phenomenologists "loosely" share "strategies for the descriptive management of the mental entities relating to such a world." But in this respect, too, phenomenologists differ greatly. Only Husserl and his disciples in the Göttingen and Munich Circles adopt a strictly descriptive approach to what Berrios calls "mental entities" (Spiegelberg 1960). Heidegger and his followers not only reject Husserl's descriptivism and replace it with hermeneutics, but they also deem it a mistake to focus on mind rather than on the more inclusive reality of human being-in-the-world (Sartre 1956, Heidegger 1962).

Regarding the question of what phenomenologists "loosely share," the most that can be said, we think, is that Husserl's own approach induced philosophers to "return to the 'things themselves'" (*auf die Sachen selbst zurückgehen;* cf. Husserl 1968, Spiegelberg 1960). What this means is that Husserl taught his students that they need not adopt and continue some pre-established philosophical or scientific approach. Whatever one sought to study could be studied simply through a faithful rendering of how the phenomena presented themselves to one in the various forms of experience. Of course, it would prove necessary subsequently to reflect upon the "method" that one had at first employed naively and uncritically, and this subsequent self-reflection and self-criticism would have to explicate, test, revise, and improve one's procedure. But at first the main point was to focus and report on what one directly observed when one experienced the phenomena under investigation. This, we suggest, is precisely why phenomenology spawned so many different approaches, doctrines, and methods and, therefore, why it remains so difficult to specify what it is that phenomenologists hold in common: Husserl taught that the thinker's first duty was to remain faithful "to the things themselves" and not to remain faithful to some pregiven method, concepts, theory, or orientation. Jaspers' approach, we think, is "phenomenological" in this broad sense. Jaspers captures Husserl's spirit precisely when he writes, "The source of knowledge always remains living intuition" (*Quelle unserer Erkenntnis bleibt immer die lebendige Anschauung*)[2] (Jaspers 1963a, p. 37, 1965, p. 32).

In order to evaluate Berrios' article, we must recognize that it harbors two different aims, although these are not clearly distinguished by Berrios himself. (A) The first aim is historical: Berrios seeks to determine whether the "descriptive method" that Husserl employed in his early writings significantly shaped Karl Jaspers' discussions of "phenomenology" and "description" in the *General Psychopathology* (Berrios 1989, p. 425). (B) The second aim is methodological: Berrios wants to know whether "phenomenology was, is (or ever will be) just a sophisticated method of description,..." (Berrios 1989, p. 427). As he explains further,

"From a technical viewpoint, the issue is whether it is possible to find in phenomenology anything that can meaningfully be recognized as a pure (atheoretical) 'method' of description" (Berrios 1989, p. 427).

It is important to recognize that these are two separate aims because Berrios' reasoning becomes faulty when he himself fails to keep them distinct. Berrios considers only four thinkers: Franz Brentano, Gottlob Frege, Wilhelm Dilthey, and Edmund Husserl. And Berrios' discussions of each of these men remains extremely sketchy; we read only about the barest rudiments of their views. Brentano, Frege, and Dilthey, however, can be deemed at the most only "precursors" of the phenomenological movement that properly begins with Husserl (Spiegelberg 1960). Unfortunately, when Berrios does discuss Husserl, he limits himself to the most elementary points in the phenomenologist's early writings (Berrios 1989, pp. 426-427). Berrios justifies restricting himself to only Husserl and then to Husserl's early works because the early philosophy of Husserl, "according to many writers (and indeed Jaspers himself), is the intellectual source of what has since been called Jaspersian phenomenology" (Berrios

---

2 We have usually substituted our own English translations of Jaspers' *General Psychopathology* for the translation by J. Hoenig and Marian W. Hamilton. This does not in any way suggest that we do not believe the translations by Hoenig and Hamilton to be a fine one. We have employed our own translations only because we are thereby able to highlight certain terms that Jaspers uses which are important for our arguments here.

1989, p. 425). In other words, the first aim mentioned above, i.e., the question of Husserl's influence on Jaspers, justifies Berrios in his consideration of no other phenomenologist than the early Husserl. And yet on the basis of this self-imposed limitation Berrios draws conclusions regarding the relevance of phenomenology in general for psychiatry in the past, present, and future. Berrios concludes,

> "...there is little in the philosophical movement called phenomenology (as developed by Husserl and continued by his followers) which is conceptually useful to the construction of a modern theory of description applicable to the signs and symptoms of mental or physical illness" (Berrios 1989, p. 427).

This is a striking conclusion since Berrios has said nothing whatsoever regarding the phenomenology "continued by (Husserl's) followers" and he has penned very little concerning Husserl's mature philosophy. In other words, on the basis of a limitation imposed regarding his first aim, Berrios draws unwarranted conclusions regarding his second aim.

In Berrios' essay, however, matters are worse than this. His discussion of phenomenology remains very superficial. He gives the most elementary definition of Husserl's early notion of intentionality, and he sketches in the briefest way Husserl's early struggles with and rejection of "psychologism" (Berrios 1989, pp. 426-427). About Husserl's notion of description—supposedly a central topic of Berrios' essay—we learn merely that it applies to "subjective experiences" and that it "relies on the exercise of special human faculties such as intuition and empathy" (Berrios 1989, p. 427). Berrios fails to explain what "intuition" means in a phenomenological context. Nor does Berrios provide any indication of Husserl's extensive attempts to justify the role of intuition in his philosophical method (Husserl 1982). Moreover, if Berrios were truly interested in the influence of Husserl on Jaspers, he should at least point out that, according to Jaspers, "intuition" *(Anschauung)* is essential to the method of psychiatry and to the methods of the empirical sciences in general: "The source of knowledge always remains living intuition" (Jaspers 1963a, p. 37, 1965, p. 32).

3. C. Walker on the Relationship of Jaspers's Phenomenology to Husserl's

C. Walker has summarized what he takes to be the relationship of Jaspers' phenomenology to Husserl's in his recent article, *Philosophical Concepts and Practice: The Legacy of Karl Jaspers' Psychopathology* (Walker 1988). Walker claims that, despite appearances to the contrary (even in Jaspers' own mind!), there is in reality no such relationship. Walker writes,

> "It is clear that Jasper's (sic) phenomenology (the study of what patients actually experience) has nothing in common with Husserl's phenomenology (the study of timeless and culture-free essential structures of consciousness). Jaspers himself was slow to realise this. He misunderstood Husserl's early work and, throughout his life, continued to think of it as similar in intent to his own phenomenology. Unlike

Husserl, Jaspers argued for a radical distinction between philosophy and science, and rejected any thought of a scientific philosophy. He was later to describe Husserl's efforts towards such a scientific philosophy as 'the most naive and pretentious betrayal of philosophy'" (Walker 1988, p. 626).

Notice that, in order to deny the influence of Husserl's phenomenology on Jaspers', Walker is compelled to claim that Jaspers *misunderstood* Husserl's work. Walker is compelled to make such a daring claim because he must at the same time concede that Jaspers throughout his life continued to think of Husserl's phenomenology as similar in intent to his own. Walker would have us believe that Jaspers was simply mistaken when in the mid-1950's he recalled,

"My own investigations as well as my reflection about what was being said and done in psychiatry (in 1911) had led me on tracks which were new at that time. Philosophers gave me the impetus for two essential steps. As method I adopted Husserl's phenomenology, which, in its beginnings, he called descriptive psychology; I retained it although I rejected its further development into intuition of essences (*Wesensschau*).[3] It proved to be possible and fruitful to describe the inner experiences of patients as phenomena of consciousness. Not only hallucinations, but also delusions, modes of ego-consciousness, and emotions could, on the basis of the patients' own descriptions, be described so clearly that they became recognizable with certainty in other cases. Phenomenology became a method for research" (Jaspers 1957, p. 18).

Jaspers is obviously convinced here that, with the exception of "intution of essences", he adopted and fruitfully employed in psychiatry the phenomenological method developed by Husserl. This method allowed Jaspers "to describe the inner experiences of patients as phenomena of consciousness." Jaspers is undeniably referring to his own appropriation of Husserl's approach when he asserts: "Phenomenology became a method of research." Walker contends that Jaspers was "slow to realise" that his own phenomenology had nothing in common with Husserl's. From the above quotation one must rather say that Jaspers *never* realised this because Jaspers himself flatly says, "As method I adopted Husserl's phenomenology" and "I retained it." Granted, Jaspers did explicitly reject that part of Husserl's method that Husserl called "intuition of essences" (Jaspers 1957, p. 18, 1963a, p. 55). But, as we shall demonstrate in detail below, Jaspers retained Husserl's notion of "intuition" (*Anschauung*). Jaspers simply recognized that psychopathology as an *empirical science* had to attain an intuition of *empirical* concepts and not the intuition of *essential* concepts that was required by Husserl's philosophy.

Walker makes it appear that the distinction between Husserl's and Jaspers' phenomenologies is greater than it in fact is by importing—what is actually irrelevant here—Jaspers' quite different conception of *philosophy*. When Jaspers—*after* his work in phenomenological psychopathology—

---

3 We prefer to render *Wesensschau* as "intuition of essences" rather than retain "insight into essences" used by Paul Arthur Schlipp and Ludwig B. Lefebre in their translation of Jaspers' *Philosophical Autobiography* (Jaspers 1957, p. 18).

came to develop his own existentialist *philosophy,* he conceived of it as extremely different from science. For Jaspers, philosophy was a kind of "thinking" that resembled Kierkegaard's notion of religious faith. (Jaspers 1970). Husserl strongly opposed this and insisted that philosophy be a "rigorous science" (Husserl 1965). Jaspers had had no trouble agreeing with Husserl when he had earlier appropriated Husserl's "rigorous science" for the scientific field of *psychopathology.* But Jaspers had subsequently to disagree strongly with Husserl's rigorous science when it came to the question of the nature of *philosophy.* It is this wide gap between Jaspers' existentialist conception of philosophy (as a thinking akin to religious faith) and Husserl's rationalist conception of philosophy (as a cognitive undertaking resembling science) that is heatedly expressed in Jaspers' condemnation of Husserl's notion of philosophy as "the most naive and pretentious betrayal of philosophy." This disagreement regarding *philosophy,* however, implies nothing regarding Jaspers' *psychopathology* and its reliance on Husserl's phenomenology.

It should be apparent to the reader by now that much needs to be done in order to clarify the issues surrounding the relationship between Husserl's phenomenology and Jaspers' psychopathology. We shall try to sort out some of these complex issues.

4. Some Basic Concepts of Husserl's Phenomenology

Let us first focus on a topic mentioned by both Berrios and Walker, *intuition.* We today are likely to dismiss intuition as a reliable cognitive tool because, for us, "intuition" typically means something like what pops into one's head without much careful thought. This contemporary trivial connotation of intuition is, however, entirely foreign to the meaning the term possessed in the tradition of Modern philosophy from Descartes through Kant, and it was from this tradition that Husserl and Jaspers acquired the term. For Husserl, as for most Modern philosophers, "intuition" signified any *direct awareness* of something. Intuition is an experience in which the object of which one is aware is *itself directly given* "in person" (Husserl 1973a, 1982). The sense perception of a physical object provides one commonplace example of intuition. When I perceive an object standing in front of me, the object is directly given "in person" to me. This can be contrasted with merely remembering the object later. In memory I am aware of the object although the object is not itself directly given to me. The object remembered is not presented to me "in person." Perception is intuitive. Memory is non-intuitive. Sense perception, however, is only one illustration of intuitive experience. Philosophy, according to Husserl, must base all of its claims on the intuition of the objects about which it speaks (Husserl 1973a, 1982).

Philosophy must base all of its claims on intuition because philosophy, according to Husserl, has the task of seeking knowledge that is *certain* to the highest degree attainable (Husserl 1969, 1973a, 1982). Not all the sciences seek certain knowledge because the various subject matters or object-domains of the various sciences do not permit them to obtain *certain* knowledge. Philosophy alone aspires to certain knowledge. Certain knowledge is attainable, Husserl thinks, only if that knowledge arises from the full direct givenness (the "intuition") of the objects one is studying. The only "objects" that can be fully and adequately intuited are *one's own* "mental processes" *(Erlebnisse)* and their intended objects (Husserl 1973a, 1982). Therefore, in order to attain knowledge that is certain, philosophy must take as its subject matter mental life *(Bewusstsein)* and the objects of mental life precisely and solely as they are intended by mental life.

Because Husserl has been frequently misunderstood on this point it is important to explain what Husserl means by "intentionality." Husserl's mature philosophy—his "transcendental phenomenology"—has been misconstrued by some interpreters as a "subjectivism." By the word "subjectivism" let us understand any philosophy or psychology which examines exclusively mental life and its (mental) contents (Gurwitsch 1966). Subjectivism, in other words, is a theory exclusively of mental events and realities, whether these mental entities be ideas, emotions, impressions, sense data, or mental representations. Husserl's mature phenomenology is not such a subjectivism, and it escapes from such subjectivism through its unique concept of "intentionality." The term "intentionality," for Husserl, expresses the peculiar capacity of mental processes to provide access to the extra-mental. "Intentionality" means that it is precisely subjectivity, the mind, that gives us direct and immediate access to objectivity, the real world (Husserl 1982). Intentionality expresses a direct relationship between subjectivity and objectivity. Husserl chose to call this a relationship between "noesis," mental process, and "noema," intended object (Husserl 1982). The intended object, for the mature Husserl, is nothing intra-mental; it is not a "mental content." The objects which mental life apprehends are extra-mental; i.e., they are "objective," except, of course, when mental life intends other mental processes. Phenomenology, then, is not confined to studying what Aron Gurwitsch has called "the closed sphere of interiority", the mind and its contents (Gurwitsch 1974). Phenomenology rather studies intentionality, the direct access that the mind has to the world.

If the phenomenologist seeks to study intentionality intuitively, however, he or she must proceed through *self-reflection,* i.e., through reflection upon one's own mental processes as exemplars of mental life in general (Husserl 1973a, 1982). For it is only my own mental processes and their objects that can be directly given, i.e., intuitively given, to me. A philosophy which employs this intuitive and reflective approach can and must be "descriptive." "Description" means, for Husserl, statements which express nothing but what one directly observes; descriptive statements report intuitions. Descriptive statements in phenomenology should thus depict exclusively what one directly observes when one reflects upon one's own mental life and its objects (Husserl 1973a, 1982).

Husserl propounds this descriptive method because he opposes theories of mind which either reduce subjective experiences to less than they observably are or else account for subjective processes by postulating unobservable mechanisms underneath them (Husserl 1968, pp. 19-22). Husserl seeks a philosophical exploration of mind that does full justice to human experiences precisely as they are lived through by the subjects whose experiences they are. Consequently, Husserl's phenomenology refuses to go beyond what can be directly observed when one reflects upon one's experiences. Husserl spoke, accordingly, of a "bracketing" or "setting aside" of all presuppositions and concepts that are not fully justified by what one can directly observe in self-reflection (Husserl 1973a, 1982). As Husserl writes, "The principle (of presuppositionlessness) means nothing more than the strict exclusion of all statements that cannot be fully and completely implemented *(realisiert)* in a phenomenological fashion". While carrying out descriptive phenomenology, all explanatory theories, whether psychological, natural scientific, or metaphysical, are systematically excluded. Phenomenological understanding consists, not in explaining *(erklären)*, but rather in clarifing *(aufklären,* cf. Husserl 1968, pp. 19-22). What is clarified are the concepts of the subject matter under investigation, concepts which are otherwise employed in a vague and indefinite fashion. These concepts are phenomenologically clarified through the intuition *(Anschauung)* of directly given individual exemplifications of them. In the intuition of particular examples I directly see their details, subtleties, and nuances. Because I have now directly seen these details, nuances, and subtleties of objects designated by the concept, I now know what the concept *means;* i.e., I have rendered the meaning of the concept clear, precise, and distinct to myself. Husserl calls such an intuition a "fulfilling intuition" *(erfüllende Anschauung)* because it fills in the precise meaning of the concept: it is a direct seeing of the exact and definite meaning of the concept. Through such intuition the phenomenologist "clarifies" concepts but never "explains" the occurrence of events. Jaspers will speak subsequently of the need to "fulfill a concept" through a seeing *(sehen)* or intuiting *(schauen)* of psychological phenomena (Jaspers 1963b, p. 319).

Having described what one directly finds in self-reflection, the phenomenologist cautiously generalizes his or her findings through a method that Husserl calls "free variation in phantasy" (Husserl 1982). The purpose of this imaginative variation is to reach universal features of mental life that are necessarily invariable. These necessarily invariant features Husserl, following the philosophical tradition, called "essences" (Husserl 1982). The phenomenologist distinguishes between essential and empirical laws and concepts. Essential laws and concepts hold for any possible or conceivable world; empirical laws and concepts apply solely to our actual world. Phenomenological psychiatrists may elect to determine the essential features of psychopathologies along with their empirical features (for a more detailled account, see Uehlein, this volume).

Berrios, on the other hand, believes that the phenomenological notion of "essences" will find little place in psychiatry. He writes, "From the point of view of the clinician, perhaps, the more difficult point to deal with relates to 'immutable essences'..." (Berrios 1989). He explains that if essences are interpreted as "metaphysical entities," they "might prove to be too high a metaphysical price to pay" (Berrios 1989). In response, we would like to point out that essences, for the phenomenologist, are simply one kind of general regularity or concept (Husserl 1982). Consequently, essences have the same "metaphysical" status as any other kind of general law or concept, such as the empirical concepts of "schizophrenia," "manic-depression," or "compulsion." Consequently, the "metaphysical price" one must pay for employing essential concepts is no higher than the "metaphysical price" one must pay for using any concepts at all.

Moreover, Husserl does allow for a "psychological phenomenology" that remains factual and empirical and thus does not concern itself with essential concepts. Such a psychological phenomenology remains within the "natural attitude" of all the empirical sciences and does not adopt the "transcendental attitude" of Husserl's philosophical phenomenology. Because this psychological phenomenology studies the general factual features of real mental events (and their objects), it is not a philosophy at all but rather an empirical science (Husserl 1982, P. xx). We shall see that, from a Husserlian point of view, Jaspers' phenomenology can be viewed as precisely such a phenomenological empirical science.

Before we address Jaspers' appropriation and modification of Husserl's phenomenological method, let us look at the topic of "empathy." Contrary to what Berrios writes, Husserl never deems empathy a component of his philosophical method. Husserl does devote numerous pages (that he himself never published) to describing the role of empathy (Einfühlung) in everyday (non-philosophical) intersubjectivity (Husserl 1973b). Empathy could never form a part of Husserl's philosophical method because the term "empathy" means one person's experiences of another person's experiences; and another person's experiences can never be directly presented to me. For Husserl as for Jaspers, I can never directly observe another person's experiences. Therefore, I can never be certain of what the other person is experiencing. Empathy can, therefore, never provide certain knowledge of mental life, and empathy precisely for that reason can never become a component of Husserl's philosophical method (Husserl 1973b). It will remain for Jaspers to recognize that empathy, despite its lack of complete certainty, must be a part of the method of phenomenology as an empirical science.

5. Karl Jaspers' Phenomenological Method

We can now examine Jaspers' view of phenomenology in psychiatry. Referring to his departure from Husserl, Jaspers takes psychiatric phenomenology to be an empirical method (ein empirisches Verfahren, cf.

Jaspers 1963a, p. 55, 1965, p. 47). This signifies that, in Jaspers' hands, it is *not* a philosophical method. It is rather a method of empirical science that attempts to describe the subjective experiences of the psychiatric patient (Jaspers 1963a, p. 53, 1965, p. 45). Because Jaspers' phenomenology is an empirical method, it disregards Husserl's procedure of free variation in imagination that finally leads to an intuition of essential features *(Wesensschau)* (Jaspers 1963a, p. 55, 1965, p. 47).

The crucial methodological question for Jaspersian phenomenology thus becomes this: By what scientific method can the psychiatrist attain valid knowledge of the subjective experiences of another person, namely, the experiences of his or her patient? Since through this method one person is experiencing another person's experiences, the method will remain some form of empathy; and Jaspers repeatedly characterizes his phenomenological procedure as empathy *(Einfühlen)* and understanding *(Verstehen, cf.* Jaspers 1963a, p. 55, 1963b, pp. 314-328, 1965, p. 47). What Jaspers views as phenomenology in empirical science will thus differ from what Husserl sees as phenomenology in philosophy because Husserl, for the reasons cited above, never thought of phenomenology as involving empathy or understanding.

This difference in method is required, however, by the differences in subject matter. Jaspers, unlike Husserl, seeks to explicate precisely the peculiarities of *pathological* experiences (Jaspers 1963a, p. 53, 1963b, pp. 314-328, 1965, p. 45). The individual facts from which such an explication must start are not, therefore, the experiences of the psychiatrist which can be directly given to him or her in self-reflection. The initial facts are rather the psychopathological experiences of the patient, and these experiences cannot be given to the psychiatrist in self-reflection—unless obviously the psychiatrist also happens to be ill in the same way. The psychiatrist must foresake, then, the intuitive self-reflection of the Husserlian philosopher. Instead, according to Jaspers—and this is the crux of his phenomenological method—the psychiatrist seeks to "intuitively represent" *(anschaulich vergegenwärtigen)* the pathological experiences of his or her patient (Jaspers 1963a, p. 55, 1963b, pp. 314-328, 1965, p. 47). Based on Jaspers' own characterization of his phenomenological method, we shall now venture an interpretation of it.

Jaspers remarks several times that it is the patient and the patient alone who has direct access to his or her subjective experiences (Jaspers 1963a, p. 55-56, 1965, p. 47-48). Only the patient can directly intuit—in Husserl's sense—his or her pathological experiences. How, then, is the psychiatrist able to gain cognitive access to these experiences? Through "representation" *(Vergegenwärtigung)* of them (Jaspers 1963a, p. 53 & 55, 1963b, pp. 314-328, 1965, p. 45 & 47). We must consequently provide an interpretation of this difficult German term, *Vergegenwärtigung.* In "representation" the object of which one is aware is not itself directly given; it is not itself directly present to one's mind. But the object is experienced *as if* it were itself directly given, *as if* it were directly present. In representation I am examining the object of my awareness as if it were directly given to me although in actual fact it is not.

But if the object is not in fact directly given to me in representation, how can Jaspers require that such representation be "intuitive" (anschaulich)? (Jaspers 1963a, p. 55, 1963b, pp. 314-328, 1965, p. 47). In addition to signifying the direct experiencing of an object, Anschauung in German sometimes carries another connotation. Anschauung occasionally has the connotation of "experiencing an object in graphic detail" (Wildhagen & Heraucourt 1965, p. 60). Now usually, of course, we experience an object in graphic detail only when it is itself directly given to us. When, for example, I simply think about some state of affairs in its absence, I usually do not have it before my mind in great detail. In visual perception, by contrast, the objects I directly see can be seen by me in marked and ample detail. Thus "intuition" in the sense of direct givenness can also carry the connotation of "experienced in graphic detail" because experiencing something in graphic detail usually seems to characteristize the direct givenness of that thing.

We can now offer an interpretation of the phrase which, for Jaspers, defines the phenomenological approach in psychiatry, "intuitive representation." When the psychiatrist "intuitively represents" to him- or herself the experiences of patients, these pathological experiences are not and cannot themselves be directly given to the psychiatrist. But the psychiatrist must graphically represent them to him- or herself in great detail. The psychiatrist must graphically represent them to him- or herself as if they were directly given. In sum, then, "intuitive representation" means a detailed and graphic awareness of the features of another person's actual experiences.

We can now mark an important difference between Husserl's and Jaspers' phenomenologies. Husserl would require the *direct presentation* of experiences in order to describe them phenomenologically. Jaspers, however, admits the *intuitive representation* of experiences in his phenomenology because the psychopathological experiences of patients can never be directly presented to the observing psychiatrist. Jaspers recognizes that intuitive representation is the closest one person can come to the "direct presentation" of another person's experiences.

It will perhaps clarify Jaspers' notion of intuitive representation if we contrast it with its opposite. Psychiatrists can have merely a vague and indeterminate awareness of the manifold features of their patients' experiences. This is the opposite of intuitive representation (Jaspers 1963a, p. 56, 1965, p. 48). Jaspers would probably say that in such cases the psychiatrist is not aware of the patient's experiences at all. The psychiatrist is rather aware of the vague and indeterminate meanings of psychopathological *concepts,* and the obscure meanings of these concepts are being mistaken for the experiences to which they refer. The phenomenological psychiatrist, for Jaspers, must break through this vague and indefinite awareness of patients' experiences and achieve instead a graphic, definite, and detailed cognizance of their features. In other words, the psychiatrist must break through dealing merely with the meanings of psychopathological terms and directly see the patient's experiences themselves as if these experiences were directly given to the psychiatrist's mind. Only when psychiatrists directly examine through intuitive represention the features of patients' experiences can they then recognize what the psychopathological concepts truly mean (Jaspers 1963b, p. 318).

How can the psychiatrist begin to attain this distinct, detailed, and graphic representation of a patient's experiences? Jaspers claims that the best help for attaining these representations comes from the patient's own self-depictions (*Selbstschilderungen,* cf. Jaspers 1963a, p. 55, 1963b, p. 320, 1965, p. 47). These self-depictions can be provoked and tested in conversation with the patient. Moreover, the clearest and most complete self-depictions by a patients are written ones. Jaspers is convinced that,

"the person who has the experience is the one who can most easily find the appropriate depiction of it. The psychiatrist who merely observes the patient would struggle in vain to formulate what the patient can say about his or her own experience" (Jaspers 1963a, p. 55, 1965, p. 47).

Because it is patients, and not psychiatrists, who alone can directly observe pathological experiences through self-reflection, psychiatrists must rely on patients' communications. Nothing can substitute for patients' self-reports. Psychiatrists should, of course, continually test the credibility of patients as well as their powers of judgment. And Jaspers is cognizant of the mistakes the psychiatrist can make in accepting a patient's statements as all too reliable. But Jaspers also warns of the reverse mistake of remaining radically skeptical of patients' reports (Jaspers 1963a, p. 55, 1965, p. 47).

6. "Presuppositionlessness" in Jaspers' Phenomenology

We can now broach the issue of the "presuppositionless" or, as Berrios prefers to designate it, "atheoretical" character of phenomenological descriptions. In Jaspers' phenomenology, it would be erroneous to ascribe to the patient anything he or she is not actually experiencing (Jaspers 1963a, p. 55-56, 1963b, p. 317, 1965, p. 47-48). Jaspers writes,

"Only that which actually exists in (the patient's) mental life should be represented; everything that is not actually given in (the patient's) mental life does not exist" (Jaspers 1963a, p. 56, 1963b, p. 317, 1965, p. 48).

Jaspers, following Husserl, wants to do full justice to what the patient is actually experiencing; he does not want to overlook any real features, however complex, of the patient's experiences. Yet at the same time Jaspers does not want to impute to the patient anything that he or she does not actually experience; Jaspers wishes to describe *exclusively* what is present in the patient's own lived experience. This is precisely what Husserl's "descriptive phenomenology" had sought to do: to describe the features of mental processes *fully* but *exclusively* as they are lived through by the experiencing subject. This means that it would be erroneous to postulate the efficacy of causes, motives, or other origins of the patient's experiences unless those causes or motives are themselves *actual* mental processes of the patient. This is why, for Jaspers as for Husserl, concepts and theories taken over from prior sources pose dangers. Concepts and theories carry connotations and implications that may not apply to the real experiences of a particular patient or of any patient at all. As Jaspers writes about phenomenology,

"We must set aside all received theories, psychological constructions, or materialist mythologies of brain processes. We must apply ourselves purely to what we can understand, apprehend, distinguish, and describe in its actual existence" (Jaspers 1963b, p. 317).

Jaspers is here guarding against an "explanatory" psychopathology that would postulate underlying mechanisms which are not themselves experienced by the patient but are nevertheless supposed to produce what the patient does experience. A "descriptive" psychopathology is distinguished from such an explanatory psychopathology because the former restricts itself to explicating the patient's experiences precisely and exclusively as the patient actually lives through them. For this reason, the phenomenological psychiatrist must learn to bracket or set aside all interpretations (*Deutungen*) and prejudgments (*Beurteilungen*) and purely describe what is actually occurring in the patient's mental life. The phenomenological method is accordingly characterized by its "presuppositionlessness" (*Vorurteilslosigkeit*)[4] (Jaspers 1963a, p. 56, 1963b, pp. 317-318, 1965, p. 48).

Jaspers acknowledges that achieving this prejudgment-less attitude is not simple or easy. He warns,

"As experience teaches us, this is a very difficult task. This peculiarly phenomenological presuppositionlessness is not an original possession. It is rather a laborious acquisition after long critical work and often futile efforts in constructions and mythologies. Just like we as children first count things not as we see them but rather as we think them, so we as psychologists and psychopathologists go through a stage in which we somehow *think* mental processes to the stage of a presuppositionlessness, immediate apprehending of mental processes just as they *are*. Always renewed efforts are required, and we must repeatedly overcome prejudgments in order to earn this prize (*Gut*): this phenomenological attitude" (Jaspers 1963b, pp. 317-318).

Jaspers' phenomenology is thus "presuppositionless" or "atheoretical" in the sense that it does not impute features to mental processes just

---

4   The reader should be aware that the German terms which we have translated simply as "presuppositionlessness" and its cognates are different in Husserl's and Jaspers' texts. Husserl prefers the term *Voraussetzungslosigkeit* and Jaspers prefers *Vorurteilslosigkeit* although Jaspers does use *voraussetzungslos* in at least one place (Jaspers 1963b, p. 322). We have felt that it is permissable to translate the two German terms as "presuppositionlessness" for two reasons: (1) it is simply too awkward in English to speak of "prejudice-lessness" or "prejudice-less"; and (2) Husserl and Jaspers employ their respective terms in order to make fundamentally the same point. We suspect that Jaspers used *Vorurteilslosigkeit* because *Vorurteil* connotes the more emphatic term "prejudice" and Jaspers sought to make plain his condemnation of the power of prejudgments to mislead. Husserl chose to employ the more neutral term "presupposition."

because some theory or set of concept implies those features. It rather ascribes features to mental processes only if those features can be intuitively represented on the basis of the evidence of the patient's speech or behavior. And it is precisely features of mental processes that can be intuitively represented on the basis of this direct evidence that shall serve as the tribunal for deciding the adequacy and validity of all psychopathological theories and concepts.

Later in the *General Psychopathology* Jaspers introduces additional methods to deal with aspects of the patient's life that phenomenology systematically "brackets" or sets aside. He will then describe (1) a "psychology of understanding" *(verstehende Psychologie)* that will furnish scientific access to the various motives or meaningful sources of the patient's experiences (Jaspers 1963a, pp. 302-413); (2) an "explanatory psychology" *(erklärende Psychologie)* that will investigate causal mechanisms that shape experience (Jaspers 1963a, pp. 451-552); (3) a "somatopsychology" for studying bodily events in the patient that can be seen or detected by an outside observer (Jaspers 1963a, pp. 222-250); and (4) methods for intepreting the objective expressions or products of the patient's mental life, such as writing, physiognomy, or conduct (Jaspers 1963a, pp. 251-297). But prior to the employment of these methods, Jaspers deems it essential to appreciate the patient's actual experiences cautiously and fully and not to precipitously leap beyond what the patient is actually living through.

Why does Jaspers in his phenomenology emphasize this descriptive procedure free from pre-established concepts, judgments, and theories? If there are to be any useful concepts in psychopathology, they must be built on a sound evidential base. Any psychopathological concepts which do not pay strict attention to the details, subtleties, and nuances of patients' experiences will fail to do full justice to its subject matter. Moreover, psychopathological concepts that imply more than is actually present in the patient's own lived experience cannot serve as a reliable foundation for theory-formation. *Jaspers thinks, accordingly, that the evidential basis for any conceptual constructs in psychopathology must be phenomenological; i.e., the evidential base must be a graphic and detailed representation of the manifold features of patients' pathological experiences precisely as the patient lives through them.* Intuitive representation, while remaining a form of understanding and empathy, is the closest the psychopathologist can come to direct observation of his or her subject matter (Jaspers 1963b, p. 319). As Jaspers writes,

"For the *representation (Vergegenwärtigung)* of all of these phenomenologically ultimate qualities I have already used several expressions like *seeing, intuiting, empathizing, understanding,* and the like. With all of these expressions I mean for the same *ultimate experience* to be understood. It is this experience which alone fulfills our concepts. It is this experience which in the psychological domain plays the same role as sense perception does in the natural scientific domain" (Jaspers 1963b, p. 319).

It has become, however, a commonplace in philosophy of science nowadays to insist that all observation is "theory-laden." If this current thesis holds, it would appear that Jaspers' championing of a "presuppositionless, immediate apprehending of the mental" (*vorurteilslosen unmittelbaren Erfassung des Psychischen*) is unrealistic (Jaspers 1963a, p. 56, 1965, p. 48). For it would appear that any "apprehending of the mental" would remain unavoidably informed by presupposed concepts and theories.

We submit, however, that such an objection to Jaspers' phenomenology would do little damage to it. For when Jaspers worries about the influence of concepts and theories on psychopathological inquires, he need not contest the theory- or concept-ladenness of psychiatric observation and description. Jaspers worries that psychiatrists, when they interview patients, will rest content with only a vague, indefinite, and indeterminate awareness of the patients' pathological experiences. Jaspers worries, in other words, that psychiatrists will content themselves with merely an awareness of the pre-given meanings of concepts and theories that the patients' reports bring to mind. What Jaspers demands, by contrast, is a detailed, definite, and graphic awareness of the experiences that patients actually undergo; and this detailed and graphic psychiatric awareness must be firmly based on what the patient says and how the patient acts. Jaspers expresses all of this quite clearly himself:

> "In histology it is required that, when examining the cerebral cortext, we should account for each fiber and each cell. Phenomenology places upon us entirely analogous demands: *we should account for each mental phenomenon, each experience* which comes to light in the exploration of patients and their self-depictions. We should in no case remain satisfied with a global impression (*Gesamteindruck*) and a few details selected ad hoc, but we should know each single particularity and how to apprehend and judge it" (Jaspers 1963a, p. 56, 1963b, p. 318, 1965, p. 48).

Intuitive representation, the method of Jaspers' phenomenology, is precisely this detailed, determinate, and graphic apprehension of the manifold features of patients' experiences grounded in the evidence provided by patients themselves.

To say that a description must be "presuppositionless" is to refer, then, to the basis upon which the terms of the phenomenological description receive their legitimate significations. The meanings of psychopathological concepts are not simply to be taken over from some pre-given taxonomy, theory, or school; the meanings of the terms are not to be "presupposed." Psychopathological concepts are rather to be tested, revised, and redefined by what psychiatrists can intuitively represent to themselves on the evidential basis of communication with patients. For these reasons Berrios is mistaken to claim,

> "Descriptions in phenomenology are not meant...to form the basis for empirical statements of the kind that might be considered as relevant to science or scientific psychopathology" (Berrios 1989, p. 427).

Contrary to what Berrios says, Jaspers' phenomenology can provide the basis for empirical statements that are directly relevant to scientific psychopathology because this phenomenology provides a detailed and graphic description of the mental processes of the psychiatric patient.

7. Components Common to Husserl's and Jaspers' Phenomenologies

As a brief summary of the rather complex points we have been at pains to make, let us now simply list those features shared by Husserl's and Jaspers' phenomenologies:

1) The phenomenologist *describes mental processes fully and exclusively* as they are lived through by the person whose mental life is under investigation.

2) *The definition of phenomenological concepts is based exclusively on the intuition of the phenomena which the concepts designate.* This is what makes phenomenology "descriptive." (Negatively stated: phenomenological concepts never refer to mental processes that cannot be intuited; i.e., phenomenological concepts never refer to mental processes whose existence and features can only be inferred.)

3) Phenomenology "brackets" or sets aside all explanatory theories of mental life insofar as these theories refer to explanatory factors that are not themselves experienced by the person whose mental life is under study. This is what renders phenomenology *"presuppositionless"* or *"atheoretical."*

8. Features that Distinguish Husserl's Phenomenology from Jaspers'

Similarly, we shall now list the differences between Husserl's and Jaspers' phenomenologies:

1) The concepts developed by the Husserlian phenomenologist are essential concepts while the concepts defined by the Jaspersian phenomenologist are empirical concepts. Husserl's phenomenology is an eidetic philosophy; Jaspers' phenomenology is an empirical science.

2) The Husserlian phenomenologist takes his or her own mental life as one example (among many other possible examples) of mental life in general. The Husserlian phenomenologist thus employs self-reflection. The Jaspersian phenomenologist studies psychiatric patients as individual examples of psychopathological mental life in general. The Jaspersian phenomenologist therefore employs empathy and understanding (*Verstehen*).

3) Husserl's methodological notion of "intuition" is the notion of a direct, self-reflective, and detailed presentation by the phenomenologist of the mental processes under study. Jaspers' notion of "intuition" is the notion of a less direct, empathetic, and detailed representation by the phenomenologist of the mental processes under study.

9. Other Influences on Jaspers

We have responded to G.E. Berrios' and C. Walker's reviews of the relationship between phenomenology and psychiatry because we believe that this relationship remains extremely important for psychiatry, historically, methodologically, and substantively. Fortunately Rickman has done much to illuminate Jaspers' indebtedness to one thinker whose importance Berrios correctly recognizes: Wilhelm Dilthey (Rickman 1987). In this regard we might also note that to appreciate Jaspers' *General Psychopathology* it remains crucial to evaluate the decisive influence of Max Weber on it (Schwartz & Wiggins 1987, in press).

We have sought to contribute to a clarification of this relationship between phenomenology and psychiatry by examining only small part of it, Jaspers' conception of a phenomenology. Investigations regarding the methods of hermeneutics and interpretation by more recent phenomenologists could also point the way to a critical re-working of Jaspers' concept of *verstehende Psychologie.*

10. Jaspers' Phenomenology and the DSM-III-R

In one important respect Jaspers' phenomenology resembles the "descriptive psychiatry" propounded in *DSM-III* and *DSM-III-R.* Like this more recent descriptive psychiatry, Jaspers' phenomenology is "atheoretical." Both, Jaspers' phenomenology and *DSM-III'* s descriptive psychiatry, bracket or set aside causal (or etiological) theories. This must be done because at present we possess few well-justified etiological theories. When causal theories are developed and grounded in sufficient evidence, they can then be employed to account for the patient's psychopathological experiences.

In another important respect, however, Jaspers' phenomenology differs markedly from the descriptive psychiatry of *DSM-III-R. DSM-III-R* delimits signs and symptoms through "operational definitions." Elsewhere we have criticized such definitions along with the methodology of logical empiricism that *DSM-III* and *DSM-III-R* implicitly presuppose (Schwartz & Wiggins 1986, Spitzer 1988). Here, in relation to Jaspers' phenomenology, we would like to extend our earlier criticisms by pointing out such definitions compel psychiatrists to remain content with a very impoverished psychopathology. The operational definitions of *DSM-III-R,* because they rely on no "theories," employ for the most part commonsensical characterizations of mental processes. With few exceptions, the psychological terms used in *DSM-III-R* come relatively unrefined from the "folk psychology" of everyday, nonscientific understanding. This, of course, avoids the terminology of any particular psychiatric school or "theory," but it does so at the price of accepting poorly examined and ill-defined psychopathological concepts (Spitzer 1990).

A much richer, more precise, and far more useful psychopathology could be developed employing a phenomenology like Jaspers'. And this psychopathology could be developed while remaining strictly neutral regarding etiological concepts and theories. What present-day psychiatry needs, we suggest, is an honest recognition of the inadequacies that necessarily accompany the determination to adopt, however implicitly, a logical empiricist methodology in psychiatry.

11. Phenomenological Descriptive Psychiatry

The psychopathology that could be developed through a continuation of Jaspersian phenomenology could furnish concepts that serve in psychiatric diagnosis, research, and nosology. If the term "descriptive psychiatry" refers to a descriptive approach to the signs and symptoms of mental disorders, such an approach ought to utilize the concepts defined by a Jaspersian phenomenology. For Jaspers has fashioned and employed a scientific method for developing precise and detailed conceptualizations of psychopathological experiences. Descriptive psychiatry would have no use for Jaspersian phenomenology only if this psychiatry elected to be strictly behavioristic or to remain content with a "folk psychology" taken over from commonsense. But to the extent that descriptive psychiatry "describes" the patient's experiences as precisely and fully as possible, it should employ the concepts carefully defined by a phenomenology of the Jaspersian kind.

Jaspers' phenomenology, however, is not the only kind of phenomenology that could assist a descriptive psychiatry. Jaspers, always scrupulous in distinguishing the many methods and subject matters of psychiatry, limited his "phenomenology" to only a part of his general psychopathology. In particular, Jaspers' phenomenology is not concerned with the non-mental features of the patient's illness. Jaspers certainly did not merely ignore these non-mental features of illness. He rather devised other ways of approaching these "objective" phenomena of mental illness (Jaspers 1963a, pp. 222-297). But if we understand phenomenology in the broader way in which Husserl conceived it, we need not restrict it to a study of the patient's *mental life*. Phenomenology can also provide a method for investigating the objective phenomena that make up the patient's disorder. Phenomenology, as Husserl envisioned it, can furnish a *Wissenschaftslehre*, a scientific methodology, for each of the empirical sciences (Husserl 1969), including a descriptive psychiatry which, among other things, examines the signs and symptoms of mental illness.

We need only notice the abstraction under which Jaspers' phenomenology operates in order to see how this could be so. Jaspers' phenomenology purposefully and systematically abstracts from the objective features of the patient's illness in order to focus exclusively on its subjective or mental features. But the patient's experiences are in reality never given to the psychiatrist apart from the objective aspects of the disorder. Indeed, in order for the psychiatrist to apprehend the patient's experiences, these experiences must be, as Jaspers himself writes, *manifested* or *expressed* through objective aspects of the patient's life. Subjective and objective features of the patient's disorder are co-presented to the psychiatrist as parts of a whole, as related aspects of the same human phenomenon, the patient's illness. This point deserves emphasis: the patient's illness is in the first instance *a unified whole* composed of mental and bodily components. For this reason, an abstraction is required in order to separate out the patient's subjective experiences and systematically distinguish them from other aspects of the patient's disorder (Husserl 1970b). Such an abstraction is precisely what Jaspers' phenomenology demands. If one's aim is solely to describe pathological experiences, this kind of abstraction is methodologically justified.

It is equally possible, however, to refrain from making such an abstraction and to study the patient's illness precisely as it is given to the psychiatrist *in its wholeness*. It is necessary then to employ a psychiatric method for studying the patient's subjective experiences *and* objective behaviors as these appear together. The psychiatrist could then devise well defined concepts of the objective aspects of the patient's illness, such as tremor or soft neurological signs, as well as of the pathological experiences. We would simply like to stress that the patient's pathological experiences would need to be studied precisely as Jaspers required: psychiatrists would have to intuitively represent the graphic details of these experiences to themselves and then define their concepts to capture these graphically "seen" details. In short, Jaspers' approach is not faulty; it merely needs supplementation. Instead, it is a "descriptive psychiatry" that elected to proceed without Jaspers' phenomenology that would remain faulty.

What, however, would make this more inclusive approach that we have envisioned "phenomenological"? Phenomenology is a descriptive account of that which is directly given to the observer exactly and exclusively as it is directly given. The phenomenologist brackets or sets aside all explanations of the non-phenomenal causes of phenomena and purely describes the phenomena themselves. The phenomena of mental illness which are thus described precisely as they appear can be subjective and objective phenomena; i.e., they can be both mental and bodily components of the patient's disorder. The methodology which such a descriptive approach involves would have to delineate the evidential bases of the descriptions and the ways in which the descriptive claims could be proven true or false. Only if we were sure of this evidential basis could we be sure that our phenomenology was genuinely scientific. This is the task of a phenomenological *Wissenschaftslehre,* a task which Edmund Husserl already has done much to fulfill (Husserl 1969, 1970b)

Berrios is correct, then, to maintain that "phenomenological descriptions apply only to subjective experiences" (Berrios 1989, p. 427) only if he means exclusively the "phenomenology" of Jaspers and does not refer to those other methods that Jaspers' devised for studying the objective aspects of mental illness. Berrios' statement, however, does not hold for the broader phenomenology of Husserl. Husserlian phenomenology can readily examine the patient's illness in its unified wholeness, encompassing both its subjective and objective aspects. About Husserlian phenomenology, one could never write,

> "objective clinical changes, such as psychomotor retardation, tremor, catatonia or soft neurological signs, fall beyond its epistemological and methodological scope" (Berrios 1989, p. 427).

12. The Need for a Detailed and Systematic Psychopathology

Since Jaspers wrote, psychopathology has grown less subtle and sophisticated rather than more (Spitzer1990). For some time psychiatrists have felt little need to develop and extend psychopathology actively, forcefully, and systematically. Such development and extension could significantly advance present-day psychiatry, however. Contemporary psychiatry has certainly refined its methods, concepts, and hypotheses regarding the biological and neurological determinants of mental illness. But this biological psychiatry would profit from supplementation by psychopathology.

A more sophisticated psychopathology would delineate differences, details, and variations in patient's experiences which could serve as clues and indicators for the selection of patients for investigation as well as for the actual research into causes. A more subtle map of patients' experiences, in other words, could guide researchers in their quest for a more subtle map of patients' brains. Moreover, a more refined psychopathology could perform some of the clinical work that is now left to biology. With a more precise understanding of the patient's psychopathology, the psychiatrist would possess a more exact basis for the selection and use of psychopharmacology. And with a more refined psychopathology, the clinician could make diagnostic and treatment decisions even prior employing far more expensive brain imaging studies and other technological devices. There are, for example, two different kinds of delusions, one found in schizophrenia and the other in delirium, whose psychopathology could profit from more thorough and detailed descriptions (Schwartz & Wiggins, this volume). A more complete phenomenology of these forms of delusions could advance both clinical and research goals.

13. Conclusion

In closing we would like to emphasize a point we mentioned earlier. Psychiatry must employ a variety of methods and draw on numerous sciences. Prominent among such sciences is neuroscience. Psychiarists can only profit from the fast moving breakthroughs in neuroscience. Indeed, we can look forward to revolutionary advances from this quarter. But, in order to do justice to psychiatric disorders, accomplishments in neuroscience require supplementation from psychopathology and psychological and sociological disciplines. At the end of the our century it is a rigorous and tough-minded *expansion* of psychopathological investigations that is required, not a defensive and dogmatic contraction. Discussion of these different but complementary methods and concepts remains part of the crucial responsibility of philosophers and psychiatrists who would grapple with the manifold problems of the discipline of psychiatry.

Summary

The terms "phenomenology" and "descriptive psychiatry" are re-examined from a methodological and historical point of view. What appears to remain especially obscure to many writers today is the nature of Karl Jaspers' phenomenology and its role in his general psychopathology. Even more opaque is Jaspers' debt to Edmund Husserl's phenomenology. The obscurity surrounding these ideas has led G.E. Berrios to claim that Jaspers' phenomenology has no fruitful relevance for present-day psychiatry, and C. Walker to maintain that Jaspers' dependence on Husserl is spurious. We clarify Jaspers' appropriation of, and departure from, Husserl's early phenomenology. This requires first an explication of some central components of Husserl's method. This leads to an account of Jaspers' phenomenology, focusing especially on the role of "intuitive representation." The significance of Jaspers' adoption of Husserl's notion of a "presuppositionless" method is explained and related to the "atheoretical" stance of *DSM-III-R*. Jaspers' phenomenology is shown to be important for present-day psychiatry because it provides a fruitful method for developing a much needed psychopathology.

References

American Psychiatric Association: Diagnostic and Statistical Manual of Mental Disorders, Third Edition, Revised (DSM-III-R). American Psychiatric Association, Washington, DC, 1987

Andreasen NC: Reply to "Phenomenology or Physicalism?". Schizophrenia Bulletin 17/2: 187–189, 1991

Berrios GE: What Is Phenomenology? A Review. Journal of the Royal Society of Medicine 82: 425-428, 1989

Gadamer H.-G: Truth and Method. The Seabury Press, New York, 1975

Gurwitsch A: Studies in Phenomenology and Psychology. Evanston, Northwestern University Press, 1966

Gurwitsch A: Phenomenology and the Theory of Science (ed. by Embree L), pp. 210-240Evanston, Northwestern University Press, 1974

Heidegger M: Being and Time (transl. Macquarrie J, Robinson E). London, SCM Press Ltd., 1962

Heidegger M: Discourse on Thinking (transl. Anderson JM, Freund EH). New York, Harper & Row, 1966

Heidegger M: Poetry, Language, Thought (transl. Hofstadter A). New York, Harper & Row, 1971

Husserl E: Phenomenology and the Crisis of Philosophy (transl. Lauer Q). New York, Harper & Row, 1965

Husserl E: Logische Untersuchungen, Vol. II, 1st part. Tübingen, Niemeyer, 1968

Husserl E: Formal and Transcendental Logic (transl. Cairns D). The Hague, Martinus Nijhoff, 1969

Husserl E: Philosophie der Arithmetik. The Hague, Martinus Nijhoff, 1970a

Husserl E: The Crisis of European Sciences and Transcendental Phenomenology (transl. Carr D). Evanston, Northwestern University Press, 1970b

Husserl E, Cartesian Meditation: An Introduction to Phenomenology (transl. Cairns D). The Hague, Martinus Nijhoff, 1973a

Husserl E: Zur Phänomenologie der Intersubjektivität (3 volumes). The Hague, Martinus Nijhoff, 1973b

Husserl E: Ideas Pertaining to a Pure Phenomenology and to a Phenomenological Philosophy, First Book (transl. Kersten F). The Hague, Martinus Nijhoff, 1982

Jaspers K: Philosophical Autobiography (transl. Schlipp PA, Lefebre LB). In: Schilpp PA (ed.): The Philosophy of Karl Jaspers, 3-94, La Salle, IL, Open Court, 1957

Jaspers K: General Psychopathology (transl. Hoenig J, Hamilton MW). Chicago, The University of Chicago Press, 1963a

Jaspers K: Die phänomenologische Forschungsrichtung in der Psychopathologie. In: Jaspers K: Gesammelte Schriften zur Psychopathologie. Berlin, Springer,1963b

Jaspers K: Allgemeine Psychopathologie. Berlin, Springer, 1965

Jaspers K: Philosophy, 3 volumes (transl. Ashton EB). Chicago, The University of Chicago Press, 1970

Pfänder A: Logik, Tübingen, Max Niemeyer, 1963

Rickman HP: The Philosophic Basis of Psychiatry: Jaspers and Dilthey. Philosophy and Social Science 17: 173-196, 1987

Ricoeur P: The Conflict of Interpretations: Essays in Hermeneutics (ed. Ihde D), Evanston, Northwestern University Press, 1974.

Rotov M: Phenomenology or Physicalism?. Schizophrenia Bulletin 17: 183–186, 1991

Sartre J-P: Being and Nothingness: An Essay on Phenomenological Ontology (transl. Barnes H), Philosophical Library, New York, 1956

Schwartz MA, Wiggins OP: Logical Empiricism and Psychiatric Classification. Comprehensive Psychiatry 27: 101-114, 1986

Schwartz MA, Wiggins OP: Diagnosis and Ideal Types: A Contribution to Psychiatric Classification. Comprehensive Psychiatry 28: 277-291, 1987

Schwartz MA, Wiggins OP: The Phenomenology of Schizophrenic Delusions. This volume, 1992

Schwartz MA, Wiggins OP: Ideal Types and Psychiatric Diagnoses. In Sadler JZ, Schwartz MA, Wiggins OP (eds.): Philosophical Perspectives on Psychiatric Diagnostic Classification. Baltimore, Johns Hopkins Press, in press

Spiegelberg H: The Phenomenological Movement: A Historical Introduction, Vols. 1 & 2. The Hague, Martinus Nijhoff, 1960

Spitzer M: Psychiatry, Philosophy, and the Problem of Description. In Spitzer M, Uehlein FA, Oepen G (eds): Psychopathology and Philosophy, pp. 3-18, Berlin, Springer, 1988

Spitzer M: Why Philosophy? In Spitzer M, Maher BA (eds): Philosophy and Psychopathology, pp. 3-18. Springer, New York, 1990

Uehlein FA: Eidetic Variation in Husserl's Phenomenology, this volume, 1992

Walker C: Philosophical Concepts and Practice: The Legacy of Karl Jaspers' Psychopathology. Current Opinion in Psychiatry 1: 624-629, 1988

Wildhagen K, Heraucourt W: The New Wildhagen German Dictionary. Chicago, Follett, 1965

M. Spitzer, F.A. Uehlein
M.A. Schwartz, C. Mundt
(eds.): Phenomenology
Language & Schizophrenia.
Springer-Verlag, New York, 1992

Phenomenology: Intentionality, Passive Synthesis, and Primary Consciousness of Time

F.A. Uehlein

In the following essay main concepts of Husserl's phenomenology, viz., the life-world, intentionality, emotion and sensation, passive genesis, association, the temporality and synthesis of consciousness, and the formation of habits are introduced and worked out in their mutual relationship. The essay does not present a set of clear-cut definitions and subsequent applications and illustrations, but follows a rather different method. The concepts in question are *developed* in a course of descriptions and reflections, so as to form a preliminary, but highly condensed, introduction to phenomenology. Readers who are mainly interested in the application of these concepts within psychiatry may skip over this chapter.

1. The life-world

We take the existence of the world for granted. At least in everyday life we do so. Moreover, the world is not just one fact among others; the world is objectively given in advance of all possible facts. Actual events and natural things, e.g. landscapes, animals, plants, and cultural, technical things, occur and are encountered within the world. We live together with other persons, share the same place, share our work, and, to a certain extent, our lives as well—within the world. The *life-world* is given in perceptions; it is discovered, experienced, and experiencable in any situation in which we find ourselves.[1] We continuously accept it as the spatio-temporal world of persons, living beings, and things.

---

1 Husserl's description and exposition of the life-world is contained in *Die Krisis der europäischen Wissenschaften und die transzendentale Phänomenologie*. For central passages cf. pp. 49-58 and §§ 28, 29, 36, 37, 38. Husserl is quoted from the collected works, Husserliana, using the following short titles:
Cart.Med.: Cartesian Meditations
E&J: Experience & Judgment
Ideas I: Ideas Pertaining to a Pure Phenomenology and to a Phenomenological Philosophy
Intersubjectivity III: On the Phenomenology of Intersubjectivity, 3rd vol.

This in no way implies, however, that space, places, regions etc. are geometrized; that time is essentially measured time and, in turn, the measurement of processes; that things are idealized into physical bodies; and that cause and effect are brought into an exact mathematical relationship. Rather, the flow of time exhibits its special articulation according to the events of a life-course. It does not pass uniformly and in mathematical, infinitesimal continuity, but streams rhythmically in an epochal sequence. Space is not yet set at a certain distance, conceptualized into a system of dimensions or vectors, and objectified in physico-mathematical and technical measurements. The life-world incorporates a more fundamental and primitive experience of space: The wide or narrow bounds of vision and horizon, for instance; the environs of a place, or a central locality, centered in a cluster of trees, a building, a landmark, which unify a whole landscape; the direction into which one moves and out of which something approaches; clearing and thicket, void and fullness, etc., determine the original experience of space (cf. Bachelard 1975).

"All categorical structures of the life-world bear the same name but do not care for, as it were, the theoretical idealizations and hypothetical substructions of geometers and physicists. ... physicists, being people like other people, living self-knowingly within the life-world, the world of their human interests, have—under the heading of physics—put a certain kind of question and ... they have practical intentions toward the things of the life-world; their *theories* are the practical results. Like other intentions, practical interests and their realizations, the sciences, too, belong to the life-world, presuppose it for their basis and enrich it by their activity" (*Crisis*, pp. 142-143. Cf. pp. 112-113).

Forming in this way the all-embracing horizon of experiential and intentional life in general, the world turns out to be the (often forgotten or concealed) sense-bestowing fundament of the sciences in particular.

Whether we live in the natural attitude of everyday practical life or whether we transform the categories of the natural attitude into exact laws and the rules of technical mastery, it is still the life-world in which we live and work, and to which our interests, aims and actions refer. (The destruction of the environment—sad to say—proves this very point.) Whatever we experience, whatever the correction and enlargement our former experiences will eventually find, to whatever the results our scientific questions and intentions may be, they all subserve the *confirmation* (*Bewährung*) of the life-world (*Crisis*, pp. 50-51). Factual existence and co-existence within the world seems to be the fundamental and ultimate fact. Phenomenology emphasizes this fact as the almost trivial, often forgotten, sense-bestowing fundament of the sciences. However, is it just a fact, and to whom is it a fact? The world is the all-embracing horizon given in advance of any particular experience. But to whom is it given? How could we state that fact and qualify it as fundamental, if it had not been for

Crisis: The Crisis of European Sciences and Transcendental Phenomenology
Log.Invest.: Logical Investigations
Pass.Synth.: Analyses on Passive Synthesis
Lectures: The Phenomenology of the Consciousness of Inner Time.

us? Phenomenology emphasizes the fact, but also asks how it has become a fact, and how it has, moreover, become a fact to be taken for granted and even forgotten. It asks for the genesis of everything that is for us, inclusive of matter-of-course facts.

Factual existence and co-existence within the world is a "fact" which we live through, feel, sense, gradually become aware of in the events of streaming consciousness, experience half-consciously in objective states of affairs, and grasp finally in mental concepts, judgments and our practical, interpersonal life. In short: the "mere fact" given in advance has been constituted as such, has *become* an objective fact for us in the course of subjective experiential and intentional life. This constitution of objectivity, or, in other words, the inner correlation of subjectivity and objectivity has been described by Husserl under the headings of *intentionality* and *passive synthesis*. The following paragraphs trace this dynamic interrelation and thus the constitution of everything which can be for us at all, of anything which has sense for us; or to say it in Husserl's own words: the constitution of "every type of existent conceivable for us ... and specifically as regards the transcendency actually given to us beforehand through experience: Nature, culture, the world as a whole" (*Cart.Med.* p. 119).

2. The Objective Correlate of Intentional Acts

When we look at something, the thing seen is no sensation. When we touch something, the thing felt is not a feeling. When we mean something, the object meant is not an act. A general structure, exemplified in these cases, begins to emerge. Intentional acts are psychic events, and what they produce is strictly correlative to them. Each specific act leads to and ends in a specific result. But even so, this result, which is produced and owned by the act, cannot be considered as a psychic event itself. It stands out from the subjective activity in its own typical form of being: its objectivity. Specific subjective acts constitute and have their specific objects.

This structure holds obviously true for perception. Perceptive acts are interwoven with direct intuitions and their sensual data, and thus constitute real things. (For a discussion of sensual intuition see the next paragraph on passive genesis.) In this case the subjective act and its objective correlate certainly cannot be mixed up nor be reduced one to the other.

But how about more complex acts such as remembrance and expectation, imagination, signification, stating and judging, etc.? An act of judging results in a unitary meaning. This unit, i.e., the judgment, is distinguished from the psychic act and event in which it arises. It is an ideal object, which claims a specific judicial truth (*Urteilswahrheit*), and can be shared and discussed by virtually every person. An act, on the contrary, is a private event. It is performed, it occurs, it does not claim any truth. When we state something, the intentional object becomes manifest outwardly. We can return to those objects and retain them in completely different acts of recognition, reproduction, correction, and manifold evaluations, such as belief, doubt, enjoyment, and disgust. To make matters even more complex, signification presents a sign (*Zeichenvorstellung*), and the object, signified and re-presented mediately, may be a real thing of the natural world, which can be perceived, or an ideal object, seen directly in mathematical intuition, or a unitary meaning, or a state of affairs, which is simply stated or also evaluated, hoped for, or feared, etc. The act of promising constitutes an object within a field of real conditions and accompanying acts of confidence, even if we do not hold to it. It is not the act we hold or break. The obligation to hold one's promise and the accompanying possibility of breaking it depend upon the specific object constituted interpersonally in the act, viz., the things to be done or to be left undone. The fictitious world of a novel can neither be given—per definitionem—in fulfilling intuitions of sensual perception, nor can it be identified with the *acts* of a poetic imagination. It is constituted as a "pure intentional object" and expressed and made public by the manifold speech acts of narration and writing. It can be shared, evaluated, and judged by the community of readers and may become a formative link in literary history.[2] The correlation of the manner of intentional givenness (*Gegebenheitsweise*) and an object of experience holds true as well for objects and happenings desired, hoped for or feared, even if they may prove to be ungrounded and cannot be fulfilled in reality. Psychpathologists vividly appreciate the haunting objectivity and devouring reality such intentional objects can achieve. Those delusional objects are definitely not the manifold, passing acts in which they arise and are elaborated, reinforced and lived through.

If we reflect on our own acts as performed in the foregoing sentences, we see that the point in question is also proved by reflective acts. In the natural attitude of practical life we focus on things perceived, statements made and promises given, things and events desired or feared, etc. We focus on objects, while our intentional acts normally remain unattended to. In the foregoing paragraph we have reflected on the intentional acts and have seen their essential correlation to those objects. Husserl's concise formula for this relationship is:

$$\text{ego—cogito—cogitatum.}$$

Each consciousness is consciousness *of* something; in every mental act we mean something. The formula applies to each act both specifically and individually; specifically, with reference to its type of intention, and individually as an actual or possible event of mental life. The typical character of reflection on mental life consists of the objectification of the very mental acts themselves. We mean such and such a thing, but we can also mean the act of meaning itself. Applying the essential structure of

---

2 Roman Ingarden has analyzed the "pure intentional objects" of narration and the correlative, constitutive acts in his monograph *Das literarische Kunstwerk*. Highly relevant to the point in question are also his remarks on music, painting, architecture and film in *Untersuchungen zur Ontologie der Kunst*.

intentionality to reflective acts, there follows: the object intended is never identical with the act intending it; and this holds true even if the object intended is itself an intending act. The act of meaning is objectified by a reflective act.[3] We see the act of meaning in its general structure, viz., the constitutive character of intentionality. Furthermore, we see the specific performance of this special act of meaning: it gives its object in direct intuition of perception or reflection; it assumes something to be true or doubtful, or imagines it without any respect to its existential and logical status; it remembers, expects, evaluates, etc. Finally, we see this particular act of meaning as a real event within the streaming mental life and grasp it as a single case of the general structure and of that specific character. Reflective acts of meaning, too, produce their specific kind of intentional objects. They render acts of meaning objective, inclusive of (other) acts of their own reflective kind.

One last trait of intentional acts which has so far been mentioned only in passing should be emphasized. Intentional acts relate to their objects in typical regularity. Each specific act constitutes (a) its specific object, just this one and no other. (A person seen; something promised; a plan worked out and executed, etc.) (b) The intentional object is produced in its particular form and determination. (Hector seen just now, face to face; the paper I promised Hector yesterday; the plan to work on the paper and have it ready by next Monday, etc.). (c) Finally, the intentional object is constituted in a certain mode. Thus one and the same determined object can be stated, doubted, negated, imagined and meant with certain evaluations. Each *noesis* (act) has its *noema* (object), and vice versa. This mutual relationship does not just form an empirical fact. On the contrary, it is the condition of all experience and facts, and in this sense it is a priori. It is not *inferred* from empirical life nor *constructed* epistemologically, but can be directly intuited in each noema and each noesis.[4]

If we were not capable of intentional acts of meaning, then there would be—literally—no meaning for us. We might live through manifold states of being, though without knowing what we encounter. We would not perceive anything as such, nor be conscious of something as this or that. We would live in streaming states without objectivity and thus without a world. When we translate this object-less experiential life into Husserl's formula ego—cogito—cogitatum, the far-reaching consequences of (the lack of) intentionality become visible. With the absence of the constitutive cogito the cogitatum disappears: ego — ~~cogito~~ — ~~cogitatum~~.

---

3 We need not go further since reflection is not a new thing altogether but a specific kind of meaning.

4 "The universal a priori correlation of experiential objects and their manner of givenness" fascinated Husserl throughout his career. As late as 1935 he mentions the shock with which *das universale Korrelationsapriori* had struck him in 1898 during the elaboration of his *Logical Investigations* (cf. *Crisis*, p. 169, note). Intentionality in its active and—as we presently shall see—passive, receptive side has accordingly become a constant theme of phenomenology. This can be seen from the following passages, in which Husserl concentrates almost exclusively on this topic: the Vth and VIth *Log. Invest.*; the IIIrd and IVth section of *Ideas* I; *Cart.Med.*, §§ 17-29; *Crisis*, §§ 45-50.

Whether the subject of such an object-less experience could know and name herself *I*: "I, this human, I, this person existing in body", is questionable.

3. Passive Genesis

There are events of experiential life which seem to contradict the structure of intentionality. When we are in a certain emotional state, when we laugh or cry, we do not intend and mean anything; and still there is something for us. In sensation we do not objectify anything and still there is something presented to us in immediate awareness. Do we speak adequately? Can the distinctions of the foregoing sentences grasp sensation/feelings? What is it that is for us? And from what standpoint, from what level of consciousness and constellation of acts can we see and say that there is *something for us in feel* something to us. The relationship of the feeling person and her feelings—taken in the double meaning of "act" and "object"—is too intimately related to appear in distinction and emerges only in accompanying or subsequent acts of reflection. "A SENSATION = a Feeling referring to some *Thing,* and yet not organized into a definite *Object* nor separated from the sentient Being" (Coleridge, *Notebook II,* 3605).[5]

Feelings and sensations are traits of experience. They belong to the spontaneous life of subjectivity. Though they do not constitute objects they are a peculiar kind of activity: we receive, we suffer. Our activity here consists in a spontaneous reception (a *passive activity* as Coleridge called it). In feelings and sensations we live through certain states of being (*Erleben*) within our streaming experiential life. *Erleben* (living through) and *Empfinden* (sensation/feeling[6]) are non-intentional, spontaneous acts of reception. Husserl therefore calls them *passive genesis* in contrast to the active genesis of intentional acts.

Though feelings and sensations do not constitute objects they present data in immediate awareness (*Empfindungsdaten*). These data—sensations, feelings, affections—are the stuff (*hyletische Daten; Materie*) for the intentional acts of perception and are "rendered objective by them."[7] Acts

---

5 The well-known poet and virtually unknown philosopher S.T.Coleridge has jotted down in his voluminous notebooks a wealth of philosophical reflections. Some of them bear surprising phenomenological overtones. I do not hesitate to quote some of his remarks, even though they belong to a different historical context: Coleridge, one of the earliest and most subtle of Kant's English readers, combines critical, transcendental philosophy and classical metaphysics. Notwithstanding this historical difference his reflections are pertinent to our question from a systematic point of view. His notes on the *passive activity* of feeling and sensation exhibit an—admittedly fragementary—theory of passive genesis (cf. Uehlein, 1982, pp 33-51).

6 Cf. Coleridge's explanation: "the German word for sensation or feeling is Empfindung, i.e. an *inward finding."* (Coleridge 1976, p. 180). "Vorstellung versus Empfindung [representation versus feeling/sensation]. Both are Excellent words—A Sensation, a Feeling, is what I *find in* me *as in* me." (Coleridge, *Notebook III,* 4443; cf. Uehlein 1982 pp. 46-49).

7 "Sensation" and "feeling" obtain a different meaning here. One aspect of the original constellation of a threefold meaning stands out) intentional consciousness in statu nascendi, and (c) the sensuous datum for perceptual consciousness. The following quotation from Coleridge's notebooks points the

of perception constitute intentional objects and fulfill themselves in corresponding data presented in immediate non-objectifying awareness: we perceive a real thing. Meaning, as we have seen, is constituted in mental acts, which result in intentional objects.[8] The acts that constitute the intentional objects are interwoven with data of sensation and conversely, those data are permeated by the objectifying acts and related to the intentional objects. Thus we distinguish what we feel and perceive what has affected us in primary sensuous intuition: the intentional object is given 'in person' (*VI.Log.Invest.*, § 26). In passive genesis emerges an "outer sphere of objectivity" (*Pass.Synth.* p. 104). Apart from perceptions, acts of judgement in particular participate of this sphere. Judgements press for realization. We claim the objects and states of affairs to be real and, logically spoken, to be true. Judgements and their claims find realization and verification or suspension and falsification in this sphere.

"Syntheses of fulfilling, interweaving again and again, go through the passive life. Again and again a striving after intuitions, which realize the intended Self—again and again, the word obtrudes itself, verification [*Bewahrheitung*]" (*Pass.Synth.* p. 102).

Objects, states of affairs and the world they foreshadow can only arise in objectifying acts, perceptions and judgements. Without them we would live in the associative and streaming states of direct awareness. No meaning, no objectivity, no world would there be for us. We would live along speechlessly. Without the passively received, sensed and felt "fulfilling Self" (*Pass.Synth.* p. 102), on the other hand, those objectifying acts would press for realization and seek verification in vain. Whatever we intend and the way we intend it in judgements, negations, doubts, expectations and evaluations, etc., refers ultimately to the passive genesis of a "fulfilling Self".

---

direction of further elaborations: "Again, an Intuition, or Present Beholding, combines actively, Activity & Passivity, [but any object is act. + pass. combined—] therefore the Object or Presence beheld, is the Spirit itself in this combination—But the Spirit merged in an Intuition cannot at the same [time] distinguish it from itself—Hence the absolute Identity of the Thing and the Perception, of the present Beholding and of the Presence beheld—& a compleat Confutation of physical or spiritual Influx, intermediate Images, &c —... However, we yet do distinguish our Self from the Object, tho' not in the primary Intuition—Visio visa—now this is impossible without an act of abstraction—we abstract from our own product—the Spirit snatches it [self] loose from its own self-immersion, and self-actualizing distinguishes itself from its Self-realization—" (Notebook III 4186 f35-f35ᵛ).

8 The difference between a real and a non-real object, be it remembered, expected, imagined, signified or purely intentionality, i.e. fictitious, or the object of a wrong statement, a false judgement etc., depends on the fulfilling sensations and feelingsand is specifically denoted. In the state of primary intuition act and object cannot be distinguished. Feeling and sensation mean an immediate awareness, which at this stage of consciousness cannot be described as awareness *of* something. Husserl's apparently simple statement: "Sensations and feelings are rendered objective by the acts of perception" ("Die Empfindungen erfahren eine gegenständliche Auffassung in den Wahrnehmungsakten" V. *Log. Invest.*, § 15 b) moves swiftly over an intricate concurrence of acts. Primary intuition is set through and discriminated by acts of abstraction and self-distinction. The so far indistinct complex of *feeling—something felt—sentient self-awareness* undergoes differentiation and decomposes into the *relationship* of constitutive moments: cogito-cogitatum-ego. Feeling now denotes the presentation *of a sensuous datum* (cogitatum). The common usage of feeling/sensation branches out and covers the different levels of (a) primary intuition, (b of passive genesis.

One is tempted to believe that in passive genesis we encounter the real world directly. This opinion, however, engages in a half-truth. The direct awareness and immediacy of feeling is well observed. But how has a world become real, so that it appears to be given in advance, unless it had been constituted by intentional acts and the fulfilling acts of spontaneous receptivity? Right from the pre-conscious beginning of experiential life receptive and productive acts are interwoven. These acts become habitual. Their correlates, being retained in constant acceptance, gradually compose an "outer sphere of experience" (*Pass.Synth.* p. 104). In conscious thought we already operate with the results of objectified passive genesis, viz., the affections and feelings of something given beforehand. Thus the life-world has been built up step by step, whereas our productive life (*leistende Leben*) remains anonymous. For this reason, in the natural attitude of practical, everyday life, we do find ourselves within a world given in advance. Phenomenological reflection uncovers our productive life and its anonymous constitution:

"the objectivity and existential sense of the life-world given in advance has been *produced subjectively*, it is constituted by the pre-scientific, experiential life. ... Not the matter-of-course existence of the world is the first and principal in itself ... the first and principal in itself is [interpersonal] subjectivity, more particularly, subjectivity as giving the world in advance, naively, and then rationalizing it or—what amounts to the same—objectifying it" (*Crisis* p. 70).

4. Synthesis

Intentional acts do not follow each other indifferently nor stick together from the outside. They are not linked like pieces of matter in the spatio-temporal world but "united into one consciousness" and "their unity is the unity of synthesis" (*Cart.Med.* p. 79). This unity of synthesis becomes evident in each act and succesion of acts we make stand out from the streaming consciousness. When we, for instance, perceive a thing of the natural world in our experiential field and see its coloured front, we anticipate its back and background, we may walk around it and encounter it in an uninterrupted change of perceptive acts and corresponding data. We can pass from aspects seen to aspects remembered and blend them with certain expectations, which we hope or fear to find. Acts of *perception, remembrance, expectation, imagination* and *evaluation* are unified. *Questions* involve both *judgements*, which we *assume* to be valid, and *fulfilling answers*. *Promises* involve a sphere of real things, given in *experience*, a situation of possible *activities*, acts of *expectation* and *mutual confidence,* etc.

"Synthesis, however, does not occur just in every particular conscious act and its object, nor does it connect one particular conscious process with another only occasionally. On the contrary,...the *whole of conscious life is unified synthetically*. Conscious life is therefore an all-embracing "cogito", synthetically comprising all particular conscious processes that ever become prominent, and having its all-embracing cogitatum, founded at different levels on the manifold particular cogitata.

...The all-embracing cogitatum is the all-embracing life itself, with its openly endless unity and wholeness" (*Cart.Med.* pp. 80- 81).

4.1 Criticism and Refutation

Husserl's concept of a consciousness unified synthetically has been widely discussed and criticized. Several strands of contemporary philosophy, as for instance Derrida's deconstructivism, originate from such a critique. The "death of the subject" and "the disappearance of subjectivity" have even become slogans.

The unity and wholeness of the I form the stumbling-block, even more so since the ambiguity, which lurks in "unity" and "wholeness", has caused misunderstandings. "Unity" and "whole" have been taken to denote a harmonious whole and a unity in which all experiences and epochs of an individual life are happily brought into unison. The formal structure of consciousness has been mixt up with a certain course of life, a certain happy realization of this synthesis. The disparate experiences of self-estrangement, of a life falling apart and the corresponding lack of personal "unity" (taken in an evaluative sense) seemed to contradict the "one Self" and the synthetic unity of her life. But how can these certainly disturbing experiences become prominent, how can they be lived and suffered through, unless they are "particular conscious processes synthetically comprised" with other contrasting experiences within one conscious life? Even if experiences result in "trace of traces" (Derrida) and do not constitute objects and a real world, such as experienced naively in everyday life, those "trace of traces" and the flight of "substitutes" and *suppléments* of an evanescent reality necessarily occurs within the synthesis of one conscious life, otherwise they could not be stated, asserted and assumed to replace the persons and real things of naive experiential life. Derrida's impressive and intriguing philosophy, which endeavours to rule out *the one* on all levels of reality (inclusive of the experiencing and thinking I) rules out at the same time its own possibility (cf. Derrida 1967a, especially the first part; 1967b; 1972).

Husserl conceives of the synthetic unity of life to be open endlessly. In other words, this unity is in becoming; it *is* a synthesis. Yet experiences, however disparate, are not entities floating freely somewhere. They do belong to the experiential life of a person and thus to a unity in becoming. In his *Analyses of Passive Synthesis* and elsewhere Husserl reflects on the disturbing experiences "of a wild confusion, in which all percieved order of the worl disintegrates" (*Pass.Synth.*, 106) and on the corresponding "many-coloured self" (*vielfärbige Selbst*) and "the decomposition of the I" and a "transformation into madness".

"Even then", he proceeds, "I am the identical I of an identical habituality, even then I retain my lasting possession—not an 'objective' surrounding world, to be sure, but the unity of my life, the manifold data of sensation and feeling within the unity of inner time. I am, but I am not with reference to nature, to a world, and I am not in the world, I am worldless. There might well be several other I, might be in the world and be persons to each other. But they are not for me [...]" (manuscript writings quoted from Marbach 1974, p. 331).

The "death of the subject", the "disappearance of subjectivity", or less modishly, the fleeting substitutes of reality, and the disturbances of objectivity can only *be experienced* as well as understood and stated by an identical person within the synthetical unity of her experiential life.[9]

5. Passive Synthesis and Association

The fundamental form of synthesis is temporality, i.e. the inner consciousness of time. Mental acts "present themselves as temporally ordered, temporally beginning and ending, simultaneous or successive" (*Cart.Med.* p. 81). In the following we concentrate on passive synthesis.

The acts of passive reception do not occur indiscriminately nor in isolation. On the contrary, they are structured temporally and can therefore be synthesized. Sensations, feelings, affections and their sensuous contents are set apart and at the same time brought into contact by their successive occurence. Furthermore, they present themselves in the field of direct sensuous awareness and hence border on other simultaneous sensations of comparable clearness or less impressive character. The same is true of their beginning and ending. An immediate impression (*Urimpression*) lasts for the moment of its "durational presence" (see section 6), sinks into retention and is succeeded by other impressions. In its beginning it succeeds a former sensation and in its ending it is succeeded by a later one. In succession as well as in co-existence we find the phenomenon of a border which sets apart and at the same time brings into contact. Such a border implicates a wider field, a continuous extension, in which it can distinguish and connect what is bordered by it: simultaneous and successive sensations occur a) within the field of sensuous awareness and b) within streaming consciousness. They co-exist and follow each other without interspace[10] and at the same time well-distinguished. William James had talked of the *fringes* of experience to describe the dialectical character of that border. Husserl quotes him with approval (cf., e.g., *Crisis* p. 267). He speaks of the halo and horizon of each mental event and of the horizonedness (*Horizonthaftigkeit*) pervading experiential life on all levels. The horizonedness is grounded deeply within us, it springs from the temporality of mental life.

In order to understand passive synthesis more fully, its fundamental form is to be supplemented by the contents of those acts, or better, by the character of their material data. What we live through in presentational immediacy (*Erlebnis*) and "find in us" by virtue of spontaneous reception

---

9 Cf. Hegel's remarks to the point in question in his *Enzyklopädie der philosophischen Wissenschaften im Grundrisse* (1830), § 408.
10 I borrow this term from Coleridge's description of the horizonal character of experience, cf. Uehlein, *Eidos and Eidetic Variation* etc., this volume, note 3.

(*Empfindung*) does not fall into a jumble nor into isolated bits. Moreover, sensations do not just occur simultaneously and successively, and then sink back and vanish without any trace; they form sediments. What does that mean? Sensations are epochs within the course of experiential life. Experiential life realizes itself in such individual sensations and data and bears their stamp. With each sensation our experiential life receives a certain determination. Acts and sensations pass by, but "from now on I am abidingly the I of such and such an experience."[11] Further acts and sensations are performed before the background of such determinations. Sensations interplay with the sediments of former sensations. They relate in form of "sensuous configurations" (*Cart.Med.* p. 114). They associate.

Association means that sensations arouse other sensations. A present feeling "awakens", as Husserl says, a sedimented, former feeling. Or in other words, a present feeling receives some datum, not yet objectified, and re-produces, re-presents a former feeling, and the latter may arouse a third one, etc. The whole life of past experience is awakened indirectly and brought into interplay with the present sensation, though in an unconscious manner (*Pass.Synth.* p. 121). For example, a portrait by Titan in the Pinakothek museum may arouse a dim association with the Galleria degli Uffizi, and suddenly, unpredictably, there stands out from this sensuous configuration the *custode* yawning in front of Boticelli's *Magnificat*.

This *genesis of reproduction* is the primary kind of association (*Pass.Synth.* p. 119). At the lower level of receptivity and in the form of still sensuous configurations it constitutes the preliminary stage of active remembrance, the consciousness of the past and the sense of duration. According to the double horizon of time, viz., retention and protention, past and future, association works as well into the opposite direction and produces a "genesis of expectation"[12]. Sedimented sentiments and the correlative passive acts of feelings and affections are associated, repeated, repeatedly synthesized, until the become customary and even habitual. Feelings of a particular kind and the habitual association of those feelings will therefore awaken feelings of imminent sensations. This secondary kind of association forms the preliminary stage of our sense of the future and of "all active logical processes, which fall under the heading of inductive inference" (*Pass.Synth.* p. 120). Passive synthesis in both its reproductive and expectant shape becomes habitual and produces a "sphere of outer experience" (*Pass.Synth.* p. 104), in which intentional acts find their fulfilling intuitions. When I look up I *am used to see* the shelves with the Greek philosophers. I need not compose this sight again and again, step by step in the course of many sensations and acts.

---

11 Cf. *Cart.Med.* p. 100. The sentence there refers to the act of decision.
12 *Pass.Synth.* p. 119. Concerning the double horizon of time see section 6. "The phenomenology of associations develops the doctrine of the original constitution of time on a higher level. Through associations this constitutive performance is augmented by all grades of apperception" (*Pass.Synth.* p. 118).

"The 'ready-made' objects that confront us in life as existent mere physical things ... are given, with the originality of the 'it itself', in the synthesis of passive experience. As such things, they are given beforehand to 'spiritual', intentional activities, which begin with active grasping." (*Cart.Med.* p. 112).

The structure of passive synthesis can be summed up in two terms: temporality (co-existence and succession) and association. Temporality refers to the acts, association to the sensuous configurations of material data. Temporality is the fundamental form, association the "universal principle" of passive synthesis (*Cart.Med.* p. 113, l. 28). Since it structures the configurations, association cannot be just an empirical fact. Husserl considers of it as an a priori, essential law of experiential life (*Wesengesetzlichkeit*).

Sensuous configuration originates with feelings of affinitive and contrasting sensations. In the course of repetition and habitualization thesefeelings will increase. They rise in ascending degrees of intensity (*Steigerungsreihe*). Simultaneous and successive sensations and sediments thus brought into constellation exhibit a tendency towards unification. (a) *Affinity* and *constrast* are (b) *heightened* to (c) *similarity* and *dissimilarity*. Similar data within the present sensuous field are felt to blend. They (d) *grow together*, arouse similar sediments of past sensations and form *concrescent* wholes. Dissimilar data are felt to stand out. This sensation of *concrescent* wholes and their *discrete* counterparts is (b) *intensified* into the apperception of (e) *homogeneous units* of sensuous data within *heterogeneous* surroundings.[13] Since the units are associated in syntheses of homogeneity and discretion, there arise connexions of comparison (*Vergleichungszusammenhänge*). Common and discrete features can be thrown into relief and the *possibility* of objectifying, conceptual predication is foreshadowed.

Temporality is the fundamental form, association the "universal principle" of passive synthesis. They

"govern a passive forming of perpetually new syntheses (a forming that, in part, lies prior to all activity and, in part, takes in all activity itself). We encounter a passive genesis of the manifold apperceptions [of homogeneous units], as products that persist in a habituality relating specifically to them. When these habitual apperceptions become actually operative, when they affect the central I and motivate it to activity, they do appear as formed objectivities given in advance. Thanks to passive synthesis (into which the performances of active synthesis also enter) the I always has an environment of *objects*." (*Cart.Med.* p. 113).

---

13 For a most elaborate discussion of association cf. the third section of *Pass.Synth*, pp.117-191. The ascending series of unification obviously tends towards identity. This tendency, however, cannot be fulfilled within the sphere of passive synthesis. Identity cannot be intuited as such within the feelings of affinity and contrast, similarity and dissimilarity, concretion and discretion, homogeneity and heterogeneity. By reflection only, we can see that these concepts are implied and work, as it were, implicitly within associative syntheses. Configurations of data are felt to be similar and equal to others and are synthesized with others into homogeneous and discrete units by virtue of the still hidden identical "essence" in which they partake. This essence, however, cannot be sensed, even though it is dimly felt along with the reception of its individual cases anf the associative synthesis of such particular matters. The identical essence is to be grasped mentally: it is intuited in "eidetic intuition". For details, see my *Eidos and Eidetic Variation in Husserl's Phenomenology* (this volume).

5.1 Habit and Personality

So far we have concentrated on the *noema* of passive synthesis. A short glance into the opposite direction will reveal what an important role passive synthesis plays in the formation of the experiencing I itself. Thanks to passive synthesis the I always owns an environment of objects. As we have seen before, experiential life realizes itself in individual sensations and their data, and bears their stamp. With each sensation we receive a certain determination. "From now on I am abidingly the I of such and such an experience" (*Cart.Med.* p. 100). Those determinations and sediments of former feelings enter into the performance of further sensations. Hence experiential life has its *history*. The sensations and associations, the *geneses* of reproduction and expectation grow together and form concrescent wholes of *attitudes*: accustomed series of feeling, customary ways of production, habits of constituting. The sphere of outer experience bears the stamp of a certain life-history, and in correlation, the I, which has passively constituted this sphere, develops habits of constituting the material for an objective world. In short: the I develops into a concrete, individual person.

The importance of this concretion of subjectivity, i.e., the formation of personality cannot be limited to the sensuous life. Its full consequences appear only in active, intentional and even moral life. It is no matter of indifference what we feel, sediment, associate and synthesize into units of sensuous apprehension. On the contrary, the material richness or poverty of the world we are able to objectify will ensue from it. And again seen from the side of the experiencing person: the feelings which we engage in habitually, the kinds of associations we are accustomed to run through, in short, the *habits*, through which we synthesize the material data of sensation, foreshadow what sort of person we are. On the preliminary stage of sensuous life the life-style of the moral character is anticipated.[14]

Husserl's phenomenological description of intentionality and passive synthesis reveals the   necessary mutual relation of subjectivity and objectivity. All that exists is not a mere fact to us (*factum brutum*), but is constituted anonymously, as it were, in passive genesis and synthesis and in consciously performed intentional acts. And in counterpoint, subjectivity does not exist insulated in itself—another *factum brutum*—, but exists as world-constituting, intersubjective, personal life. The relationship is primary and fundamental: the pole of subjectivity and the pole of the world are embraced within it.

6. Primary Consciousness of Time

We talk of events, actions, facts and intentions, of meetings, persons met and things and events dealt with during those encounters; we say *now*,

---

14 Husserl emphasizes the importance of habits to such an extent as have only Hegel and Aristotle, so far as I can see, done before him (cf. Funke 1958).

then, just now, for the time being and *for good.* Actions and happenings are dated by the day and the hour. It may easily be overlooked what happens and what we do when we are conscious of processes, use such temporal words and phrases, and date occurrences and facts. The awareness of goings-on seems to be founded in the measuring of time; using these words and phrases we indicate the time-point and temporal extension of episodes. To all appearance consciousness of events and processes and the application of temporal words can easily be explained: we locate events in a generally agreed upon time-scale and we measure processes.

But how do we obtain such a time-scale and how do we measure processes? Processes are measured by the (temporal) succession of their (temporally extended) phases. The time-scale, on the other hand, is the (temporal) succession of such (temporally) extended phases brought to rest, spatialized into one continuous extension, and seen together, at least partly so, in one glance. The awareness of events and processes and the use of temporal words refers back to the primary consciousness of time. The original differences of temporality, presence, past, and future, are intuitively constituted in consciousness (*Lectures* § 2).

The cast shadow of the gnomon slipping over the dial, the rotation of the minute and the hour hand sliding over the face indicate time passing. In our attention we retain the span which has been slipped over while the shadow glides on. The spot which it leaves and the span which it has left are taken together as if they were a stretch tinged by the gliding shadow-line and seen at once in one glance. While it seems to rest we foresee the span into which it is gliding. We hold fast what has happened and hold out and stretch forth our attention towards further goings-on. Without this retention (i.e., retaining) on one hand and that protention (i.e., anticipating) on the other movement, processes and events would remain unperceptible.

Minute hand and second hand skip. In following their movement (the span they have skipped held fast) we foresee their next station with hightened attention or even suspense. This tension can be poignantly felt when the timepiece breaks and then stands still. The attention is sharpened for the foreseen skip. The second hand may jerk but does not clear its station, the minute hand rests, the liquid crystal readout persists in showing one cypher: we are aware of the protentive character of experiential life.

Reading a timepiece is only a single example. Each experience incorporates this structure.[15] Experiential life is retentive and protentive. The self, the active subject of experience, thought and intention, lives through what is given to it, thinks its own thoughts, pursues its intentions etc., spreads out and spans its own durational presence by virtue of its

---

15 Who hears a sound has already heard it and is still listening. Cf. Husserl's famous analysis in his *Lectures*. This internal temporality finds striking expression—and inevitably discovers itself—in the temporal structure of language: the tenses, the temporal words; the formation of phrases and sentences and the very process of speaking and listening, writing and reading.

double-faced attention. It spreads out and spans, distends, time within the double temporal horizon of retention and protention.[16] *Time* here means the primary consciousness of time: the constitution of the durative presence of experiential and intentional life. Within this internal temporality the self can suffer affections, obtain dates, and live through what is given to it. Apart from this durational presence, nothing could possibly be sensed, experienced, perceived, thought and intended. The constitution of this durative presence is one of the fundamental traits of experiential and intentional life. This sphere of immanent time therefore furnishes the basis of the awareness of *now, just now, no more, not yet,* and of the measurement of processes, the formation of a continuous time-scale, and the location of events.

When we consider the time-point *now* to be a durationless moment, time shrinks and tends to dwindle into an illusion. In a durationless *now* nothing can happen, nothing can be experienced, thought and intended. *Now* signifies a boundary dividing happenings which are no more from those encountered not yet. Still, the boundary seems to separate and connect durative events. But how has the past event been lived through and how shall the future occurrence be encountered, perceived and grasped mentally when the durative presence of experiential life is reduced to a sudden transition? The mere boundary *now* appears to be an abstraction, a mark on the time-scale that nonetheless has been formed on the basis of the durational presence. It is true that this boundary cannot constitute the continuous extension of the scale, and that the durationless transition can neither be, nor substitute, the presence constituted by the double-faced activity of the self; but still we do find such boundaries and transitions in our experiential life. Self spreads out its own duration, it distends and spans its present time *now* and in the same instance distinguishes its time past and what it *then* has lived through. The self itself sets the boundary by differentiating between its active presence and the past life-span which it can re-enact and re-present (*Lectures* § 14). It experiences and suffers the transition from the immediacy of its presence to its own past which can only be remembered.

---

16 Retention and protention "distend the consciousness of the *now*" (*Lectures* § 11, p. 45, l. 27.) In his Introduction to the *Lectures* (p. 3) Husserl refers to Augustine's *Confessiones*: "Chapters 14-28 of the XIth book of the *Confessions* must needs be studied thoroughly by anybody who engages in the problem of time." A few sentences pertinent to our considerations will prove him right. "This is why I have come to think that time is simply a distention. But of what is it a distention? I do not know, but it would be surprising if it is not that of the mind itself. ... What then am I measuring? Time as it passes but not time past? [XI,26,33] In process of passing away it was extended through a certain space of time by which it could be measured, since the present occupies no length of time. [27,34] So it is in you, my mind, that I measure periods of time. ... The impression which passing events make upon you abides when they are gone. That present consciousness is what I am measuring, not the stream of past events which have caused it. When I measure periods of time, that [present consciousness] is what I am actually measuring. [27,36] But how does this future, which does not yet exist, diminish or become consumed? Or how does the past, which now has no being, grow, unless there are three processes in the mind which in this is the active agent? For the mind expects and attends and remembers, so that what it expects passes through what has its attention to what it remembers. ... None can deny that present time lacks any extension because it passes in a flash. Yet attention is durational [*perdurat attentio*], and it is through this that what will be present progresses towards being absent. [28,37]."

Within itself the durational presence is a *continuous* extension shading off within the double *horizon* of retention and protention. But it is *discrete* as well, showing a double temporal *limit*. On the one hand it stands out from experiences which can no more be held fast and retained but may be re-enacted, re-presented, and remembered. (A past life-span without any experiential contents might hardly be recovered.) On the other hand it differs from a presence that can no more be protended and integrated into the present time-span. The self detaches itself from a future *now* that can only be expected.

Retention should neither be confused with remembrance (*Wiedererinnerung*) nor protention mixed up with expectation. They are part and parcel of the durational presence of any experience and act. What has been constituted just now, and what might be constituted just now in consciousness is held fast and kept up by retention and protention. Remembrance and expectation, on the contrary, are particular acts performed within their own presence. They possess their own retentive and protentive halo (*Zeithof; Lectures* § 14, p. 35. Cf. §§ 16, 17, 19).

The durational presence extends undivided and indivisible.[17] Division originates when the self distinguishes its durational presence from its past life-span and a future presence only to be expected.[18] Self sets the boundary and suffers the transition and thus divides and connects the many time-spans—the history—of its experiential and intentional life.[19] Being undivided and indivisible its durative presence spans an immeasurable extension and consequently forms the basis of the continuous time-scale and of measurement. Differentiating its life, self can posit any boundary of time passed to be the point zero from which the measuring of time commences.

The constitution of temporal objectivity, e.g. the awareness of alteration, duration and succession, the measuring of processes, and the location of events *now*, *no more* and *not yet*, is grounded in the internal temporality of the self: the durational presence, the transition and differentiation of experiential life.

---

17 The attempt to divide it results in a sudden transition and change of attitude: retention has not been detached from the *now* but stepped over, as it were, and replaced by remembrance and re-production; protention has been substituted by expectation.

18 We become aware of this distinction when we persist in one experiential attitude, e.g. when we go on perceiving one and the same phenomenon (cf. *Lectures* § 18 the interplay of retention and remebrance in the constitution of duration and succession), or one and the same object in its different sides and features, or when we consciously change attitudes and intertwine intuition with remembrance, expectation, imagination etc.

19 Cf. the striking passage in S.T.Coleridge's *Friend*: "If we listen to a symphony of Cimarosa, the present strain seems not only to recal, but almost to *renew*, some past movement, another and yet the same! Each present movement bringing back, as it were, and embodying the spirit of some melody that had gone before, anticipates and seems trying to overtake something that is to come: and the musician has reached the summit of his art, when having thus modified the Present by the Past, he at the same time weds the Past in the Present to some prepared and corresponsive Future. The auditor's thoughts and feelings move under the same influence: retrospection blends with anticipation, and Hope and Memory (a female Janus) become one power with a double aspect" (Coleridge 1969, pp. 129–130; cf. Uehlein 1982, pp. 80–82).

Summary

A Husserlian analysis of human life is given with emphasis on those aspects which may be of particular interest to psychiatry: Passive (automated) synthetic processes, intentional (conscious) acts, the formation of personality, and the consciousness of the flow of time. Phenomenology starts its analysis with the life world: It is still the life-world in which we live and work, and to which our interests, aims and actions refer, whether we live in the natural attitude of everyday practical life or whether we transform the categories of the natural attitude into exact laws and the rules of technical mastery. In Husserl's phenomenological account of how lived human experience is possible in this life world, three concepts are of fundamental importance: Intentionality, passive synthesis, and the primary consciousness of time. Husserl argues that there is a necessary mutual relation of subjectivity and objectivity. All that exists is not a mere fact to us, but is constituted in passive synthesis and in consciously performed intentional acts. Passive syntheses and intentional acts constitute the world. The relationship is primary and fundamental: the pole of subjectivity and the pole of objectivity are closely mutually related. Passive syntheses and intentional acts are performed by a person living with other persons. The history of such syntheses and acts will influence the way in which future syntheses and acts will be performed—personality and habits are formed. The awareness of alteration, duration and succession, the measuring of processes, and the location of events *now*, *no more* and *not yet*, i.e., the constitution of temporal objectivity, is grounded in the internal temporality of the self: the durational presence, the transition and differentiation of experiential life.

References

Augustine: Confessiones (transl. by H Chadwick). Oxford University Press, 1991
Bachelard G: Poetik des Raums (French original: La poétique de l'espace). München, Carl Hanser, 1975
Coleridge ST: The Friend (BE Rooke, ed). The Collected Works of S. T. Coleridge 4, London, Routledge & Kegan Paul, 1969
Coleridge ST: The Notebooks (K Coburn, ed) vols. II and III. London, Routledge & Kegan Paul, 1961/1973
Coleridge ST: On the Constitution of Church and State (J Colmer, ed). The Collected Works of S. T. Coleridge 10, London, Routledge & Kegan Paul, 1976
Derrida J: De la grammatologie. Paris, Les Éditions de Minuit, 1967a
Derrida J: La voix et le phénomène. Paris, Presses Universitaires de France, 1967b
Derrida J: La différance. In: Marges de la philosophie. Paris, Les Éditions de Minuit, 1972
Funke G: Gewohnheit. Archiv für Begriffsgeschichte 3: 518–546 , Bonn, Bouvier, 1958
Hegel GFW: Enzyklopädie der philosophischen Wissenschaften im Grundrisse (1830). German-English ed. by MJ Petry: Hegel's Philosophy of Subjective Spirit. Dordrecht, Reidel, 1978

Husserl E: Cartesianische Meditationen und Pariser Vorträge (*Cart.Med.*). Biemel W (ed), Husserliana vol. I. Den Haag, Nijhoff, 1965

Husserl E: Erfahrung und Urteil (*E&J*). Landgrebe L (ed). Hamburg, Meiner, 1985

Husserl E: Ideen zu einer reinen Phänomenologie und phänomenologischen Philosophie (*Ideas*), Erstes Buch. Biemel W (ed), Husserliana III. Den Haag, Nijhoff, 1950

Husserl E: Die Krisis der europäischen Wissenschaften und die transzendentale Phänomenologie (*Crisis*), Biemel W (ed), Husserliana vol. VI. Den Haag, Nijhoff, 2nd ed, 1962

Husserl E: Logische Untersuchungen (*Log.Invest.*), Zweiter Band, I. Teil. Halle, Niemeyer, 2nd ed, 1913

Husserl E: Zur Phänomenologie der Intersubjektivität (*Intersubjectivity*). Texte aus dem Nachlaß, Dritter Teil (1929-1935). Kern I (ed), Den Haag, Nijhoff, 1973

Husserl E: Analysen zur passiven Synthesis (*Pass.Synth.*), Fleischer M (ed), Husserliana vol. XI. Den Haag, Nijhoff, 1966

Husserl E: Zur Phänomenologie des inneren Zeitbewußtseins (*Lectures*) (1893-1917), Boehm R (ed) Husserliana vol. X. Den Haag, Nijhoff, 1969

Ingarden R: Das literarische Kunstwerk, (4th ed). Tübingen , Max Niemeyer, 1972

Ingarden R: Untersuchungen zur Ontologie der Kunst Tübingen, Max Niemeyer, 1962

Marbach E: Das Problem des Ich in der Phänomenologie Husserls. Den Haag, Nijhoff, 1974

Uehlein FA: Die Manifestation des Selbstbewußtseins im konkreten »Ich bin«. Endliche und Unendliches Ich im Denken S.T.Coleridges. Hamburg, Meiner, 1982

M. Spitzer, F.A. Uehlein
M.A. Schwartz, C. Mundt
(eds.): Phenomenology
Language & Schizophrenia.
Springer-Verlag, New York, 1992

Eidos and Eidetic Variation in Husserl's Phenomenology

Friedrich A. Uehlein

1. Introduction

Eidetic variation, eidetic intuition and the descriptive science of essences are elements of reasoning which are in constant implicit use in scientific work.

Husserl's term, *Eidetic intuition*, denotes the constitution of a certain kind of knowledge, which is rather different from the awareness of *this* and *that*, from the acquaintance with things of everyday life, and from empirical knowledge. Eidetic intuition, or catching sight of what things are themselves essentially, lies at the very heart of phenomenology and is therefore knit together with phenomenological reduction and other central features of this philosophy.[1] To name only two: (1) intentionality and (2) the horizonal character of experience. Intentionality means the active life of each individual person, and, more generally, the activity inherent in the general structure of subjectivity, of which the person an individual case. Intentionality means that special character of our experience that there is something for us, that there are *objects* (in the most inclusive sense of the word), whether they be given in pre-conscious affections, vague feelings, sensual awareness, or in conscious experience and practice, scientific research or phenomenological intuition.[2]

The second feature I wish to intimate is the horizonal character of experience. Objects are given within specific horizons in which we

---

1 Husserl is quoted from the collected works, Husserliana, using the following short titles:
Cart.Med.: Cartesian Meditations
E&J: Experience & Judgement
Ideas I: Ideas Pertaining to a Pure Phenomenology and to a Phenomenological Philosophy
Crisis: The Crisis of European Sciences and Transcendental Phenomenology
Log.Invest.: Logical investigations
Intersubjectivity III: On the Phenomenology of Intersubjectivity, 3rd vol.

2 Cf. Spitzer & Uehlein; Uehlein; Wiggins et al. (all in this volume). Substantial passages in Husserl's oeuvre: *V. Logische Untersuchung*: Über intentionale Erlebnisse und ihre 'Inhalte'; *Cart.Med.* §§17-20 and *Crisis* §§ 37-54 [In his article *What is phenomenology? A review*—cf. the critical discussion by Wiggins et al., this volume—G.E.Berrios styles *The crisis of European science* "the almost mystical book" (p. 426). I should think he is talking of a different book which happens to have the same title as Husserl's late work.]

encounter, experience, and explicate them, passing forward to new aspects of the same object and further to new objects, and reaching back to already experienced traits and objects, and taking them together into growing objective units. When we, for example, encounter a thing of the natural world in our experiential field and see its colored front, we anticipate its back. We may walk around it and experience it in an uninterrupted change of data in changing horizons. We can inspect the thing in detail and be sure that new data and new anticipations in these "inner horizons" will never fail us. We may concentrate on the place in which it is situated, anticipate its background while viewing its foreground, and go on to another thing next to the first one within one and the same "outside horizon" of their mutual togetherness in one environment. In our experience, there is never a hard edge, an ultimate limit, where it breaks and objectivity ends without any horizon for further possible data and further possible intentional activity. Horizons distinguish and connect phenomena, things and inclusive unities of things. In short, horizons differentiate and connect objectivity within the all-inclusive horizon of the World.

The same is true of intentional life: Horizons—of inner time and of kinds of activity, like being affected, being aware of, perceiving, signifying, remembering, doubting, etc.—differentiate, articulate and connect the manifold actions to the one stream of experiential life (cf. *Crisis* §§ 44-48).

2. The Pre-conception of General Concepts in all Items of Experience

Whatever we meet up with in experience is in some way already familiar to us. We encounter it and events in the horizon of a typical familiarity: it is something, this or that, here and now, of a certain (perhaps not quite distinguishable) shape, similar and strikingly different to things we are already acquainted with. What is experienced displays inner and outer horizons in which it gives itself to further familiarity. We can enter any horizon and enquire "what lies in it", we can uncover, enfold and clarify what begins to appear in strange familiarity.

How does such familiarity arise? It arises in the pre-conscious intentional life of affections and passive constitutions (passive genesis, cf. Spitzer & Uehlein, this volume). Whatever we live through forms sediments; as Leibniz put it: the soul does not forget anything. All sediments are effective, continuously so; they associate and arouse each other by virtue of association. Therefore, even the *novel* experience arises in typical familiarity, however unspecific these types may yet be. Affections and their sediments and—on a different level of consciousness—perceptions in various modes, and finally the content of intentional acts associate in presentational immediacy as well as in expectation and remembrance. Affections, appearances and things given never occur in the form of single impressions, which are products of an abstractive analysis. On the contrary, they affect, they appear, and they are 'for us' within the the experiental field and the plurality of other phenomena equally given[3]. A plurality of things can even operate as a single affection by virtue of the type of familiarity they share. Right from the beginning items of experience are given in the framework of general features, viz. the types of familiarity, by which they associate, remind us of each other and affect in a similar way or even as one overall affection. At a later stage of his argument Husserl writes of the pure essence of a thing:

"It is passively pre-constituted [right from the incidental beginning of our experiental life], and the envisagement of the eidos is achieved by the active glance and grasp comprehending it in its pre-constitution." (E&J, p. 414).

In being affected, in passive genesis of appearances and associative synthesis of events and objects, we already operate with eide[4], i.e., (at this stage of our argument) peculiar types of familiarity and resemblance, without having any declarative, explicit knowledge of them. We need to anticipate familiarity and resemblance, some kinds of generalities (eide, as it were) when we experience things and events to be manifold, connected and comparable, when we experience them as similar and different items. To make these implicitly functioning general features explicit, to seize them out of their preconstitution, is the aim of conceptual comprehension in general and of eidetic reduction in particular.

3. Empirically General Concepts
Individual and General Judgement

Individual judgements are of the form: S' is p'; S" is p"; S'" is p'". p', p", p'" are individual features (constituent elements) of S', S", S'". We may stick to their types of familiarity, by which they associate and affect in a similar way. We overlap and superpose those things of our experience with respect to those common features. We may find out that p' and p" and p'" are equal: they are equal with respect to a general character p. Their equality points to one identical p. The identical p is one only, and over and over again in repetition of comparison and superposition one and the same. p', p" and p'" etc. are individual items of the *form p* (e.g. *house, computer*, but as well *red*, perhaps *delusion, person*). This form is no part of the various objects, otherwise they should hang together and intersect in that identical section that they share. The general form p is, as Husserl says, the unity of the species [*die Einheit der Species*]. Proceeding on the guideline of equality we glance through the superposed objects and envisage the one and identical p, the unity of the species, on the back (so to say) of those

---

3 Cf. *Crisis*, p. 165. With respect to mental life (*Bewußtseinsleben*) a particular item of experience is neither insulate nor separable. Husserl describes in this short and implicative passage the synthetical transition from the field of perception (*Wahrnehmungsfeld*) to the field of things (*Dingfeld*) and to the universe of things perceptible, the world (*Welt als Wahrnehmungswelt*).

4 "In truth, everybody sees 'eide', 'essences', sees them, as it were, all the time, operates with them in his thought." (*Ideas* I, p. 49)

objects, but not as one of their parts. Individual objects partake of the general form, and by virtue of their participation in this identical one they are equal. Equality can neither be isolated and understood by itself, nor should it be conflated with participation. It is related to the general form. Equality refers to the identical, the one and same *eidos*.

4. Experience and the General Form

Our awareness of the general forms originates in experience. But even though the general forms become visible by the association and the conscious and intentional overlapping and superposition of phenomena of experience, they are not limited by experiential data. The operation of seeing things together and comparing them can be repeated with other data. It can even be imagined beyond the limits of casual experience. In fact, the *general form* transcends those particular operations and individual cases and demands an open, illimitable horizon of application. Thus it becomes evident that it is not confined to experience and does not depend upon any singular fact. Even the more so, to be truly general, the concept has to go beyond any particular instances of experience.

We now have reached an important station on our way to Husserl's idea of pure knowledge of the essence of things, i.e., the eidos.

A short reminiscence of the empiricist conception of the general form may help to clarify the argument. According to the empiricist, the general form is a mere *collection of ideas*, which are found to be equal in certain items of experience. This collection of ideas is bound to experience and has to be checked over and again against single items of renewed experience. Hence, the unity of a general concept—*the unity of the species* in Husserl's terms—is always endangered by possible new data. At its best it is a general concept not yet falsified. Therefore, we never know for certain *what* it is that we experience. We never know what the singular features, the symptoms, characteristics and qualities newly experienced, amount to. Are they still unknown aspects of the same thing, or features indicative of a new thing altogether? Since we cannot measure out the entire range of experience and encounter all potential objects of a certain species, our general concept of that species remains uncertain. Furthermore, by what criterion can we decide that single features, characteristics and qualities newly experienced belong to the species in question, so that they can falsify and re-inforce it? No criterion can be found if the specific features won so far depend on particular instances of renewed experience. In case there are no specific features, which transcend their momentary, casual occurence and may be seen along with all data right from the beginning of experiential life, experience turns out to be an illusion: indifferent singular impressions and ideas of 'I don't know what' flit by in an indiscriminate sequence. How can we properly talk of experience and *renewed* experience and of *novel* data at all? How could we hope to falsify, correct and improve on a general concept won so far?

Husserl avoids this dilemma. Intentional life does not set out from single ideas and simple impressions, but from experiences in the horizon of typified similarity, and by implication from the one and same unity of the species. We do not see mere, unspecified pixels, but rather grey elephants and red roses. Our grasp of things as of such-and-such kind, belonging to sets of things, as defined by a general form, is implicit in the immediate affections and presentations. In the first steps of perceptual awareness we become aware of that general form but we may not see it clearly. Our concept of that form is certainly under correction all the time. Such corrections and completions, however, are directed by the growing awareness of that unity of the species, and belong to the widening horizons of objectifying experience and thought. That the entire range of experience cannot be measured out does not endanger the unity of the general, since each general concept by its very nature exhibits an open, illimitable horizon of application.

General concepts of experienced items, however, may still include traits of particular things, i.e., unanalysed remains taken over from incidentally given things. To give an example:[5] We may have encounterd a lot of shapes made up by three strait lines as their boundaries but all of them may have had certain paculiar features (for example, the angles between the lines may always have been greater than 20°). In other words, while at this stage we have some kind of general concept of a triangle, this concept is still tinted with the incidental feature of "all three corners form angles of more than 20°. Such a concept is neither simply false, nor does it represent a different collection of ideas, but it is "impure": essential features, invariants, and still variable determinations are interwoven to form a *hybrid conception*. Of such kind are normally our general concepts. The notion of the pure eidos has not yet been reached.

5. From the Empirically General Form to the Eidos

All concepts of every-day life are realized—notwithstanding their general character—in individual things, at least potentially so. We do mean things and events in the real lived world. Empirical concepts undergo revision, correction, re-inforcement. They integrate new types of qualities on the basis of newly experienced individual qualities. They are enlarged and become richer and more complete in areas which so far have been antici-pated only vaguely. However, it is important to realize that those changes do *not* change the concept as such and the object intended, so that another concept would arise instead of the originally intended one. Each new quality [*Merkmal*] opens up the anticipation of further qualifications. All

---

5 For the sake of simplicity of the argument, we adhere to a long lasting philosophical tradition and take an example from geometry. This does not imply, however, that similar examples, though more complicated ones, cannot be made up in the realm of psychiatry. Is the concept of hallucination pure? Does it include the notion of impaired reality testing? Is a delusion necessarily always a wrong statement?

changes occur within the open horizon of unfulfilled qualification and completion. Thus, qualities and qualifications, determinations and changes grow together into one concrescent whole. They tend towards a completion beyond the hybrid unity which had been gained so far.

Empirical, general concepts have an extension of actual and potential singular entities (objects, events). They do not only include the countable number of real items of experience, from which they took their origin, but exhibit a horizon of presumptive further experience. Their extension therefore is indefinitely open towards possible, *real* data. Their unity, however, is still casual and incidental: from incidentally given things (particular triagular shaped objects, certain cases of hallucinations and delusions, etc.) the conceptualization started and was pursued through equally incidental data and is still open towards further real, and for that reason, casual data of experience.

6. Eidetic Variation

We can transcend the associative nexus and the intentional superposition of *real* things and pass on to free imaginations of things. By means of the process of free imagination, general concepts become indifferent towards real cases. Imagination, as it were, cuts general concepts loose from casual data. Such data, as we have seen, may make contigent facts appear essential. In order to attain truly general concepts, untinted with casual empirical data, we need the process of free imagination.

A comparison of perceptual intuition and eidetic variation might be helpful in order to understand the function of eidetic variation. Perception receives and apprehends its object on the basis of passive syntheses, i.e., automated processes, independent of conscious acts. Inner and outer horizons prescribe the course of experience. Each further step and each further piece of experience and the whole course of data have to be brought into unison with the beginning and all intermediate steps if the object is to become real to us. A house we see or imagine cannot be tiled and thatched, round and cubical, bungalow and six-storied, etc. Certainly, the red house here can be painted blue, it can be rebuilt with a semicircular front and slated roof, etc. But then we see exclusive alterations and different individual houses. Eidetic variation is not under such restrictions. It leaves behind the prescribed course of a particular experience and its unison of data. Alterations and individual cases, which exclude each other in particular experience, are the very matter of variation. It actually aims at that unity which *includes* all *possible* alterations and all *possible* individual cases.

Firstly we feign individuals equal to those experienced, then, as much as we please, new ones, individually different things at random. Variation means that we even leave the identity of the individual behind and transform one possible individual into another one. (Not only one house, one delusion altered, but other houses, other delusions altogether!) In free variation we superpose possible individuals, which cannot co-exist but exclude and supplant each other. The eidos proves to be one and the same in all variations, alterations and contradictions of mutually exclusive individuals. Imagining things as *potential* singularities we grasp the eidos. It is to be conceived as an object which has a purely ideal being independent of the real existence of corresponding individual things. As Husserl says in *Experience and Judgment* (p. 396), it is what it is, even if the corresponding individuals would exist only potentially.

Free variation liberates from the empirically given data and the casual comparison and equalization of data. It enables us to see the eidos or idea (E&J, p. 411) free from all contingent differences. The experienced objects from which the empirically general concept originates become arbitrary examples of an endless manifold of variants. In the variety of such variants, imagined ad libitum, we can catch sight of an identical "it is what it is", which runs through the whole variety unvariably. The random sample of the incidental beginning and the whole process of variation and all variants are unimaginable and unthinkable without this identical one. The process renders the eidos explicit: we have been operating with it, implicitly, from the reception and association of affections and their sediments, according to their family-likeness and familiarity, to the awareness and perception of phenomena within the widening horizons of intentional, objectifying acts, from the comparison and superposition of objects to the free imaginative variations of things and events.

All the differences of the variables become a matter of indifference and the absolutely identical is thrown into relief; what cannot fall into indifference and withstands all variations stands out: the invariable identical features, in Husserl's words, the essence/the *eidos*. We even strain the variation to its limits, where it breaks down, and envisage the necessary invariable form which sets the limit to all variability and renders variations and variants possible.

Eidetic variation owns a critical impetus, too. If it starts from theory-laden observations, as for example from signs and symptoms which have been interpreted already within a certain etiology, the variation will lead to that particular etiology and not to the conception of the experiences lived through by the patient. Consequently, the etiological preconceptions have also to undergo variation. Generally speaking, the conditions which are responsible for a certain acceptance (*Geltung*) of phenomena have to be put the test of free imaginative variation. This holds true even of the words and phrases of ordinary language and "language games" in which we name phenomena and talk about them. Those sedimented meanings are too easily taken for granted. They form a layer of hidden modes of acceptance which tinge phenomena almost imperceptibly and are therefore the more in need of critical variation.[6]

---

6 Husserl has worked out a fairly elaborate analysis of meanings, e.g., in the second and fourth *Logical Investigation*. He not only describes how we use the language factually; he introduces critical variation to linguistic presuppositions (cf. Wittgenstein, *Philosophische Untersuchungen*, p. 124). "The eidos is prior to all concepts, in the sense of verbal siginifications; indeed, as pure concepts, these must be formed to fit the eidos." (*Cart.Med.* p. 105). Even so, his analysis of meaning borders on the

The contents of the general concept comprises a yet incidental and presumably hybrid unity; the contents of the eidos is the unity of invariables. Empirical concepts reveal themselves to be indefinitely open step by step, subsequently—*posteriorly*—by opening up the horizon of presumptive experience. The eidos, on the contrary, "reveals itself as the unity of determinations without which an object of that kind can neither be thought or imagined as such" (*E&J*, p. 411). Consequently, there can be worked out "laws of necessity, which determine the necessary features of an object, if it is to be a object of that kind" (*E&J*, p. 426). The eidos is the general and necessary essence of all potentials of this kind. It decides, as it were, what a given thing is.

An individual of that kind has to be such and such since we have seen that it cannot be different, and essentially so. In this sense eidetic knowledge is a priori.

7. Envisagement (*Ersehen/Wesensschau*)

Envisagement means that an object itself is given. It is not only represented by an image or mediated by a sign or symbol, but presented directly. All representation refers finally to an original intuition, all proxies presuppose ultimately the immediate presence of the thing 'in person'.[7] Sensual awareness presents 'something' which has been pre-constituted in the manifold affections and associations of passive genesis. Perception gives the object in direct intuition. Remembrance gives the thing, once experienced, in its typical modification of intuition, etc. Eidetic intuition equally gives a genuine, original object: the eidos. It is an object in its own right and directly intuited in the process of eidetic variation and intuition. It is neither a vague re-presentation, the remnants of vivid and originally given sensual "impressions", nor a mere abstraction of understanding filtered out from originally given simple ideas. In eidetic intuition we see and own the eidos in direct evidence and do not build on causal inferences or syllogistic reasoning. We do not argue from conceptual presuppositions, but *describe* essential features and their interrelation as seen in direct intuition. Notwithstanding, it must not be overlooked that it is a spontaneous activity: "The original consciousness of the general is an activity, in which the general constitutes itself originally" (*Cart.Med.* p. 111; cf. *Ideas* I §§ 23, 24). The ideal character of the eidos does not imply an existence in and by itself severed from all subjectivity. "The existence of the general in its several stages is essentially constituted in those processes [of idealization, eidetic variation and intuition]" (*E&J*, p. 397)

---

philosophy of language as exemplified by Wittgenstein, Strawson and Castañeda, and on the theory of speech acts (cf. Searle).
7 *Ideen* I, p. 15, l.18: "in seiner 'leibhaftigen Selbstheit'". Cf. *Ideas* I, pp. 52, & 24: *The principle of all principles*. "Each intuition giving [the intuited] originally is a genuine source of knowledge. Whatever appears originally in intuition and gives itself 'in person', as it were, is simply to be received and apprehended as such."

The eidos is passively pre-constituted right from the incidental beginning of our experiential life, and the envisagement [*Erschauung*] of it is achieved by the active glance and grasp comprehending it *in* its pre-constitutions. It is envisaged not as a collections of ideas—collected from incidental items of experience and in danger of being crossed out by new incidental items—but as the unity of invariable determinants. For that reason it does not stand in the flux and alteration of experiential life, even if it is singularized in the streaming events which it determines. In other words, the application of eidetic knowledge to experiential facts does not involve that unity in the stream of data. In this special sense eide are 'beyond time' (*überzeitliche Gegenstände*). Each *actual* object is at the same time a *potential* one, an example, a case of ..., a realization of a pure essence. The essence comprises all possibilities and singularizes into potential individual cases a) in the first random sample, from which the process of eidetic intuition takes off, b) in all variations, as well as in all arbitrary series of variants. All the momenta of the pure essence—and it incorporates essential features only—must needs be determinants of the actual fact. The eidos decides, as it were, what a given thing is. If ever eidetic knowledge is reached science can judge actual facts and casual data of experience according to the structure of their pure potentiality.

It need hardly be added that empirical research is not supplanted or rendered superfluous by eidetic knowledge. The particular conditions and specific situations in which any factual thing is given and apprehended, the factual occurence and co-occurence of certain phenomena and the regularity of their co-existence or sequence (the necessary or incidental character of their togetherness still left undecided) have always to be researched by the "Erfahrungswissenschaften". In the application of eidetic knowledge, however, a new status of empirical sciences could be reached. Descriptive comprehension of empirical reality could partake of rational principles, by referring empirical data to their essential potentialities [*Wesensmöglichkeiten*].

8. Eidos and Experience
The Incompletion of Eidetic Knowledge

The inquiry into essences presses for completion, experiential life is prepared and expectant to encounter new things. Both seem to fall into an irreconcilable opposition. When eidetic cognition is reached, eventually, in the process of reduction and variation, does it then blur experiential life and render it insubstatial and unimportant? The constant flux of mental processes (*Erlebnisstrom*) and their data, to be sure, could not be brought to a standstill; still new things would happen to us and would be experienced in passive and active genesis—as long as we live and live on (cf. Uehlein, this volume). But would not those experiences be reduced to indifferent cases and boring repetitions of an universally valid and perfectly known eidos? If, on the other hand, eidetic reduction does not terminate in a completed concept, is it then worth its name? Does it not thwart the end for which it has been undertaken and will therefore entangle human knowledge (and practice) into the dilemma of empiricism?

Experience is "essentially one-sided" (*Cart.Med.*, p. 96). A thing or a complex of affairs in the experiential field is intuited from a limited perspective. Though giving itself, the thing, nevertheless, gives itself only from one side. It is received, perceived and apprehended in a limited view, which opens horizonally unto further views and further sides. Eidetic reduction cuts loose from these limitations. The features—as I tried to show before—which appear in free imaginative variation and prove to be invariable, do not depend again on renewed items of experience. They are given and apprehended in their own right. In eidetic intuition we envision features which enable us to compare, distinguish, contrast and unify phenomena within the growing pattern of interpersonal experience. We refer to them when we communicate and work together, and appeal to them in points of difference. At the same time we still strive for them, since what we refer to and appeal to does not form a body of completed eidetic knowledge but a scheme of hybrid eidetic conceptions to be enlarged, refined and outstripped with respect to the unitary eidos. The novel experience—whether it may prove a new variable trait hitherto unperceived or a new invariable hitherto anticipated only within the incomplete eidetic pattern—does appear, strikes our attention and can be identified on the back, as it were, of the imperfect 'eidos' reached so far. (Strange to say, but there is no room for novel experiences within strict empiricism.)

Eidetic reduction and free imaginative variation cut loose from the empirically given in order to intuit its essence. But can they free themselves to such an extent that they are in no need of renewed experience, novel experience sharpened by variation itself, in order to accomplish their own work of envisaging essential features and their interrelation?

In the concluding section I will try to argue for two things: eidetic knowledge is incompletable, yet it still avoids the dilemma of empiricism. I preceed in three steps: 1. Eide are incompletable within their own sphere. 2. There is one extraordinary eidos which necessarily entails factual existence: the individual person 3. The starting point of eidetic reduction is lived experience.

1. The interweaving of eide.

The question, e.g., what it is to hallucinate, implies—apart from the concentration on the phenomena of hallucination itself and the ensuing eidetic variation—a truly general concept and, for that reason, eidetic knowledge of *perception*, in particular of *fulfilling intuitions* which present real things 'in person'. Furthermore, it requires a general concept of *stating* and *referring*, of *language* and *situational behaviour* (i.e., of "intentionality" as used in ordinary language philosophy). It implies, finally, a general concept of *consciousness*, *self-consciousness* and the capability to *reflect* one's own intuitions, actions and their outcome. Eidetic knowledge of hallucionation thus entails a wide range of neighbouring eide within one and the same ontological domain, as well as closely related and encompassing domains. Apart from that a new line of research may be started on the basis of the phenomena of hallucination itself but in a somewhat wider field. The gender, age, biography, the life-style, social conditions and the cultural membership of hallucinating persons are investigated on suspicion of some regularity. The variables and invariants of such a correlation (in case it could be verified) do not appertain to the essential features of hallucination proper but to the founding strata (*Fundierungen*) of individual persons, persons perceiving, hallucinating etc. This hint of the domanial interralation of specific eide is far from being precise but perhaps suggestive of the rather incompletable enterprise of eidetic cognition.

Even the relatively closed pattern of eidetic features envisaged in the intuition and variation of "fixed" things of the natural world remains ultimately incompletable since one essence relates with other essences within one domain and refers to other foundational and encompassing domains.[8]

Strong empiricism (with a nominalistic bias) considers eidetic knowledge to be impossible or meaningless or to represent an overdrawn claim, a hypothesis not yet proven or even unprovable. Such general features of experience as the temporality of experiential and intentional life, intentionality, the horizonal character and the one-sidedness of perception, corporality, intersubjectivity and the life-world (*Lebenswelt*), however, can neither be reduced to empirical facts nor verified or falsified since they belong to the uneliminable preconditions of experience in general and verification in particular. Those traits of the individual person within the community of persons (*Monadengemeinschaft*) are a) trustworthy general features, b) attained by eidetic reduction, and c) not brought to an end, even if each of them has been brought to a certain perfection.

As one essence cannot be isolated (notwithstanding the determination of its own), but interrelates with other essences within specific domains and the composition of encompassing regions, and since it was fully constituted only within these manifold interrelations, the allegedly complete eidos would amount to a complete knowledge of the world and of (inter-monadic, world-constituting) subjectivity. Such an idea of a timeless, completed, absolute knowledge needn't be absurd. (Preposterous it would be, however, to surmise that Husserl ever held human knowledge to be capable of such a timeless perfection.) It can be conceived as the ideal of knowledge, even of the growing comprehension of finite minds: "the system of all objects of possible consciousness."[9]

---

8 Cf. *E&J* 442: "Each concept of an essence, which has been won by the genuine method and is, nevertheless, one-sided, is an integral part of universal ontology."

9 Cf. *Cart.Med.*, pp. 90-91: "That indicates in advance a *universal constitutive synthesis*, in which all syntheses function together in a definitely ordered manner and in which therefore all actual and possible objectivities (as actual and possible for the transcendental ego), and correlatively all actual and possible modes of consciousness of them, are embraced. ... But we speak more correctly if we say that here is a matter of an infinite *regulative idea*, that the evidently presupposable system of possible objects of possible consciousness is itself an anticipative idea (not however an invention, an 'as if'), and that, as regards practice, it equips us with the principle for combining any relatively

2. In his earlier, static-descriptive phenomenology, Husserl had concentrated on "fixed" kinds of objects—real things of the natural world, ideal things of mathematics and logic—and the correlative complex of constitutive mental acts in which those objects are given. In his later genetic-explicative phenomenology he emphasized the *genesis* of those constitutions which result in the correlation of acts and objects (*noeseis* and *noemata*). Genetic phenomenology pursues the history of objectifications, the history of the constitution of things, and thus the history of the objects themself as objects of possible cognition. Main themes of genetic phenomenology are: the life-world (*Lebenswelt*); horizons of experience; the transcendental I and the habitual attitudes (*Habitualitäten*) in which it is an individual person: "I, this human; this person existing in this body"; furthermore, corporality; intersubjectivity; sociality; the truly objective, transcendent nature as constituted within the community of monads. Perfect cognition of essences (which might open a gap between eidos and fact, eidetic intuition and experiential life) is out of the question here. The phenomenological self-explication of all constitutions of the ego and of all objectivities existing for the ego gives the facts their place in the corresponding *universe of eidetic possibilities* (cf. *Cart.Med.*, p. 117) Phenomenological self-explication is an "unending task ... which is to be carried on synthetically" (cf. *Cart.Med.*, p. 119).

The obviously all-embracing scope of genetic phenomenology centres upon the eidos of constitutive, inter-monadic subjectivity. The very intuition of its features and constitutive operations, the process of reduction and variation, implicate the factual existence of one particular case of the self-same eidos: a concrete person unravelling her own essence.

"Here we find a remarkable and unique case of the relationship between fact and eidos. The existence of an eidos, the existence of eidetic possibilities and of the universe of those possibilities is not bound by the existence or non-existence of any realization of such possibilities, it is independent in its existence from all corresponding reality. But the eidos of the transcendental ego is unthinkable without the transcendental ego existing in fact. ... I cannot go beyond my own factual existence and, within it, beyond the intentionally included co-existence of others etc., I cannot go beyond absolute reality." (*Intersubjectivity* III, pp. 385-386).

The inseperability of eidos and factual existence in the case of the concrete person directs our attention back to

3. The starting-point of eidetic reduction: Lived experience.

"All that exists, may it be concrete or abstract, actual or possible, real or ideal, has its own ways to give itself and to appear 'in person'. On the side of the ego it has its corresponding ways of being intended in modes of acceptance [*Modis der Geltung*] and in subjective alterations of those modes within syntheses of agreement and disagreement." (*Crisis* , p. 169).

---

closed constitutional theory with any other: by an incessant uncovering of horizons—not only those belonging to objects of consciousness internally, but also those having an external reference, namely to essential forms of interconnexions." (Dorion Cairns' translation). This idea of knowledge resembles, mutatis mutandis, the absolute mind and his wisdom (*Nous*) in the platonic tradition, and the regulative idea in Kant's *Critique of Pure Reason* (A 670-704).

Each passive awareness, each perception, each intentional act, all have their specific mode of acceptance. They are determined, limited, one-sided and at the same time horizontally open to further awareness, perceptions and acts, modes and alterations. Each act owns horizons of unfulfilled anticipations, which point to, lead to further syntheses with further intuitions and evidences.[10] Consequently each object of our experiential and intentional life is never intuited completely in all it possible features, is never received and perceived in all its possible modes of acceptance: it is never "for us", at once and for all, in the totality of its possible constitutions.[11] We cannot fix the existent in an exhaustive experience. On the other hand, neither are we given up to an indiscriminate reality which flits by in a multitude of single impressions only to be arranged into a haphazard and changing collection of facts.

Experiential life, however, is the point of departure for eidetic reduction. The incomplete synthesis of experience forms the starting point and in this manner enters into free imaginative variation.[12] The incomplete synthesis lacks certain possible features of the thing in sight, lacks them still..., they will be lacking in eidetic variation, too. (They can hardly be procured by the process of variation itself!) "Eidetic knowledge is incompletable, because right from its beginning it is no pure eidetic knowledge severed from all fact" (Waldenfels 1975, p. 75). The pattern of eidetic features, envisaged in the variation, and especially the interrelation of those features which demand each other, will show veins of indetermination and places of empty apprehension. Even so, the eidetic features won so far will not decay into makeshift abstractions, which have to be validated anew by particular cases of experience. It still holds true: "As the variation ... presents in pure intuition the possibilities themselves as possibilities, its correlate is an intuitive and apodictic consciousness of something universal" (Cart.Med., p. 105). We retain the invariants and fall back upon a renewed presentation of the same intentional object in order to procure novel individual features for further eidetic variation.

To give an illustration: A relatively coherent, 'operative eidos'[13], such as a pathological pattern (Krankheitsbild), which allows for diagnosis and treatment, requires application. With attention sharpened by the 'operative eidos', we fall back upon particular cases. We intuit their features as given 'in person' and vary them in order to envisage their essential character, and

---

10 "No imaginable synthesis of this kind is completed into an adequate evidence: any such synthesis must always involve unfulfilled, expectant and accompanying meanings." (Cart.Med., p. 96)

11 "Jedes Seiende ist in einem weitesten Sinne 'an sich' und hat sich gegenüber das zufällige Für-mich der einzelnen Akte." ("Each existing thing or complex of affairs is 'in itself'—in the most inclusive sense of the word—, and stands in contrast to its accidental being-for-me of particular acts.") (Cart.Med., p. 96). In Wesenserkenntnis und Erfahrung, Waldenfels discusses this point from the perspective of epistemology and the philosophy of language. He discusses "the difference of meaning and object".

12 "Intuition of individual things and intuitions of eide differ in principal", but at the same time they stand in an essential relationship. Eidetic intuition "is founded in individual intuition, in the appearance of an individual in sight" (cf. Ideen I, p. 15, l. 29- p. 16, l. 13).

13 "In truth, everybody sees 'eide', 'essences', sees them, as it were, all the time, operates with them in his thought" (Ideas I, p. 49).

then match the latter against the 'eidos'. In this overlaying, partial coincidence and identification, experiential intuition, variation, and eidetic knowledge are interwoven. In case the identification is successful, the application may a) complement the 'eidos' (the pathological pattern) and b) point to further neighbouring eide within the interrelation of diseases or to the foundation of this special illness in physiological and neurological etc. object-domains. The eidos still remains the guiding *aim*. In it all essential features (invariants) would be unified to such an extent that each feature demanded each other directly or indirectly, none could be lacking, none be added. Each single trait would be apprehended along with each other. The complete and perfect unity, the eidos, would include each feature distinctly and all of them in their necessary correlation.

In rare cases of ideal objects human knowledge might be capable of such a perfection. Normally we have to be content with far less, but still it seems to be the eidos that we mean, when we ask, what the case in point is, what a certain illness is, how it can be identified in countless particular cases and treated favourably.

It is true, inquiry into essences presses for completion, experiential life is prepared and expectant to encounter new things. The seemingly irreconcilable opposition resolves into a compatible contrast. Eidetic reduction has in view the determinacy of things and events and does therefore press for the thorough determination of experience. The eidos forms the directing aim of that determination. Experience within the life-world; passive and intentional, prehensive and apprehensive constitution; intuition of individuals; and eidetic variation are incompletable actions towards that goal. Without them empirical work stumbles.

In any case eidetic intuition and experience cannot be reduced one to the other. Experience may well exist without eidetic reduction (though we would not know what we are living through). Eidetic reduction, on the contrary, sets out from founding intuitions, cuts loose and operates in its own right towards the envisagement of the eidos.

To contrast the view presented here with a widely held consideration of the general, Wittgenstein's position may be briefly mentioned. Wittgenstein held "craving for generality" to be equivalent to "the contemptuous attitude towards the particular case" (Blue Book, p. 18). However, to consider the eidos at the expense of the particular case is mistaken. One is left with a rather empty set of fixed abstractions, which threaten to cover the data of experience. Instead, eidetic variation demonstrates that on the road to the eidos no individual feature is discarded as being insubstantial and unimportant. No individual trait is to be 'idealized away'. On the contrary, the invariant features are meant to include all possible variables. The unity of all invariants encompasses all possible variations and thus each realized, individual case. "In this way we can raise all reality to pure potentiality" (*E&J* p. 426). The eidos is a rich, inclusive concept.

Of course, the factual occurence, the case in sight, is a matter of experiential intuition. Neither are particular cases intuited within a definitely closed horizon and done with, nor is the unity of essential features completed once and for all. As the under-determined features and empty apprehensions within an eidetic pattern (an 'operative eidos') direct us back to new intuitions and variations, so the invariant features can serve as a guiding line a) to detect fleeting individual traits, which hitherto have been overlooked and b) to determine hard facts, which have eluded our understanding; they can function as Ariadne's thread, so to speak, leading psychopathologists to signs and symptoms which have not been expressed so far by their patients or have remained opaque. The invariant can keep awake curiosity and sharpen attention in the search for novel or familiar traits, hidden so far in uncommon and exotic disguises. Furthermore, by means of the invariant and still under-determined features of the eidetic pattern, those traits can be distinguished and determined, whether they belong to the eidos in question or to a different essence.

Craving for eidetic knowledge is definitely not "the contemptuous attitude towards the particular case", to slightly modify Wittgenstein's saying. It is rather the craving for a fuller understanding of phenomena. Eidetic reduction craves to rescue the phenomena from flitting by—unperceived or slighted. It craves to rescue what is fleeting or stubbornly opaque in experiential life into a full understanding of what it is.

Summary

The process of scientific reasoning is described in its elements: perception of particular cases and empirical general conceptualizations aiming at the unity of essential, invariable features of things, which determine what the object in question truly is.

References

Husserl E: Cartesianische Meditationen und Pariser Vorträge. Biemel W (ed), Husserliana vol. I. Den Haag, Nijhoff, 1965
Husserl E: Erfahrung und Urteil. Landgrebe L (ed). Hamburg, Meiner, 1985
Husserl E: Ideen zu einer reinen Phänomenologie und phänomenologischen Philosophie, Erstes Buch. Biemel W (ed), Husserliana III. Den Haag, Nijhoff, 1950
Husserl E: Die Krisis der europäischen Wissenschaften und die transzendentale Phänomenologie, Biemel W (ed), Husserliana vol. VI. Den Haag, Nijhoff, 2nd ed, 1962
Husserl E: Logische Untersuchungen, 2. Band, I. Teil. Halle, Niemeyer, 2nd ed, 1913
Husserl E: Zur Phänomenologie der Intersubjektivität. Texte aus dem Nachlaß, Dritter Teil (1929-1935). Kern I (ed), Den Haag, Nijhoff, 1973
Searle JR: Speech Acts. Cambridge, Cambridge University Press, 1979
Uehlein FA: Die Manifestation des Selbstbewußtseins im konkreten »Ich bin«. Endliche und Unendliches Ich im Denken S.T. Coleridges. Hamburg, Meiner 1982
Waldenfels B: Wesenserkenntnis und Erfahrung. In: Kuhn H, Avé-Lallement E, Gladiator R (eds): Die Münchener Phänomenologie, pp. 63-80. Den Haag, Nijhoff, 1975
Wittgenstein L: The Blue and Brown Book. Oxford, Basil Blackwell, 1958

M. Spitzer, F.A. Uehlein
M.A. Schwartz, C. Mundt
(eds.): Phenomenology
Language & Schizophrenia.
Springer-Verlag, New York, 1992

Eidetic and Empirical Research: A Hermeneutic Complementarity

John Z. Sadler

1. Introduction

One benefit of this book is to demonstrate the utility of philosophical inquiry in issues pertinent to clinical and research aspects of schizophrenia. Recently there has been renewed interest in the general role of philosophy in psychiatry, (Spitzer 1990, and this volume) as well as the role of phenomenological philosophy in medicine (Berrios 1989). In this paper I hope to illuminate the role of phenomenology in scientific research (particularly the human sciences), using examples from psychiatric research in psychotic illness. I will primarily describe the potential utility of phenomenological inquiry in empirical research, and secondarily, the converse: the utility of empirical research in phenomenological research. By describing the complementarity of phenomenological and empirical research, I also hope to suggest (but not really explore carefully) a complementarity between the continental and analytic philosophical traditions. In order to accomplish these goals, I will first describe some salient features of the general scientific process as I have conceived it in prior work.

In basic and clinical science I think there are at least three sources of hypothesis–generation and discovery: (1) analysis of background assumptions, (2) shifting of research exemplars from one disciplinary context to another, and (3) the formation of hypotheses of essential features and their interconnection (eidetic claims), and (4) the application of those hypotheses to exemplary cases and the test of empirical research. Let me describe these four notions and their associated processes before going on to discuss the "hermeneutic complementarity" of eidetic (phenomenological) and empirical research.

2. The Process of Science and the Hermeneutic Spiral

The notion of scientific discovery through empirical testing of hypotheses needs no review here. Discussion and examples of this process are ample in the literature. Let me spend more time reviewing the notions of background assumptions and shifting of exemplar context.

Longino, in her fine work *Science as Social Knowledge* (1990) describes the important role of background assumptions in shaping scientific knowledge. Background assumptions are taken–for–granted, common-sensical as well as technical beliefs that partly shape scientific questions, hypotheses, observations, and conclusions. For Longino, science develops not only through the usual channels of Kuhn's "normal science" (i.e. programmatic empirical research in a focused area) but develops also through the examination of background assumptions. Indeed, one could speculate that part of the obscurity of the scientific discovery process is precisely the taken–for–grantedness of background assumptions. Historically, philosophers have looked primarily to the overt hypothesizing and empirical work to uncover the genesis of discovery. In contrast, Longino demonstrates that discovery can occur in the *researcher's mind* as well as in the empirical, objective world. For Longino, a role of philosophy in science is the disclosure and critique of background assumptions. Indeed, background assumptions shape the form and content of scientific hypotheses. This suggests that exegesis of background assumptions may be (1) a fruitful area for understanding hypothesis–generation and the discovery process, and (2) a fruitful means for advancing scientific progress.

In prior work done collaboratively with Yosaf Hulgus (1989) and Frederick Grinnell (in press), we discussed the notion of a "hermeneutic spiral" (see Figures 1 and 2). The hermeneutic spiral is a variation on the familiar hermeneutic circle or round. The spiral emphasizes the developmental, evolutionary character of knowledge, and still preserves the whole/part distinction embraced by the original hermeneutic circle.[1] Figure 1 illustrates the process of scientific understanding in the clinical sphere (i.e. a doctor–patient encounter) where hypotheses are confirmed, disconfirmed, and modified after comparison with clinical evidence. The parallel axes labeled "hypothesizing" and "evidence–gathering" reflect the dialectical, whole/part reciprocity of scientific understanding. The spiral as a whole reflects the interpretive acts of the clinician, which we call "scientific understanding." Figure 2 is a variant where the hermeneutical structure of a basic science research program is illustrated. Scientific observations interact reflexively with enabling (background) assumptions to create new scientific facts and their corresponding "thought styles," roughly comparable to Kuhn's notion of "paradigm" (1970). That is, a thought style is a shared viewpoint revealed by a particular scientific community's background assumptions, preferences about research methods, theoretical committments, and foci of inquiry. The thought style evolves as research program(s) proceed, as do the components of the thought style. The enabling or background assumptions change as new

---

1 The hermeneutical circle depicts the process of understanding. Understanding is essentially a process, in which the foreign character, the difference of the matter in question and one's own preconceptions (assumptions, convictions and temporary knowledge) are worked through to an eventual fusion within the horizon of the one historicity common to both: "Verstehen ist seinem Wesen nach ein wirkungsgeschichtlicher Vorgang" (Gadamer: 1960, ch. II,1,c p. 275). Gadamer therefore has already explained the hermeneutic circle in the shape of evolving concentric circles.

knowledge supplants old views. As Hanson (1958) has described, the field of experience evolves as well, because changes in theory may reveal new sides of the experiential data or lead to entirely new phenomena.

Figure 1: Evolution of scientific understanding

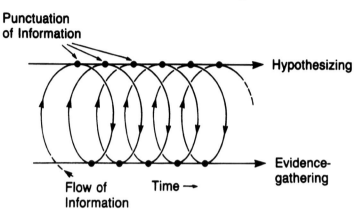

Figure 2: Discovery

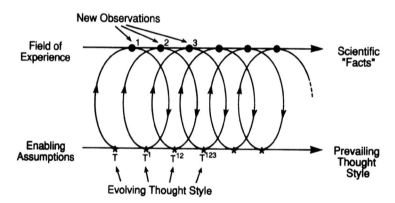

The hermeneutic spiral suggests that discoveries occur in the context of an evolving hermeneutical project, and that from the perspective of the scientist/clinician, "revolutions" do not occur, because all discoveries are realized within a hermeneutical connection. Even if one's eyes are suddenly opened up, this "revelation" actually takes place within a hermeneutical process. A conclusion of this work is that all scientific work, whether laboratory or clinical, is interpretive or hermeneutical, a conclusion borne out by others (Brown 1977, Heelan 1983, Bernstein 1983).

Another way discovery occurs within the hermeneutic spiral is by applying old or exemplar concepts to new phenomena. A new research problem is seen as resembling one in another field or "thought style." The exemplar is applied to the new thought style context, bringing a unique and new set of background assumptions, which affords the opportunity for a new, empirical "field of observation."

Psychiatric research poses unique research problems. Most psychiatric clinical phenomena pose great descriptive ambiguities compared to phenomena in the natural sciences. Even the most basic psychiatric phenomena pose descriptive and definitional ambiguities. Consider the phenomenon of hallucinations. Defining them is a riddle (see Spitzer 1990). In contrast, defining "velocity" in physics poses little difficulty. Moreover, in physics there will be strong consensus with a minimum of contextual information—i.e. for terrestrial bodies moving at low speed, use Newtonian mechanics; for celestial bodies moving at high speed, use relativity theory.

If one is to conduct psychiatric research on an ambiguous phenomenon such as hallucinations, two paths may be taken. One path is to choose a worthwhile empirical question, such as "How common are hallucinations in the active phase of schizophrenia?" and design a valid empirical approach to answering that question. This is the conventional empirical scientific approach that occupies scientists worldwide. Another path is to investigate research concepts *per se* as well as their accompanying background assumptions. The latter path can be done in a number of ways, but I will begin to explore only one in this chapter.

Let us consider the meaning of the concept "hallucinations" as it might be used in an empirical research setting. It is practically important to have a definition of hallucinations that is specific to all cases of hallucinations, yet general enough to allow for the variations in the properties of individual cases that are inevitably encountered in complex psychiatric research. Indeed, one could broadly generalize and say that understanding the relationship between general knowledge and specific knowledge of the world is the task of science. In our case, if the definition of hallucinations is too general (nonspecific), say as in "Hallucinations are unusual conscious experiences" the empirical scientist will likely "catch" all cases of hallucinations, but will have an overwhelming burden of cases to study, as well as a burden of patients with unusual experiences that most would not consider hallucinations. On the other hand, if the definition is too restrictive, individuals with (what many psychiatrists would call) "hallucinations" would be excluded from study. Clinically important varieties of hallucinations may be defined out of the research program, even perhaps defined out of clinical recognition. Therefore the research would be of limited pragmatic interest, and perhaps be misleading to the clinician. (The ongoing dispute between research and clinical psychiatrists over the utility of psychiatric research in clinical practice is a testimonial to this problem.)

How one chooses to define a research concept of hallucination will reflect the background assumptions of the defining investigator. For example, the definition "Hallucinations are unusual conscious experiences" assumes that frequency, sensory modality, personal situation, (and multiple other factors) are not critical to the concept. The most useful research or clinical definition of hallucinations will provide some way of accounting for, acknowledging, or minimizing these background assumptions. It is phenomenological work that can shed light on these issues in a psychiatric research program. Indeed, we will see that the phenomenological notion of "eidos" will provide a means for striking a pragmatic balance between generality and specificity in describing and delineating psychiatric research concepts.

3. Phenomenology and Empiricism: A Hermeneutic Complementarity

Edmund Husserl's phenomenology is an attempt to found a descriptive science of whatever becomes manifest in experience (taken in the most inclusive sense of the word). At the same time it is conceived as a descriptive, constitutive science—a science of how experience is "made up." An important method of his "rigorous philosophical science," is the method of free–fantasy variation (Husserl 1960, 1969, 1973, Zaner 1973a,b). Free–fantasy variation (FFV) reveals the "eidos" (essence) of the object intended by consciousness. For Husserl, mental life is characterized by its intentional quality—consciousness is always "of" something, hence, consciousness will have "objects," the things consciousness is conscious *of*. I will consider the method of FFV after discussing the notion of eidos as it pertains to the problem of definitional generality vs. specificity.

I have already suggested that the researcher needs conceptual precision, as well as a means for revealing background assumptions— assumptions that can constrain discovery. One aspect of scientific "progress" could be considered the differentiating of simple phenomena into more complex, interactive components. For example, the everyday concept of hallucination, when researched, is differentiated into a complex array of components that relate to each other in various ways. For instance, hallucinations could be described in neurophysiological terms. This (under certain circumstances mechanistic, reductive) approach to differentiating phenomena differs from the constitutive, eidetic approach of differentiation in phenomenology. In phenomenology, the role of research is to uncover qualities or properties of the object (of research) that are present in *all* examples of the object, and are intuited in the direct perception of the object or matter in question. This set of invariant properties is called the *eidos* of the object. Phenomenology asks how hallucinations manifest themselves to the patient and the psychiatrist directly and indirectly, concentrates on these manifestations and their internal relationship, and does not pass on immediately to possible neurophysiological processes and brain events, which might provide a more or less adequate "causal explanation". In case a connection between hallucinations and brain events can be observed, a phenomenologically oriented physiology will in turn concentrate an the manifestations of these correlative brain events as phenomena (a) of the founding organism of experiential life and at the same time (b) of the natural world. Regarding hallucinations, the eidos would be those properties that all examples of hallucinations would possess, including possible single cases that have never, and may never, exist in fact. The eidos refers to a constitutive structure that holds good for all examples of hallucinations—factual examples or imagined ones. Note the eidos is a particular kind of universal claim about the object. Eidos refers to those properties that are present in all *actual* examples, as well as all *possible* (imaginary) examples. In contrast, empirical "universality" of properties is confined to only *actual* examples. Thus, the eidos encompasses and transcends the domain of empirical general properties; it aims at the unity of the essential features.

The eidos is a peculiar conceptual entity. It is a very general concept— the eidos of hallucinations would account for *all* hallucinations. All properties or characteristics of hallucinations that are not eidetic would then be *contingent* properties—properties that are present with this particular kind (or token) of hallucination, but not necessarily in all kinds of hallucination. Yet while the eidos is very general, it is very specific in that it specifies a set of universal properties for hallucinations that set them apart from any other human experience.

It is the eidos that settles the conflicting conceptual demands of the empirical researcher. It provides a definition for the research object (hallucinations) that will (in theory) catch all cases, but will provide specificity that will exclude dubiously "hallucinating" cases.

The eidetic revelation of the invariant qualities of the objects of consciousness would bring new conceptual precision to philosophy and to the sciences as well. To describe the method very briefly, eidetic discovery using FFV would involve the following:

(1) Consideration of a particular object X of consciousness. (In this case, hallucinations)

(2) Freely varying the properties of X, and comparing to the target concept. (Imagine the conceivable varieties of hallucinations. We can only name a few here. One could have the actual sensation of the taste of green peas, one's first sexual experience, Ronald Reagan speaking, salivation, etc.—all with the absence of green peas, sexual activity, Ronald Reagan, and saliva. All of these, and innumerable other examples, are actual and possible examples of hallucinations. Examples in FFV that in fact occur are called *empirical* variations, and in this case would be hallucinations of tasting green peas, re–experiencing a first sexual experience, and hearing Ronald Reagan's voice. They may all be imagined, too. The last, hallucinating the sense of salivation, to my knowledge has not in fact occurred. This would be an example of a purely *imagined* variation.)

(3) Those properties that are preserved in (ideally) all possible variations constitute the *eidos* of object X. Indeed, conceiving the object *without* a postulated eidetic property should be impos-

sible—impossible because without the eidetic property, the object loses its identity. (In this brief and incomplete example, we might say that the eidos of hallucinations might include the following properties: (i) perceptual–like experience, (as no examples include other kinds of experience); (ii) absence of respective perception-like experiences in others; (iii) no limit to sense modality.)

(4) The process of FFV is subject to continual revision (Zaner 1973a). For example, if we were to empirically encounter a group of individuals who together experienced the voice of Ronald Reagan, (with Reagan absent), we might reconsider the eidetic validity of our claim in (3) above. Indeed, if we only imagined such a case of group hallucination, we still might want to revise our eidetic claim, as a group hallucination is possible, and would not necessarily contradict the concept of hallucination.

Having described the process of obtaining eidetic knowledge, I can now show how Husserl's FFV–based eidetic science is complementary to empirical science. Let us discuss how the problem of hallucinations could be played out in a complementary phenomenological/empirical research approach. This example is not intended to solve the problem of defining hallucinations, but rather to illustrate the ways in which the solution to the problem of hallucinations can be "discovered."

One of the editors of this volume has criticized the psychopathological concept of "hallucinations" (Spitzer 1990, and in press), as it is defined in the American Psychiatric Association's official diagnostic manual, DSM–III–R (1987, p. 398):

"A sensory perception without the external stimulation of the relevant sensory organ. A hallucination has the immediate sense of reality of a true perception..."

The conceptual problems for Spitzer are: "What are hallucinations?", "How are hallucinations to be defined?", "What constitutes valid knowledge of hallucinations?" Keep in mind that in this and any other research project the starting point is not important, because the hermeneutic spiral is "already going", i.e. one can enter the spiral at any point and embed oneself in the historical, knowledge–generating process of studying hallucinations. In our case, we can begin by reflecting on hallucinations ourselves and review the historical literature as an instructive—though not conclusive—aid.

Let us start conventionally from the perspective of a typical empirical research program. Following Hempel (1965 1966), a hypothesis is a generalization about a state of affairs. Hallucinations (as defined by DSM–III–R) fits this description, and can be taken as a hypothesis to be tested or validated. As such, we will be interested in demonstrating *empirically* general properties. In empirical research, evidence would need to be collected that would either confirm or disconfirm the hypothesis. Regarding hallucinations, we go out and study a group of schizophrenic patients with hallucinations (or, for that matter, any and all groups of people with hallucinations). Following Spitzer, let us suppose that our empirical studies show that there is a subgroup of hallucinators who *know* that they are hallucinating, so–called insightful hallucinators. This would appear to be a disconfirmation of the DSM–III–R definition of hallucinations. "The *immediate* sense of reality of a *true* perception" cannot be connected with insight into its hallucinatory character.

There is, however, another way to come to this conclusion. Again we start with the DSM–III–R definition of hallucination. Instead of an empirical study, we could conduct an eidetic FFV study of hallucination. As one can without contradiction conceive of possible examples of insightful hallucinations and as well of cases without such insight, the property of insight is *inessential*, and not an eidetic property. The advantage of eidetic research is that it is not bound to actual (empirical) examples. The eidetic researcher can provide a conceptual "head start" by providing definitions of concepts such as hallucinations that have universal properties that hold for *both* actual and imaginary examples. These properties can then be utilized by the empirical researcher as new hypothetical material to be tested, or utilized as fundamental concepts in beginning investigations of related phenomena (for example, using an eidetic definition of hallucinations in schizophrenia diagnosis).

Going back to, and assuming the validity of the empirical finding of insightful hallucinations, at least two conclusions can be drawn: (1) the DSM–III–R definition of hallucinations is wrong, or; (2) patients with insight into these perceptual experiences are not hallucinating. From the perspective of the eidetic researcher, conclusion (1) illustrates what I will call an *eidetic defect*. In *phenomenological* research, any scientific concept can be treated as an eidetic claim (within a particular technical context). An eidetic defect is a mistaken eidetic property—a property that was thought to have an eidetic universality, but later (eidetic or empirical) research shows to be a nonuniversal property. As I said, in the process of FFV, new actual or imagined variations may present themselves. Some of these variations may prompt revision if they demonstrate that what was thought to be an eidetic universal is, in fact, nonuniversal. The empiricist would simply call a defective eidos a less general concept or a mistaken or poor definition of a concept. Thus, an eidetic defect represents a failure, error, or omission in eidetic research, as well as a mistaken general definition of an empirical research program. If the eidetic defect is a newly described property of hallucinations, it is a scientific discovery. If we assume that "some hallucinators may be/are insightful" is a new finding, then this finding would be a discovery. This kind of discovery is one that occurs in the context of the attempted validation of a hypothesis in an empirical setting, or occurs in eidetic research through FFV. Conclusion (2) [that "insightful hallucinations aren't really hallucinations] suggests that a new inquiry is needed: If these perceptual experiences are not hallucinations, then what are they? This would also be a fruitful new research question that could be explored along either (empirical or eidetic) path described in this chapter.

Therefore, in research programs regarding the definitions of concepts, there are at least two paths to take: (1) do further empirical research (the empirical path) and; (2) refine or research the eidetic claim of the problematic concept (the phenomenological path). Path (1) fits into the Kuhnian (1970) notion of normal science, while Path (2) involves phenomenological research. With Path (1), defining general properties will be limited to *actual* (empirical) examples. The advantage of considering all *possible*, and therefore universal, properties is absent. Consequently, the empirical path aiming at universal properties is hampered by its piecemeal empirical testing of postulated universal properties. With Path (2), the discovery of universal properties is limited by the investigator's experience with actual and possible examples, and by the investigator's imaginative capabilities. However, Path (2) offers the empirical investigator a quicker means for building hypotheses by circumventing the piecemeal empirical testing of concepts. Therefore, each path offers the other unique advantages. The eidetic path offers a fruitful means to early conceptual precision, more efficient hypothesis generation, and more focused empirical exploration in the lab or clinic. The empirical path offers unforeseen phenomena and new actual examples for consideration by the phenomenologist's process of FFV.

I have described the relationship between eidetic and empirical research with respect to the discovery and validation of hypotheses/concepts. What role does phenomenological research have in revealing background assumptions? Eidetic analysis can be a tool for uncovering background assumptions as well. Returning to the debate over the DSM–III–R definition of hallucinations, C may be Spitzer's empirical observation that some hallucinators *do not* have hallucinations with "the immediate sense of reality of a true perception," i.e., some hallucinators know they are hallucinating. This fact makes the DSM–III–R definition of hallucinations a false claim. Let us investigate the form of reasoning through which background assumptions can be inferred:

(1) A surprising falsity F is discovered.

(2) But if A was assumed to be true, F would follow as a matter of course.

(3) Hence, there is reason to suspect that A is a background assumption of the eidetic claim F.

In this example, we could call F the DSM-III-R definition of hallucination. Eidetic, imaginative variation or empirical findings (of insightful hallucinations, i.e., C) have already revealed this definition to be false—the DSM's eidetic claim is defective. One could assign a number of possible contents to A. One example could be, A = "Perceptual systems in the human are necessarily linked to the capacity for self-reflective consciousness." Therefore a hallucinatory perception, too,—if reflected at all— would be linked necessarily to the consciousness "I perceive X; here and now X is present 'in person'" and cannot at the same time be associated with the insight "I perceive X; it is here and now as if it were present 'in person': I hallucinate X." Therefore, insightful hallucinations should be impossible. The false eidetic claim F ("a hallucination has the *immediate* sense of reality of a *true* perception") takes its plausibility from the false background assumption A. Other background assumptions than A are, of course, possible, as long as F follows from them.

This process of inferring possible background assumptions is a variation of Charles S. Peirce's logic for hypothesis generation in empirical science—a logic he calls abduction (Peirce 1955). As Peirce's abductive inference is a method for generating hypotheses for empirical research, my variation is a method for generating "hypotheses" for underlying background assumptions. Eidetic empirical or imaginary variations can "test" the core concept, and if an eidetic defect is discovered, background assumptions can be inferred from the relationship between the core concept and eidetic defect. (Suspected background assumptions can be iteratively tested through the method of FFV: Would A hold as an assumption for all possible variations of F?)

Scientific concepts can benefit from the definitional or conceptual precision of eidetic work. The sharpening of concepts with eidetic research can facilitate the empirical project, both by setting practical boundaries for ambiguous concepts, and by providing clues to background assumptions for concepts. Returning to our example, several strategies are possible for investigating hallucinations further:

(1) Empirical path: Continue empirical studies of insightful hallucinators by comparing them to routine hallucinators, normals, etc. This process could result in lawlike statistical generalizations about the ways in which insightful hallucinations differ from noninsightful ones.

(2) Phenomenological path: Re–examine the eidos of hallucinations, including the new empirical variations (such as insightful hallucinators and group–shared hallucinations).

By refining the eidetic claims of scientific concepts, refined definitions of difficult concepts can be applied to empirical research.

The above illustrates how the epistemological and scientific problems of "What are hallucinations?" could be addressed. It also illustrates the complementarity between eidetic inquiry and empirical inquiry. Eidetic studies provide a pragmatic way to define concepts for empirical testing. The inevitable exceptions or anomalous findings in an empirical research program can prompt a re–examining of the eidetic claim of fundamental research concepts. Eidetic research can also give rise to new, empirically–testable scientific concepts. The method of free–fantasy variation has its own practical limits, so empirical research can be a rich source of phenomena for phenomenological research. These reciprocal, complementary functions of eidetic research and empirical research I call a *hermeneutic complementarity* (see Figure 3). Hermeneutic complementarities are interpretive schemes that structurally and procedurally differ from each other, but when used jointly, facilitate the evolution of knowledge. Figure 3 illustrates this hermeneutic complementarity by connecting two circles by a single tangent. This tangent represents the point where the researcher can opt for phenomenological *or* empirical research of the concept. One interpretive path uses the method of FFV toward a new eidos—phenomenological research. The other uses the hypothetico–deductive method toward new facts—empirical research. As with Figures 1 and 2, this process could be visualized in three dimensions as parallel spirals intersecting through a single axis. This would then represent the evolutionary "dialogue" between the two viewpoints.[2]

Figure 3: Hermeneutic complementarity of eidetic and empirical research

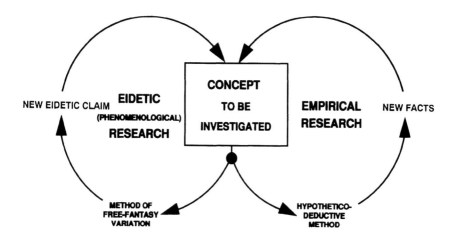

As the case example illustrates, discovery can occur with both modes of inquiry. Eidetic analysis in concert with abductive inference models a genetic process of hypothesis formation that eluded Hempel (1965, 1966) and other philosophers of science looking for a "logic of discovery." To summarize these methods briefly: What are hallucinations? Perform an eidetic variation of the phenomena of hallucination as directly experienced and reported by patients, contrast this with the received concepts, and put the latter (and their background assumptions) to the test of free variation (hyopothesis generation and logic of discovery). Then empirically test the resulting eidetic claim with a population of hallucinators (logic of verification). Defective definitions of concepts can be abductively examined and refined into new eidetic claims. New facts, eidetic claims, and contingent properties can iteratively be fed back, the whole process *aiming at* the full eidos of the matter in question.

---

2 The author appreciates the contributions of Osborne P. Wiggins, Yosaf Hulgus, Frederick Grinnell, Friedrich A. Uehlein and Manfred Spitzer to this paper.

114   J.Z. Sadler

Summary

The method of eidetic variation is applied and its relation to "normal science" is demonstrated. Using the example of hallucinations, it is shown how conceptual clarification and empirical research strategies are in no way contradictory. Instead, they both are aspects of scientific reasoning and practice.

References

Bernstein RJ: Beyond objectivism and relativism: Science, hermeneutics, and praxis. Philadelphia, The University of Pennsylvania Press, 1983

Berrios GE: What is phenomenology? A review. Journal of the Royal Society of Medicine 82: 425–428, 1989

Brown HI: Perception, theory, and committment: The new philosophy of science. Chicago, The University of Chicago Press, 1977

Gadamer H-G: Wahrheit und Methode. Tübingen, Mohr, 1960

Hanson NR: Patterns of discovery. Cambridge, MA, Cambridge University Press 1958

Heelan PA: Space–perception and the philosophy of science. Berkeley CA, The University of California Press, 1983

Hempel CG: Philosophy of natural science. Englewood Cliffs NJ, Prentice–Hall, 1966

Hempel CG: Aspects of scientific explanation. New York, The Free Press, 1965

Husserl E: Cartesian meditations (transl. by D Cairns). The Hague, Martinus Nijhoff, 1960

Husserl E: Formal and transcendental logic (transl. by D Cairns). The Hague, Martinus Nijhoff, 1969

Husserl E: Experience and judgement: Investigations in a genealogy of logic (transl. by JS Churchill & K Ameriks). Evanston IL, Northwestern University Press, 1973

Kuhn TS: The structure of scientific revolutions (2nd ed.). Chicago IL, The University of Chicago Press, 1970

Longino HE: Science as social knowledge. Princeton NJ, Princeton University Press, 1990

Peirce CS: Abduction and induction. In: Buchler JB (ed): Philosophical writings of Peirce. New York, Dover, 1955

Sadler JZ, Hulgus YF: Hypothesizing and evidence–gathering: The nexus of understanding. Family Process, 26(3): 255–267, 1989

Sadler JZ, Grinnell FG: Discovery in clinical psychiatry and experimental biology. Theoretical Medicine (in press)

Spitzer M: Why philosophy? In: Spitzer M, Maher BA (eds): Philosophy and psychopathology, pp. 3-18. New York, Springer, 1990

Spitzer M: The basis of psychiatric diagnosis. In: Sadler JZ, Schwartz MA, Wiggins OP (eds): Philosophical perspectives on psychiatric diagnostic classification. Baltimore, The Johns Hopkins University Press (in press)

Zaner RM: Examples and possibles: A criticism of Husserl's theory of free–phantasy variation. Research in Phenomenology 3: 29–43, 1973a

Zaner RM: The art of free phantasy in rigorous phenomenological science. In: Kersten F, Zaner R (eds): Phenomenology: Continuation and criticism: Essays in honor of Dorion Cairns. The Hague: Martinus Nijhof, 1973b

M. Spitzer, F.A. Uehlein
M.A. Schwartz, C. Mundt
(eds.): Phenomenology
Language & Schizophrenia.
Springer-Verlag, New York, 1992

Emil Kraepelin and Philosophy: The Implicit Philosophical Assumptions of Kraepelinian Psychiatry

Paul Hoff

1. Introduction

Probably few psychiatrists would spontaneously associate Emil Kraepelin's name with philosophy. Nevertheless, I think it is necessary to look at this relationship for the following reasons: During recent years, several authors have described a crisis in psychiatry, particularly in psychiatric diagnosis. It is not purely coincidental that in such a "critical" era, many concepts and ideas are "re-discovered" which previously have been regarded as of merely historical interest. This is especially true of Emil Kraepelin's psychiatry. The influence of what is often called the "neo-Kraepelinian movement" is well-known, an influence which manifests itself, for example, in the operationalized diagnostic criteria of DSM–III–R, and which proves the profound relevance of Kraepelinian ideas for present-day psychiatry (Blashfield 1984). Given this situation, it seems appropriate to critically re-evaluate Kraepelin's nosological positions as they changed over time (which cannot be further discussed here), and—our present topic—to highlight the philosophical implications of this nosology, although—as will be shown—they often are quite well hidden.[1]

2. Biographical Note

To begin with, a short biographical remark: Emil Kraepelin (1856–1926) never had many personal contacts with philosophers. There is, of course, one important exception. The question of whether this man, Wilhelm Wundt (1832–1920), was a philosopher or a psychologist, is closely connected with our main topic, and we will return to this later on.

---

1 A comprehensive study on Kraepelin's work, its philosophical implications and its relevance for modern psychiatry, is in preparation by the present author.

Those who regard Kraepelin as a decidedly "unphilosophical" psychia-trist[2]—as often happens—might be astonished to read the following passage in his memoirs, where Kraepelin describes the winter term 1874/75 at the university of Leipzig—he was 19 years of age:

"At the same time, I started learning philosophy and joined the academic-philo-sophical society, which was successfully headed by Avenarius at that time. I also got to know the very much older colleagues, Kehrbach, Vaihinger, Eduard Meyer and Moritz Wirth, who were members of the society." (Kraepelin 1987, p. 3)

And, during the next year, 1876, while studying in Würzburg:

"In the summer of 1876, the state examinations seemed to be a long way off and I eagerly read the philosophical works of Kant, Hume, Locke, Berkeley, Hobbes, Schopenhauer, de la Mettrie and so on. An older friend of mine, Rieck, had to write his philosophical thesis on 'Studies on the concept of necessity'[3], which gave me particular incentive to work on the origin of the concept of causality." (Kraepelin, 1987, p. 4)

These formulations might suggest a developing interest in the questions involved; but in Kraepelin's psychiatric work we do not find, for example, thorough discussions of Kant's relevance for psychiatry, nor even comments on the philosophy of Richard Avenarius (1843–1896), whom he obviously met in Leipzig and who later developed the concept of empiriocriticism. This theory was part of the positivistic and neo-Kantian movement of the second half of the 19th century with its strict opposition to metaphysics, its orientation towards empirical data and—a highly typical example of "Zeitgeist"—its profound confidence in the ideas of development and progress. All these aspects can be found in Kraepelin's writings also, but in a more or less implicit manner rather than in an explitely philosophical context.

3. The Influence of Wilhelm Wundt

Without going into detail about the personal and scientific relationship between Emil Kraepelin and Wilhelm Wundt, one point can definitely be made: It is nearly impossible to overestimate Wundt's influence on the development of Kraepelin's general conception of science and his par-ticular conception of psychiatry. A very brief summary of Wundt's philosophy is necessary to show which elements of it became relevant for Kraepelin and which did not.

Wundt's aim was to establish psychology as a kind of natural science which relied on experimental data. He criticized the highly speculative approach of the philosophy of nature, as, for example, developed by Schelling or Schleiermacher, but he also did not agree with materialism or

---

2 Of course, it is a contradictio in adiectu to talk about an "unphilosophical psychiatrist". This study provides arguments for how close this relationship necessarily is; being not interested in philosophy does not at all mean being not influenced by philosophy.
3 "Studien zum Begriff der Notwendigkeit".

with association psychology sensu Herbart (Wundt 1880). There has been a lively controversy in the literature about whether or not Wundt directly stands in the tradition of English empiricism, as represented by J. St. Mill (1806–1873) and Herbert Spencer (1820–1903) (Arnold 1980, Boring 1950, Danziger 1990, Titchener 1921, Pauleikhoff 1987, Schneider 1990). The majority of recent studies deny this relationship and emphasize Wundt's profound knowledge of and appreciation for so-called German idealism, especially in its Kantian version.

And indeed, Wundt's insistence on one of the central functions of "consciousness"—"apperception", as he calls it—is reminiscent of Kant's transcendental epistemology: For Wundt, apperception is the psychological function which intentionally connects sensory data and forms personal knowledge about them. Without apperception, which is an active mental process and not mere sensorial input nor simple additive association, there would be—according to Wundt—no knowledge and no science at all.

At least in his earlier writings, Wundt favored parallelism as his point of view in the mind-body-problem. And he postulated a certain kind of causality within mental life as well. But this mental causality must never be mixed up or, even worse, identified with physical causality.

Experimental research—and this Wundtian idea was obviously the most fascinating one for the young Kraepelin—may successfully be used in psychology as well as in natural sciences without ignoring the epistemological differences between the two fields. As a practical consequence, Wundt founded the world's first laboratory for experimental psychology in Leipzig in 1879 and Kraepelin became one of his co-workers there (see Kraepelin 1987, pp. 22 ff.).

In his later work, particularly when it came to the philosophical foundation of his monumental "Völkerpsychologie" (10 volumes, 1900–1920), Wundt broadened his views significantly: He developed a voluntaristic, not to say idealistic concept which has been criticized from the materialistic perspective as falling behind his previous views of psychology as a natural science (Arnold 1980).

In my view, Wundt's philosophy and psychology should be understood as a profound effort to combine Kant's critical impetus against metaphysical speculation and materialism with a psychology which understood itself as an empirical but non-reductionistic study of man. His roots in Kant's philosophy and his very specific, very personal development of classical philosophical concepts led to a highly complex theory which was not free of contradictions and was therefore very likely to be misinterpreted.

In turn, Kraepelin modified this complex Wundtian "Weltanschauung" by extracting what he regarded as useful for the foundation of empirical research in psychiatry. This is the reason why Wundt's psychology, viewed through the "filter" of Kraepelin's texts, seems so much more unified and straight than it really is. Kraepelin simplified and in a certain way "smoothed out" Wundt's concepts, but he did not falsify them.

4. Kraepelin's Hidden Philosophy

After these introductory remarks, I would like to formulate the main hypothesis of this paper: Kraepelin's psychiatry, though intended to be as independent from theoretical assumptions as possible, is in fact intensively connected with several philosophical theories. This, in itself is not a problem. But—and this is a problem—Kraepelin adopted philosophical theories more or less implicitly. Contrary to the steadily changing clinical aspects of his nosology, he did not call into question the philosophical implications once they had become an integral part of his theory of psychiatry as a science. In doing so, Kraepelin underestimated the implicit difficulties and contradictions within the philosophical theories themselves and "imported" these problems into psy-chiatry.

It is obvious that we have to be very cautious in simply attaching any of the common philosophical categories to Kraepelin's thinking. But, nevertheless, when looking at the basic ideas underlying his psychiatry, be they implicit or not, we have to distinguish and discuss the following four major philosophical concepts:
1. Realism
2. Parallelism
3. "Experimentalism"
4. Naturalism
   I will now discuss these points in some detail.

4.1 Realism

Once again, there is no definitive statement by Kraepelin himself on realism as a theory. Nonetheless, what he wrote about science in general and psychiatry in particular tells us that he—philosophically speaking—was a realist. However, we will hardly be able to philosophically qualify this realism in more detail: He does not discuss the ideas of empiricism or positivism apart from merely mentioning Locke and Hume in his memoirs (and not in his psychiatric writings), although especially positivism gained much influence during the last decades of the 19th century. In addition, at the beginning of our century, there was extensive philosophical discourse about the epistemological consequences of realism. Some of the protagonists, including Oswald Külpe (1862–1915), Hans Driesch (1867–1941) and Erich Becher (1882–1929), were decidedly interested in psychology and psychiatry; two of them, Külpe and Becher, were Kraepelin's colleagues at the University of Munich. Although Kraepelin—according to the historical information available at present—did not participate in this debate, there can be no doubt that he did believe in an independently existing "real world", including other people and their healthy or disturbed mental processes. Only on rare occasions, Kraepelin declared that we have access to all objects only via consciousness. However, this must not be misunderstood as an idealistic, nor even as a transcendental point of view.

Instead, this is a typical Wundtian position, stressing the importance of mental processes in generating knowledge. These processes themselves, however, are not believed to be apriorical, as Kant had suggested, but aposteriorical and subject to empirical, and particularly to psycho-physiological research:

"All things primarily exist for us as inner experience. We call the form of these inner experiences 'consciousness'; our mental life represents a string of subsequent conscious processes" (Kraepelin 1921, p. 1, translated by P.H.).

In different places in his work Kraepelin points out that the psychiatric researcher has to objectively describe what really exists and what nature presents to him—the formulations differ, but the essence is a strictly realistic philosophy:

"The raw material of experience, which is provided by sensory perception and clarified by attentiveness[4], forms the basis of all further mental acts and therefore of man's whole set of ideas. ... The less perfectly and more falsely our information about the external world is perceived, the more incomplete and unreliable will be the idea, developed in man's consciousness, of the external world surrounding him, of his own mind, and of his mind's relation to the external world" (Kraepelin 1899, pp. 126-127, translated by P.H.).

The consequences for psychiatric nosology are evident: Such realism will lead to the concept of natural disease entities which exist completely independently from the researcher. The scientist describes what he finds—or, in a stronger formulation, he describes "given things". His own activity in constructing scientific hypotheses or diagnostic systems will tend to be underestimated.

Kraepelin often speaks of the "essence" of a disease process ("das Wesen des Krankheitsvorganges"). This might lead to the assumption that his understanding of "essence" is similar to Husserl's or, as an important representative of anthropological psychiatry, Binswanger's. But this is not at all the case. Without going into detail on this specific topic, the present article illustrates that there can be no doubt about the fundamental discrepancies between Kraepelin's and Husserl's philosophical approach. Given this theoretical incompatibility, it is all the more remarkable that anthropologically oriented authors often refer to and accept the clinical relevance of Kraepelin's dichotomy of endogenous psychoses (e.g. Binswanger 1957, 1960).

4.2 Parallelism

Kraepelin held a position of psychophysical parallelism. Like Wilhelm Griesinger (1817–1868), whom he admired for his highly critical views against speculative psychiatric theories, he disapproved of reductionistic

---

4 Although Kraepelin uses the German word "Aufmerksamkeit", the term "apperception" probably represents the more appropriate translation, especially taking the specific Wundtian background of Kraepelin's psychology into consideration (see Hoff 1988, 1990).

materialism which declares mental events identical with neurophysiological processes.[5] Kraepelin characterizes two kinds of phenomena, somatic and psychological, which are decidedly different, but closely connected:

"We strictly adhere to the principle that a regular parallelism between somatic and mental processes exists. Without this principle, scientific psychiatry would definitely be impossible. However, it is important to always keep in mind that this connection is not exhaustively understood by the assumption of a simple causal relationship." (Kraepelin 1887, pp. 17–18, translated by P.H.)

Kraepelin repeatedly defended the existence of mental phenomena against various kinds of "brain mythologies" (his term). Some of his remarks on this issue do not lack polemic undertones, as for example, his ironic criticism of "the position of naive materialism":

"..., which believes that psychiatry's and psychology's work is completely done by studying the physical basis of our mental life. This position by no means merely belongs to outdated epochs of our historical development; it often still underlies— more or less consciously—the ideas of contemporary psychiatric authors. This is proven by expressions like 'moral fibre systems', 'logic of brain process', 'cortical conclusions', 'foci of emotions of innervation', 'stocks of memories'[6] and the like" (Kraepelin 1887, p. 12, transl. by P.H.).

Contrary to Wundt (1894) himself, Kraepelin, although calling himself a parallelist, did not enter the philosophical controversy about this concept. In particular, he did not critically differentiate between parallelism and interactionism. Therefore, he did not realize that any strictly defined parallelism makes it more than doubtful that mental life can still be regarded as an independent sphere and not merely relegated to a one to one relationship with the somatic level; this, of course, means determinism.

As a consequence of his somewhat ambigious position regarding the mind-body-relationship, there is an implicit tendency towards monism in Kraepelin's writings, particularly when we consider his ideas about psychology as a natural science. However, to avoid severe misunderstandings, it should be emphasized that this "monistic tendency" is definitely not a metaphysical one and especially not comparable with Eernst Haeckel's understanding of monism—this topic will be taken up again in the context of Kraepelin's naturalism. Keeping in mind Kraepelin's pragmatic attitude towards philosophy, one might speak of a weak version of methodological monism, insofar as he decidedly favored quantitative methods brought forward by the natural sciences. But, again, Kraepelin

---

5 Although Kraepelin often mentions Griesinger as one of the important forerunners of scientific psychiatry, some of his formulations suggest that he occasionally misunderstood Griesinger's point of view as a materialistic one—a position which is definitely not supported by Griesinger's textbook. For example, in his inaugural lecture as director of the psychiatric hospital in Dorpat (a town in Estonia which is now called Tartu) in 1887, Kraepelin refers to Griesinger's "well-known sentence: mental disorders are disorders of the brain" and calls it an "incorrect formulation" (Kraepelin 1887, pp. 17-18).

6 " ... moralische Fasersysteme, Logik des Hirnprocesses, corticale Schlussbildungen, Herde von Innervationsgefühlen, Vorrathsstellen von Erinnerungsbildern ... "

does not explicitly apply the term "methodological monism" nor does he refer to philosophers who had thoroughly evaluated that concept, e.g. Friedrich Albert Lange (1828-1875; cf. Verwey 1985). It may be assumed that it was Wundt's basic concepts which prevented Kraepelin from moving even closer to the materialistic and monistic point of view. In conclusion, Kraepelin's theory of the mind-body-relationship, although regarded by himself as parallelistic, is not free from certain ambiguities and therefore may create more questions than it answers.

4.3 "Experimentalism"

Kraepelin's views here are quite clear: The psychological experiment should become a major scientific tool not only for the understanding of disturbed mental processes, but also of healthy mental life—one has only to remember Kraepelin's lifelong efforts to improve his "work curve". Both Wundt and Kraepelin realized the difference between a physical and a psychological experiment, but the experimental design in both spheres did not differ significantly. The following quotations demonstrate Kraepelin's emphasis on the experimental approach and—more generally—his scientific optimism, which is so typical of the way in which many scientists in the second half of the 19th century saw themselves:

"One would be astonished, however, if suddenly knowledge which was gained by the systematic application of psychological experiments was dismissed from our science" (Kraepelin 1920, p. 359, translated by P.H.).

In cases of psychoses occuring during imprisonment, one can—as Kraepelin argues—

"follow the development of persecutory ideas under the pressure of adverse life events with the clarity of an experiment" [7](Kraepelin 1915, p. 1760, translated by P.H.).

And, in an even stronger version:

"The methods developed by experimental psychology provide us with the means to define a more precise concept of the alterations of mental life that nature produces by its harmful influences".[8](Kraepelin 1918, p. 187, translated by P.H.).

Kraepelin seems to have considered "experimentalism" to be a kind of guarantee for the scientific status of psychiatric research. Therefore, it is obvious that he rated the experimental approach higher than the mere description of clinical phenomena, although the latter method was regarded as indispensable, especially if combined with follow-up examinations. Introspection, however, was discussed critically and suspiciously by Kraepelin, as were the theoretical and practical aspects of psychoanalysis— an important topic which cannot be further developped here.

---

7   "... mit der Klarheit des Versuchs ..."
8   "... wie sie die Natur durch ihre krankmachenden Eingriffe erzeugt ..."

In summary, Kraepelin maintained a skeptical attitude towards the subjective and especially the biographically determined aspects of mental disorders which could not be studied experimentally.

4.4 Naturalism

In his early writings—especially on forensic psychiatry—Kraepelin clearly expresses the opinion that there are no such things as apriorical ideas, freedom of the will or unchangeable moral values. Everything depends upon the time and the specific sociocultural situation in which it occurs. For Kraepelin, human beings are merely a part of nature, and anything humans do is a product of this natural existence—Kraepelin as an exponent of the evolutionary approach:

> "In this context morality completely loses its absolute value and becomes a product of cultural and historical development; it is no longer something existing outside of mankind, but instead is linked to the concept of human society; it is conceptualized as developing within and founded upon manifold human relations" (Kraepelin 1880, p. 3, translated by P.H.).

As for the field of religion, Kraepelin even speaks of:

> "the idea of God, which has developed with psychological necessity" [9] (Kraepelin 1880, p. 5, translated by P.H.).

Later in his life, Kraepelin became somewhat more cautious concerning this matter, but there is no reason to believe that he substantially changed his mind. His naturalistic, "anti-metaphysical" point of view was sympathetic with Darwinistic and biologistic concepts, although—this should be stressed once more—Kraepelin always rejected simplified monistic theories as for example represented by Ernst Haeckel (1834-1919), Jakob Moleschott (1822-1893), and Ludwig Büchner (1824-1899). His naturalism, of course, is one of the topics where Kraepelin definitely departed from Wundtian psychology and philosophy, although he never discussed this fact.

5. Consequences & Conclusions

As for the consequences of Kraepelin's attitude towards philosophy for his successors, this is not the place to discuss them in detail, although two examples may give an impression:

Around 1920 there was a psychiatric controversy between the two psychiatrists Ernst Kretschmer and Heinrich Körtke. Körtke tried to improve Kraepelin's nosology by pushing it towards a strange kind of methodological dualism: He suggested the use of two different diagnostic systems, one for the somatic and one for the psychopathological level. In

9 "... mit psychologischer Notwendigkeit ..."

this way he arrived at a rather artificial and unpractical terminology, for example by separating what he calls "Morbus dementiae praecocis"—i.e. the organic side—from the psychological field of "Dementia praecox"; and in a definitely "non-Kraepelinian" manner he included very different kinds of mental disorders in his psychopathological concept of "Dementia praecox" (Körtke 1919).

Kretschmer, in his comment on Körtke's paper, severely criticized this approach. He postulated that his own biological and constitutional concept is much more in accordance with Kraepelin's intentions than Körtke's artificial terminological dualism, since it emphasizes the close relation and not the separation between organic and psychological phenomena (Kretschmer 1919).

More recent examples are DSM-III-R (APA 1987) and ICD-10 (WHO 1991) or, generally speaking, operationalized diagnostic systems, which are conceptually influenced by positivism and—even stronger—by logical empiricism (Faust & Miner 1986, Klerman, Vaillant, Spitzer & Michels 1984, Kraus 1991, Saß 1990, Schwartz & Wiggins 1986, Spitzer & Degkwitz 1986, Stein 1991).

There is a striking parallel between these new diagnostic systems and Kraepelin's concept: Being based upon empirical observations, both of them develop a tendency—quite outspoken in Kraepelin's case, but at least implicit in DSM–III–R and ICD–10 also—to treat their "objects" (diseases, disorders, even syndromes) as independently existing "things". Kraepelin would have called these "natural entities", which are once and forever to be found. Of course, there is an important difference, too: For Kraepelin, nosological entities generally exist, no matter whether or not they are already fully understood scientifically; the authors of operationalized diagnostic systems, however, are well aware of the fact that they write about mainly psychopathologically, seldom organically defined conventions, which are subject to change according to new empirical evidence. But—and here lies the parallel to Kraepelin—, if used uncritically, i.e. without keeping these epistemological limitations in mind, operationalized diagnostic systems may be misunderstood as dealing with quasi-ontologically determined entities. From a nominalistic point of view, this phenomenon has been criticized as the "reification" of psychiatric diagnoses.

I think we should not forget Karl Jaspers' warning (Jaspers 1946) that Kraepelin's idea of natural disease entities was—and is—a useful heuristic concept, a "regulative idea" in a quasi-Kantian sense, but not more, in particular not a given ontological dogma.

We cannot go into the details of the ongoing debate on psychiatric diagnosis here; but the analysis of Kraepelin's underestimated and complex relationship with philosophy should remind any "neo-Kraepelinian" to seriously take philosophical aspects into account. Otherwise, the same problems, which were shown to underlie Kraepelin's concepts, are likely to be "imported" into psychiatry again.

I conclude: It may sound paradoxical, but especially the example of such an influential psychiatrist as Emil Kraepelin, although he was not interested in "classical" philosophical matters, proves the significance of philosophical ideas in psychiatry.

As for the relationship between philosophy and psychiatry, two extreme positions lead astray: On the one hand, to ignore philosophy or to reduce it to the methodological background of biological psychiatry—as Kraepelin at least implicitly did—will overlook the powerful philosophical influences which are necessarily at work. But, on the other hand, to underestimate clinical-empirical work by supporting speculative philosophical theories—be they romantic or materialistic—will reduce psychiatry to a mere illustration of a metaphysical doctrine.

Given the philosophical implications of any psychiatric action, especially diagnosis and therapy, we need close contact between philosophy and clinical psychiatry, surely not to replace one by the other, but to learn from one another.

Summary

The example of the influential psychiatrist Emil Kraepelin, although he was definitely not interested in subtle philosophical problems, impressively demonstrates how closely and necessarily philosophy and psychiatry are linked. Furthermore, it is argued that there will be mutual disadvantages if these two fields ignore each other; from a psychiatric point of view, the main consequence of any "unphilosophical" approach will be to—unintentionally, but all the more effectively—import severe philosophical problems into psychiatric theory and practice.

References

American Psychiatric Association: Diagnostic and statistical manual of mental disorders (3rd ed., revised). Washington, DC, APA, 1987

Arnold A: Wilhelm Wundt—Sein philosophisches System. Berlin, Akademie, 1980

Blashfield RK: The Classification of Psychopathology—Neo-Kraepelinian and Quantitative Approaches. New York and London, Plenum Press, 1984

Binswanger L: Schizophrenie. Pfullingen, Neske, 1957

Binswanger L: Manie und Melancholie. Pfullingen, Neske, 1960

Boring E: A history of experimental psychology (2nd ed.). New York, Appleton-Century-Crofts, 1950

Danziger K: Constructing the subject: Historical origins of psychological research. Cambridge, Cambridge University Press, 1990

Faust D, Miner RA: The empiricist and his new clothes: DSM-III in perspective. American Journal of Psychiatry, 143: 962-967, 1986

Griesinger W: Die Pathologie und Therapie der psychischen Krankheiten. Stuttgart, A. Krabbe, 1845

Hoff P: Nosologische Grundpostulate bei Kraepelin—Versuch einer kritischen Würdigung des Kraepelinschen Spätwerkes. Zeitschrift für klinische Psychologie, Psychopathologie, Psychotherapie, 36: 328-336, 1988

Hoff P: Der Begriff der psychischen Krankheit in transzendentalphilosophischer Sicht. Frankfurt/Main, Campus, 1990

Hundert EM: Philosophy, Psychiatry, and Neuroscience—Three Approaches to the Mind. Oxford, Clarendon Press, 1989

Hundert EM: The Brain's Capacity to Form Delusions as an Evolutionary Strategy for Survival. This volume, 1992

Jaspers K: Allgemeine Psychopathologie (4th ed.). Berlin, Springer, 1946

Klerman GL, Vaillant GE, Spitzer RL, Michels R: A Debate on DSM-III. American Journal of Psychiatry 141: 539-553, 1984

Körtke H: Ein Dilemma in der Dementia-praecox-Frage. Gedanken über die Fortentwicklung der psychiatrischen Systematik. Zeitschrift für die gesamte Neurologie und Psychiatrie 48: 354-369, 1919

Kraepelin E: Die Abschaffung des Strafmasses. Ein Vorschlag zur Reform der heutigen Strafrechtspflege. Stuttgart, Enke, 1880

Kraepelin E: Die Richtungen der psychiatrischen Forschung. Leipzig: FCW Vogel, 1887

Kraepelin E: Psychiatrie (6th ed.). Volume 1. Leipzig, Barth, 1899

Kraepelin E: Psychiatrie (8th ed.). Volume 4. Leipzig: Barth, 1915

Kraepelin E: Ziele und Wege der psychiatrischen Forschung. Zeitschrift für die gesamte Neurologie und Psychiatrie 42: 169-205, 1918

Kraepelin E: Wilhelm Wundt. Zeitschrift für die gesamte Neurologie und Psychiatrie 61: 351-362, 1920

Kraepelin E: Einführung in die psychiatrische Klinik (4th ed.). Volume 1. Leipzig, Barth, 1921

Kraepelin E: Memoirs. (eds: H Hippius, G Peters, D Ploog). Berlin, Springer, 1987

Kraus A: Methodological problems with the classification of personality disorders: The significance of existential types. J Personality Disorders 5: 82-92, 1991

Kretschmer E: Gedanken über die Fortentwicklung der psychiatrischen Systematik. Zeitschrift für die gesamte Neurologie und Psychiatrie 48: 370-377, 1919

Pauleikhoff B: Das Menschenbild im Wandel der Zeit. Ideengeschichte der Psychiatrie und der klinischen Psychologie. Volume 3. Hürtgenwald, G. Pressler, 1987

Saß H: Operationalisierte Diagnostik in der Psychiatrie. Nervenarzt 61: 255-258, 1990

Schneider CM: Wilhelm Wundts Völkerpsychologie. Bonn, Bouvier, 1990

Schwartz MA, Wiggins OP: Logical empiricism and psychiatric classification. Comprehensive Psychiatry 27: 101-114, 1986

Spitzer M, Degkwitz R: Zur Diagnose des DSM- III. Nervenarzt 57: 698-704, 1986

Stein DJ: Philosophy and the DSM-III. Comprehensive Psychiatry 32: 404-415, 1991

Titchener EB: Wilhelm Wundt. American Journal of Psychology 32: 161-177, 1921

Verwey G: Psychiatry in an anthropological and biomedical context—Philosophical presuppositions and implications of German psychiatry 1820-1870. Dordrecht, D. Reidel, 1985

World Health Organization: Tenth revision of the International Classification of Diseases, Chapter V (F): Mental and behavioural disorders. Clinical descriptions and guidelines. Geneva, WHO, 1991

Wundt W: Grundzüge der physiologischen Psychologie (2nd ed.). Leipzig, Engelmann, 1880

Wundt W: Über psychische Causalität und das Princip des psychophysischen Parallelismus. Philosophische Studien 10: 1-124, 1894

Wundt W: Völkerpsychologie. Eine Untersuchung der Entwicklungsgesetze von Sprache, Mythus und Sitte. 10 volumes. Leipzig, Engelmann, 1900-1920

M. Spitzer, F.A. Uehlein
M.A. Schwartz, C. Mundt
(eds.): Phenomenology
Language & Schizophrenia.
Springer-Verlag, New York, 1992

Schizophrenia, Delusions, and Heidegger's "Ontological Difference"
On "Poor Reality–Testing" and "Empty Speech"

Louis A. Sass

1. Introduction

By definition, all psychoses involve disturbed judgement and acceptance of some kind of altered reality. Only in schizophrenia, however, do we find delusions and hallucinations that can be described—in Karl Jaspers's words—as "mad in the literal sense," that is, as concerning situations that are not only false but virtually inconceivable or incomprehensible because they imply alterations in the most fundamental structures of time, space, causality, or human identity. Thus schizophrenic delusions will often involve cosmic or nihilistic fantasies that can only be described as bizarre: the patient may claim, for instance, that everyone else in the world is but an automaton devoid of human consciousness; that the entire universe is on the verge of dissolution; that all the clocks in the world feel the patient's pulse; or that when his eyes get bright blue, the sky also turns blue (Jaspers 1963, pp 577, 296).[1] By contrast, in the other "functional" psychoses (manic-depressive illness and pure paranoia), the prominent symptoms tend to involve beliefs or experiences that could occur in real life or that can at least be comprehended as exaggerations of normal fears and fantasies—as, for example, when patients have thoughts of being followed or poisoned or admired by multitudes (American Psychiatric Association 1987, p 202).

The sheer strangeness of schizophrenia is, in fact, enshrined at the very center of diagnostic practice. In the latest American diagnostic manual, delusions identified as "bizarre" are considered to be especially suggestive of a schizophrenic type of psychosis; while European psychiatry has long been influenced by the views of Jaspers, who believed that the most accurate indicator of schizophrenia was the feeling of alienness evoked by such patients: namely, the interviewer's intuitive but unmistakable sense of encountering someone who, in the words of the Swiss

---

1 Jaspers describes schizophrenia in its initial stages as often involving "cosmic, religious or metaphysical revelation"; quoted in Cutting 1985, p 30.

psychiatrist Manfred Bleuler, is "totally strange, puzzling, inconceivable, uncanny, and incapable of empathy, even to the point of being sinister and frightening" (M. Bleuler 1978, p 15).

The purpose of the present essay is to illuminate the phenomenology of at least some instances of this supposedly incomprehensible condition as well as to understand why it should pose such a challenge to hermeneutic understanding. (I don't claim that my reading is necessarily relevant to all patients diagnosed as schizophrenic.)[2] The main aspect of schizophrenia on which I shall focus is the nature of these patients' characteristic delusions and of the form or structure of the delusional world that is implied. A second issue is more concerned with the problem of communication, and this is the presence in their speech of what is frequently called "poverty of content" (sometimes termed "empty speech"). This quality, found in some studies to be the single most distinctive feature of schizophrenic language, involves speech that is adequate or normal in quantity and pace, but that appears to convey little information because it seems "vague, overly abstract or overly concrete, repetitive, and stereotyped" or because it sounds to the listener like "empty philosophizing" (American Psychiatric Association 1987, pp 188, 403; Andreasen 1986, p 475; also see Andreasen 1979, p 1327).[3]

In order to illuminate these phenomena, I will have recourse to a central concept in the philosophy of Martin Heidegger, that of the famous "ontological difference" (sometimes referred to simply as "the difference"). This phrase refers to an issue that is easy enough to state but exceedingly difficult to explain: the, in Heidegger's view, all- important yet easily forgotten distinction between entities and their presence as entities, or between what he calls beings and Being, the latter of which might be spelled with a capital B. While there can be no possibility here of expounding all the nuances, ramifications, and possible contradictions of the concept, we do need to consider its basic meaning and certain of its ambiguities before we can use it to understand schizophrenia.

2. Ontological Difference

In *Being and Time* (1962, orig. publ. 1927), the major work of his first period, Heidegger distinguishes between two domains of inquiry that he labels the "ontological" and the "ontic"—terms he leaves undefined but which his translators gloss as referring, in the first instance, primarily to

---

2 The interpretation I am offering might best be thought of as a kind of ideal-type analysis. The patients to whom it is most applicable would fall into the schizophrenia category in DSM III-R (though it may not apply to *all* such patients). I will not concern myself here with certain transitional types, e.g., the schizoaffective and schizophreniform categories.

3 One Russian investigation found that fifty-four percent of schizophrenics studied had a tendency toward "fruitless intellectualizing, philosophizing, and pseudo-abstract reasoning" (Gabrial, 1974, cited in Ostwald and Zavarin, 1980, p 75). As Ostwald and Zavarin suggest, however, these Russian findings may be tainted by the nature of the sample of "schizophrenics": the diagnosis of "sluggish schizophrenia" has sometimes been applied in the Soviet Union to intellectuals and political dissidents.

Being and in the second to "entities and the facts about them" (Heidegger 1962, p. 31, fn). Being, at least at this stage of Heidegger's work, refers largely to the context or mode of being, what he describes as the all-inclusive but, for this very reason, unspecifiable "horizon" or "clearing" within which the things and beings of our experience can appear.[4] In this sense, Being is something that can differ from person to person or culture to culture, and that has changed from epoch to epoch in the West (the latter being an issue that takes center stage later in Heidegger's career). Being in this sense is equivalent to the *meaning* of Being, to the general background understanding or lighting process that determines how the entities of our experience are experienced—what counts, for example, as real or unreal, living or dead, human or divine.

The sense that receives particular emphasis after Heidegger's famous "turning" that occurred in the 1930s, might, by contrast, be thought of as something more constant and in certain respects non-perspectival: not Being as the *understanding* of Being but Being as itself—the sheer, unquestionable, and, significantly enough, virtually ineffable reality or actuality of the world, the presencing, if you will, that, like the elephant for the blind men, is the real source of all the partial understandings that humans have *of* it. If Being in the first sense always reminds us of the totality in which any given entity participates, in its second sense it turns our attention away from the "what" of the entity and toward the fact that it exists,[5] or more generally, toward the wondrous fact that there happens to be something rather than nothing, a universe rather than mere absence or void. Heidegger always emphasized the difficulty of characterizing Being, and the way verbal descriptions can distort its true nature—to the point where he eventually insisted that even the word "Being" should only be written with an X crossing it out.

Being in the first sense might be thought of as at least very roughly equivalent (and here the purists, those who would describe Heidegger's views in no terms but his own, can be expected to grumble) to the structure or form of experience, as opposed to its content.[6] To forget the ontological difference would, then, be roughly equivalent to an ignoring of form in favor of content or a focussing on parts rather than the larger entities which contain them. If the second sense of Being is regnant, by contrast, the oblivion of the ontological difference refers more specifically to the failure to appreciate what, for lack of less ambiguous and contaminated terms, I will call the reality or actuality of the world, that is, its

---

4 I am indebted to the discussion in Dreyfus (1991).

5 "[I]n the 'is'" of everything that is, according to Heidegger, "Being is uttered" (Heidegger, 1977, p. xxviii).

6 This distinction should not be too misleading if one is careful to avoid interpreting "content" in a materialist or sensationalist fashion, or "form" in an idealist one. Incidentally, there is an inevitable dilemma in explaining Heidegger's views: to compare his concepts and distinctions to more traditional ones runs the risk of distortion, but adhering always to Heidegger's own vocabulary will not clarify his thinking to those not already steeped in his thought. Also, strict adherence to Heidegger's vocabulary can result in an uncritical stance toward his thought, and in a tendency to repeat his language in a litany of word magic.

pervasive and unquestionable *thereness* and its priority over the consciousness with which it is nevertheless deeply connected—something that, according to Heidegger, has been largely lost since the preSocratics; and this aspect of Heidegger's critique is more reminiscent of at least some forms of mysticism or religious revelation.[7] Interestingly enough, Heidegger's major example of writing that captures this latter kind of revelation is the late work of Friedrich Holderlin, a poet who was manifestly schizophrenic at the time of producing most of the poetry in question. And this, not incidentally, is the same writer whose work the psychiatrist Eugen Bleuler, one of the creators of the concept of schizophrenia, has called an "example of emptiness and obscurity of ideas with preservation of a certain formal technical skill" (E. Bleuler 1950, p 89).

In the course of his work, Heidegger offered various speculations concerning the reasons for this most crucial event, the forgetting of the difference between Being and beings, and for the oblivion of Being which results; this subtle interplay of revelation and concealment is a theme throughout his philosophical career, one that we shall need to take up later. For the moment, however, we can begin our analysis of the world of schizophrenia.

3. The Question of "Poor Reality Testing"

My first point will be made very briefly, since it is one that I have treated at length elsewhere, and that has, in any case, already received a fair amount of attention in the phenomenological literature (Sass 1990a; Sartre 1966, pp. 174-206). This is the fact that both the hallucinations and delusions of schizophrenic patients usually seem to be embedded in a context—a clearing or horizon, if you will—that is quite distinct from the common-sense world of everyday pragmatic understanding. The tendency to forget this, and to focus instead on aspects of the *content* of such symptoms—on

---

7 Both senses of "Being" are found in both periods of Heidegger's thought, by the way, so we are speaking here of a matter of emphasis. I should also note that my description of Being in the second sense runs the risk of oversimplifying Heidegger's views; a couple of qualifications are in order: First, it should not be thought that, on Heidegger's account, Being (in the second sense) could exist on its own, entirely apart from Man who knows or experiences it; also, Being (also in the second sense) is in some sense perspectival, for it does reveal itself in different *ways* in different epochs. The fact remains, however, that the later Heidegger often does distinguish between epochs or modes of existence which are more or less distanced from Being, or in which Being is more or less forgotten--and this implies something like a persistent essence to Being which can be approached or revealed, gained or lost (thus, in "The Age of the World Picture," Heidegger writes; "Where anything that is has become the object of representing, it first incurs in a certain manner a loss of Being", Heidegger 1977, p 142). It is this aspect which I am trying to foreground in my description of the second sense of Being. The present essay is not an exercise in Heidegger-scholarship, but an attempt to use certain of his ideas to think about psychopathology; and it serves my purpose to stress (perhaps overly much, some might say) the contrast between the two meanings of "Being" which I describe. Re. some of the ambiguities and obscurities in Heidegger's concept of Being, see William Lovitt's introduction to Heidegger (1977), and the various pages in the volume by Heidegger which Lovitt refers to in his essay. I might also add that the nature of Heidegger's famous "turning" (*die Kehre*) is an issue of considerable controversy among scholars; some would view the turning not as a reversal but only as an intensification or deepening of his thought (see, e.g., Boelen 1976).

their presumed incorrectness (as with the important notion of "poor reality-testing") or on their purported unconscious symbolic meanings (which has been the usual psychoanalytic approach)—can be understood as resulting from a failure to be sensitive to the distinction between Being and beings. Here as elsewhere, such a failure could be said to result in an unself-critical tendency to presuppose the everyday horizon, and to conceptualize schizophrenic experience by modelling it on the understanding of what are really just entities within the everyday world.

The inadequacy of the traditional view emerges clearly enough if one considers certain central concepts in psychopathology, and then compares these with either the characteristic behavior or the experiential reports of actual schizophrenic patients. The concepts I am thinking of are those of delusion, hallucination, psychosis, and—most fundamental of all because it underlies all the others—that of so-called "poor reality-testing." The official definitions of these concepts all imply that, while the *content* of such experiences is incorrect, their *form* or ontological status, the way in which the patient experiences what he experiences, is identical to that of actual perceptions and accurate beliefs. "What objectively are hallucinations and delusions are to him unassailable truth and adequate motive for action," wrote the superintendent of the asylum in a legal brief arguing for the continued involuntary incarceration of Daniel Paul Schreber, the famous paranoid schizophrenic whose bizarre experiences were the subject of Freud's only case study of a schizophrenic (in Schreber 1988, p. 282).[8]

There are, however, several features of schizophrenic behavior that are hardly consistent with this traditional picture.

One feature is the utter indifference to counterargument or counterevidence with which such patients usually maintain their beliefs. The degree of impermeability such patients manifest is so extreme—Karl Jaspers called it a "specific schizophrenic incorrigibility"—as to distinguish their delusions from other kinds of belief, since these delusions seem to be on principle divorced from any possible need for or source of corroboration. More obviously inconsistent with the traditional view is something

---

8 Schizophrenia is traditionally seen as the quintessential form of *psychosis*, a mode of being usually marked by the presence of true *delusions* or *hallucinations*. And hallucinations and delusions are, in turn, defined by the presence of *poor reality-testing*, a psychopathological concept that corresponds more or less to lay notions of madness as being a matter of seeing or hearing things that are not there or believing things that are not true. Thus, the current diagnostic manual of the American Psychiatric Association defines "delusion" as "a false personal belief based on incorrect inference about external reality and firmly sustained in site of what almost everyone else believes and in spite of what constitutes incontrovertible and obvious proof or evidence to the contrary"; while "hallucination" is glossed as "a sensory perception without external stimulation" and having "the immediate sense of reality of a true perception" (American Psychiatric Association 1987, pp 395, 398). One might, incidentally, wish to criticize the cognitivist implications of the phrase "reality-testing," which seems to imply some explicit process of confirming or disconfirming a representation of or hypothesis about the external world. According to Heidegger, reality is normally taken for granted in a much more immediate fashion than this—one is simply *attuned* to it—and explicit testing is a more unusual event. Generally, however, this distinction is not made in medical-model psychiatry, where "poor reality-testing" can refer to either kind of mistakenness. A critique of the Cartesian and cognitivist implications present in the concept of "poor reality-testing" is beyond the scope of this essay, however.

that may seem surprising in the light of the incorrigibility: the general failure of such patients to take action on the basis of these very delusions to which they so firmly adhere—a characteristic Jaspers described as their "peculiarly inconsequent" attitude (Jaspers 1963, p 105; also see E. Bleuler 1950, p 129).

The personal accounts that many schizophrenics give of their hallucinations and delusions cast further doubt on the traditional conception of these phenomena. In the famous memoir of his psychosis, for example, Daniel Paul Schreber describes what he calls his "so-called delusional system" in terms very different from those used by his psychiatrist. He does not, in fact, make claims about actual characteristics of the objective, external or consensual world—the sort of statements that could be shown to be false by reference to evidence independent of the experiences in question. Thus, when he describes a delusional belief about himself, he typically says not "I am a scoffer at God" or "I am given to voluptuous excesses," but, rather, I am *represented* ["dargestellt"] (Schreber 1988, p 120) as one of these things. Similarly, another patient described the objects he hallucinated as appearing in "their own private space peculiar to themselves"; the sight of such objects could not, he said, be blocked by real objects, nor could they appear simultaneously with real ones (Jaspers 1963, p 71).[9]

The suggestion of these and many similar accounts is that such patients do not in fact experience their hallucinations and delusions as having the same quality of reality as do their actual perceptions or realistic beliefs. These seem, in fact, to have a different sort of Being (in Heidegger's first sense of the term)—as if they existed in some kind of subjectivized or merely representational domain, appearing only as images or merely ideational entities rather than as actualities with an independent or substantial form of existence. (Thus they could be said to *lack* Being in Heidegger's second sense of the term.) In some cases, in fact, the delusions and hallucinations are experienced in the context of a kind of solipsism, with the objects of attention being felt to exist only for the self.[10]

This subjectivized domain can, incidentally, coexist or alternate with a relatively normal mode of perception, but it may also come to preoccupy the patient to such an extent that even realistic perceptions begin to seem derealized. Thus reality, as one patient said, may "pass inwards"— leading to a situation in which, to quote another patient: "Reality, as it was

---

9 Another illustration can be found in *Autobiography of a Schizophrenic Girl* (Sechehaye 1968, p 54), where the patient Renee describes a quasi-solipsistic sense that the world depends on the observer. Renee also mentions the feeling of isolation that tends to accompany this orientation: "at that time, according to my concept of the world, things didn't exist in and of themselves, but each one created a world after his own fashion. ... The question of social relationships did not touch me in the slightest degree."

10 This phenomenological hypothesis is consistent with a recent proposal by Manfred Spitzer, who suggests the following definition of "delusions": "statements about external reality which are uttered like statements about a mental state, i.e., with subjective certainty and incorrigible by others" (1990 p 391). Spitzer's argument is based on purely linguistic and logical considerations, however, and he does not speculate about the mode of experience that underlies delusions.

formerly, no longer exists. Real life has suffered a decline" (quoted in Cutting 1985, p. 390; Werner 1957, p 418; also see M. Bleuler 1978, p. 490). The quality of unreality pervading the world of delusions does not, however, make patients like Schreber treat this domain as unimportant or "merely" subjective, for they may be obsessed with it to the exclusion of any interest in The Real. But their failure to act on the basis of these experiences (patients who claim to be surrounded by poisoners, for instance, may nevertheless sit down happily at lunch), or to show even the slightest interest in potential corroboration or disconfirmation (which according to Jaspers are distinctive features of true schizophrenic delusions) suggests that this is a domain where reality-testing simply plays no role, a domain to which neither belief nor disbelief of the usual kind is of any relevance.[11]

Let us now turn to a closely related point, the fact that certain classic schizophrenic delusions do not just imply but actually thematize this quality of derealization—expressing in their very content the pervasive but difficult-to-specify ontological status of their world.

4. Epistemological Delusions

Although paranoid delusions are common in all types of psychosis, certain types of such delusions seem to be especially characteristic of schizophrenia; these are not primarily concerned with the *content* of reality—with, say, fear of a burglar who is imagined to be lurking somewhere in real space, spying and waiting to attack. Instead of issues existing within the world, the delusions in question primarily involve the overall ontological status of the world itself, which seems to the patient to be somehow unreal, dependent for its existence on being an object of knowledge for some consciousness or representational device that records or represents events.

"Then it started in the living room," said one patient. "I kept thinking I was being watched by videocameras ... I had a tremendous feeling of claustrophobia. I felt trapped. ... It was all like a story" (Cutting 1985, p. 291).

In their written memoirs, two other schizophrenics recount remarkably similar experiences of what might be called epistemological delusions. A schizophrenic nurse describes "a most disturbing experience. I saw everything I did like a film camera..."; and another patient writes:

"I was myself a camera. The view of people that I obtained through my own eyes were being recorded elsewhere to make some kind of three-dimensional film" (Wallace 1965, p 23; Coate 1965, p 101, also p 103).

---

11 Eugen Bleuler offers an interesting example of the kind of misunderstanding that can occur when the patient "takes symbolically what the physician understands in its literal sense." One schizophrenic insisted, for example, that he was unable to see, that he was blind, when it was obvious his eyesight was not impaired; what he meant, says Bleuler, is that he did not experience things "as reality" (1950, p. 56).

Such delusions seem to express (and perhaps, to rationalize) a pervasive feeling of subjectivization—the sense that all one's perceptions involve not realities but only images or representations.

The full significance of this kind of epistemological delusion will, I think, be missed if, as so often occurs, the patient's claims are interpreted as essentially analogous, except for the fact of their erroneousness, to everyday statements about objects in the real world—as if, for instance, the first patient quoted just above were imagining that a real videocamera trained on him existed somewhere in actual space, or even in the same space that contains the *unreal* objects being filmed. I would argue, in fact, that such delusional phenomena function as something like symbols for subjectivity itself, for the self-as-subject, and thus that they are not objects within the world, whether real or delusional, so much as expressions of the felt ongoing process of knowing or experiencing by *which* this world is constituted. If this is true, such phenomena would be expected to be doubly ephemeral and unreal—difficult to locate not only because they have no existence in the objective world independent of the subject's consciousness, but also because, like the eyeball that sees, they are unlikely to appear even as immanent objects within their own (subjectivized) fields of vision.

And it is, in fact, true that the knowing, representing, or recording devices or persons in the "epistemological" delusions so characteristic of schizophrenia often have an especially shadowy mode of being: there is a videocamera "somewhere" but the patient doesn't actually see it in his mind's eye and he cannot tell you where it is. Such entities often seem to be everywhere and nowhere, existing only as unspecifiable, almost atmospheric presences that pervade the universe like a miasma of unreality. Like Being as understood by Heidegger, such phenomena are difficult to locate because they veil themselves precisely by the sheer pervasiveness of their presence.[12]

Such delusions are, we might say, concerned with ontological rather than ontic questions, with the general metaphysical status of the entire universe or the most fundamental issues involving the relationship of knower and known, rather than with objects or events existing within such a universe. Blindness to this fact—which is enshrined in the widely accepted "poor reality-testing" formula—has, in my view, been one of the most important sources of misunderstanding between schizophrenics and those who treat them. A patient who says that "everything from the largest to smallest is contained within me" should not, it seems to me, be taken literally or ontically, as if he meant that things exist within him in just the same *way* that furniture exists within a room or pencils inside a drawer. A patient who says his eyes and the sun are the same is unlikely to mean that the sun has been removed from the sky and inserted into his skull, or even

---

12 Heidegger speaks of Being as: "both nowhere and everywhere," having no place since it is "the placeless dwelling place of all presencing" (1977, p 43).

that his eyes burn as brightly as the sun. (In the typical case, he does not deny, after all, that there is still a sun above him.)

A patient who speaks of objects and people coming out of her eyes ("Many things come out of my lovely blue eyes, ... bedsteads, commodes, baskets, thread, stockings of all colors, clothes from the plainest to the most elegant"; E. Bleuler 1950, pp 111-112) is unlikely to be referring to the plane of physical reality, to a material producing or a spatial emerging of objects, as if it were a matter of watching objects spill miraculously from one's head in the manner of toys from a bag. For a patient to believe such a thing would imply a profoundly altered conception of the everyday physical world—of those laws of gravity, object constancy, or spatial organization that preclude material objects from flying about, materializing instantaneously, or existing inside one's skull. And if such were the case, one would expect profound confusion or mistakenness about the physical world; whereas in fact schizophrenics are usually well- oriented and quite capable of practical activity when this is called for. Such statements, which may seem to involve the most egregious mistakenness about material reality, are better understood as having an ontological or epistemological import, as being ways of claiming to be the consciousness for which all objects exist, of saying that one's own perceiving (symbolized by the eyes) does not simply reflect but somehow vivifies or makes possible the perceptual universe (as the sun does).

A more reasonable view, then, is that such delusions amount to a sort of epistemological claim, akin to that of the philosophical solipsist who draws back into an acute awareness of his experience-as-such and, as a result, feels and declares the world to be his own idea.[13] This is not to say, of course, that there is nothing abnormal or pathological about such experiences—obviously there is something very deviant about becoming so preoccupied with, and living out, a solipsistic or quasi-solipsistic attitude. But to think of such a form of existence as essentially involving "poor reality-testing" is to equate this ontological mutation with the *kind* of mistake that occurs within the common-sense world. And this is not only to overestimate the patient's proneness to error but, even more importantly, to miss the profound way his form of life differs from the normal.

5.   Ineffability and the Ontological Dimension

One way to defend the traditional view against the interpretation I have been suggesting would be to call attention to the rather literal and physical nature of the vocabulary that such patients do employ: is it likely, one might ask, that schizophrenics would speak of, say, objects and people "flying out" of their eyes if their real concerns pertained to quasi-philosophical issues of an abstract and ontological nature? Would a patient

---

13 An this, incidentally, seems less a reversion to the infant's ignorance of ego boundaries, as psychoanalytic theory would suggest, than the result of an exaggerated awareness of the role of consciousness in constituting its world.

speak of "containing" all things if he really meant to express not a spatial but an epistemological relationship?

To answer this objection one needs to recognize certain subtle but crucial facts about language and its relationship to the human condition; and to appreciate the inherent difficulty—indeed, the near impossibility--of describing or conceptualizing experiences or insights of an ontological kind without resorting to a vocabulary or repertoire of concepts derived from the physical and everyday world. This, incidentally, is an issue to which Heidegger devoted considerable attention; he argued, in fact, that many of the major errors, obscurities, and controversies in Western philosophy derive from the tendency, even on the part of the greatest thinkers, to adopt language and conceptual imagery applicable to objects within the world when attempting to characterize the world in its totality or in its fundamental relationship with consciousness.[14]

Perhaps the most important criticism which Heidegger directed at Descartes, his major *bete noir*, for example, is that the latter's philosophy makes the category mistake of treating the experiential subject as if it had the same ontological status as its objects, as if it were an entity within the world rather than the transcendental ground *of* the world (this is the implication of Descartes's notion of *res cogitans*, a thinking substance). Both Kant and Husserl also made this criticism of Descartes; yet, according to Heidegger, neither of these critics was really able to liberate himself from the same misleading way of thinking, which their own philosophies only reproduced in subtler forms. Thus Heidegger argues that the Kantian and Husserlian tendency to conceive of the transcendental subject as if it could, at least on principle, exist prior to or in the absence of its world, also stems from conceiving of subject and world on the analogy of two objects existing side-by-side within the world. Such a way of thinking, says Heidegger, obscures the essential inseparability of consciousness and its objects, and it can lead to the error by which the mind's epistemological constituting of experiential objects comes to be conceived on the model of some kind of actual generation or production of one object by another.[15]

Heidegger considers this tendency to interpret, understand, or express ontological issues regarding the fundamental nature of existence or the world on the analogy of empirical facts within the world (the latter being what he calls merely "ontic" issues)—or, as he sometimes says, to confuse presencing with a thing that is present—to be the deepest and most treacherous source of confusion in the entire history of Western thought.[16] It is for this reason, he says, that the study of Being as such has either been forgotten or else confused with thought about particular—that is, ontic—

---

14 As Heidegger puts it, "The Interpretation of the world begins... with some entity within-the-world, so that the phenomenon of the world in general no longer comes into view" (1962, p 122).
15 Re. this tendency in Husserl, see Olafson (1987, pp 19ff).
16 See, e.g., Heidegger (1975, p 50) where Heidegger writes that "The oblivion of Being is oblivion of the distinction between Being and beings." In a forthcoming book, I discuss the relevance to schizophrenia of an analogous point made by Ludwig Wittgenstein: his argument that solipsism, subjective idealism, and other forms of metaphysical thinking stem from a confusion of empirical with transcendental issues (to be published by Cornell University Press).

beings. If Nietzsche and other philosophers have considered Being to be nothing more than "a fallacy and a vapor" (Heidegger, 1961, pp 29- 30), this is because Being is so difficult to conceive in its own terms. Like the light by which we see, it is everywhere and nowhere, closer to us than anything else yet at the same time always eluding our grasp.

On Heidegger's view, then, the oblivion of the difference between Being and beings is no mere accident, nor something that could be avoided without great difficulty, if at all. If this analysis has any truth to it, we ought not to be surprised that schizophrenic patients, who are hardly to be expected to be more subtle or careful than most philosophers of the Western tradition, should also succumb to this same nearly irresistible temptation. We should not be surprised that they should speak of spatial and physical relationships like "containing" the universe, or of objects "flying" out of their eyes, when they are, in some sense, responding to ontological experiences of their own epistemological role, their centrality as knowers, in their experiential worlds.

It seems, in fact, that some patients may actually have a certain awareness of the potentially misleading nature of their (ontic) modes of description, an awareness that may well involve at least an inkling of what Heidegger called the ontological difference. Daniel Paul Schreber—a patient who had elaborate delusions concerning what might sound like a rather literal cosmos of entities called "nerves" and "rays"—was, for example, quite conscious of the difficulty of communicating the specific quality of his lived-world, in this case a subjectivized one, to people who had not had such experiences themselves.

"Again it is extremely difficult," he wrote, "to describe these changes in words because matters are dealt with which lack all analogies in human experience and which I appreciated directly only in part with my mind's eye..." (Schreber 1988, p 117, also see pp 137, 227).[17] "To make myself at least somewhat comprehensible," he says, "I shall have to speak much in images and similes, which may at times be only *approximately* correct" (p 41).

His concern about being misunderstood sometimes caused him to describe his hallucinations and delusions in what his translators call "involved and endless sentences contain[ing] clauses within clauses" (p 26).

I do not mean to imply that schizophrenics will usually be cognizant (as Schreber may sometimes have been) of the potentially misleading effect of using ontic imagery to speak of ontological concerns or experiences. The tendency to neglect the ontological is, after all, deeply rooted in the very structure of human experience; and one should hardly expect that schizophrenics, any more than other people (including most pre-Heideggerian philosophers), will always maintain a vigilant awareness of the merely metaphoric nature of the ontic vocabulary and imagery which they are inclined to use. The patient's own understanding of his experience

---

17 "mit meinem Geistigen Auge" (Schreber, 1973, p 123, in original pagination).

may, in fact, be plagued by some of the same errors as are found in psychoanalysis and medical-model psychiatry, for the patient too may, in reflecting upon his experiences, be inclined to understand in ontic terms what is in fact an ontological issue.

There is also another possibility to be considered: this infection of the ontological by the ontic might occur not only at the level of vocabulary and self-conceptualization but also at that of prereflective experience itself. A remarkable passage by the writer and man of the theatre, Antonin Artaud, who was most certainly schizophrenic, illustrates this very well. With images of the spatial universe shaking and disappearing, he invokes a cataclysmic sense of ontological catastrophe, of the threatened disappearance of the All that can accompany schizophrenic solipsism. And, in the midst of this catastrophe, he has an uncanny vision: what he describes as the "rootlets which were trembling at the corners of my mind's eye" detaching themselves "with vertiginous speed" from the mass of space now heaving and collapsing before him. This image of the rootlets at the corners of the mind's eye, which at one level demands to be read as having an ontological import (it seems to convey the sense of the world being contained by, or dependent for its Being and its stability upon, his own consciousness, the eye that sees) is at the same time highly ontic in nature, since the rootlets show up as entities within the perceptual universe. And, though it is impossible to be sure, one certainly gets the impression that this was more than a manner of speaking for Artaud: an ontological awareness of the self-as-subject seems, impossibly enough, to have invaded the field of awareness, so that he actually sees, pulsating in this concretistic image of the eyeball's capillaries, the emblem of his own being as a constituting consciousness (Artaud 1976, p. 60).[18]

The traditional, ontic understanding inherent in the poor reality-testing formula may not, then, be entirely mistaken. For, while it is true that the delusions of schizophrenics often pertain to an ontological dimension that is all too often overlooked, it is also the case that their experiences will sometimes involve a curious mixture of the ontic with the ontological—a mix that, from a theoretical standpoint, is difficult to

---

18 Incidentally, there are certain kinds of at least quasi-ontic entities that Heidegger sees as bodying forth the ontological in a legitimate fashion. These include "emblems" like a Greek temple or Gothic cathedral, both of which manage to focus and epitomize the mode of Being of their respective cultures. Presumably, in the case of such emblems our attention and understanding does not remain focused in a literal way on the ontic as such, but is somehow turned toward the ontological dimension. It is difficult to prove the case, but I am inclined to view the "rootlets" example as something rather different—not a symbolizing of the ontological in worldly terms so much as a distortion whereby it seems actually to *have* an ontic mode of existence. It is also interesting to consider the paradoxical ontological status that ontic/ontological beings like the rootlets have, and to notice how problematic this would make any attempt on the part of the patient to determine whether they are "real" (an extremely ambiguous question, but one frequently arises because of the poor reality-testing formula). The rootlets do of course have a quality of reality insofar as they are ontic, i.e., specific and in a certain sense concretely existing entities. But this of course is also what makes them in another sense unreal, since the mind which they symbolize is not itself an ontic entity. On the other hand, the mind, as something ontological (without concrete specificity) is real, but the least misleading representation of it would therefore have to have an ephemeral quality, and thus would be, in another sense, unreal.

characterize yet seems nonetheless to be experientially quite real. The patient who speaks of objects issuing from her skull or of the sky turning the blue of his eyes, cannot, therefore, be taken simply as being either literal or metaphoric, since neither of these readings does full justice to what appears to be the actuality of the experience. Perhaps it is better to say that the patient speaks in both modes at the same time, or, at least, in rapid succession. This contradictory mix may, in fact, be one of the reasons for the hybrid quality of both over-concreteness and over-abstractness which schizophrenic experience can have (see Weiner 1966, pp. 85-94, 100-102), and, more generally, it may contribute to the observer's general impression of bizarreness, contradiction and ineffability.

6. Poverty of Content

The near-ineffability of ontological concerns or of an ontological trans-formation may also help to account for another kind of misunderstanding between schizophrenics and those who treat them—this time a misunder-standing that, unlike the usual "poor reality-testing" interpretation, results not from the patient's giving in to but from his resisting, or being indif-ferent to, the temptation of ontic modes of expression. I would argue that some instances of so-called "poverty of content" of speech—a psychiatric sign defined as "speech that is adequate in amount but conveys little information because of vagueness, empty repetitions, or use of stereotyped or obscure phrases" (American Psychiatric Association 1987, p 403)[19]— may actually be the result of attempts to give more purely ontological, and in this sense more direct, characterizations of mutations of the lived-world that are experienced in an essentially ontological fashion. It should be evident that, because of their very nature, such mutations cannot be described by any but the most abstract or indirect phrases—phrases that, especially to the unsympathetic listener, may well seem vague, obscure or empty, but which the speaker, in the absence of any alternative, is likely to repeat again and again in his (usually vain) attempt to convey the over-whelming importance of his theme.

Such a quality of vagueness or hypergenerality is present in the fol-lowing passage by Antonin Artaud—an excellent example of the sort of statement that tends to be dismissed as an instance of pseudo-philosophizing and poverty of content:

"Like life, like nature, thought goes from the inside out before going   from the outside in. I begin to think in the void and from the void I move toward the plenum; and when I have reached the plenum I can fall back into the void. I go from the abstract to the concrete and not from the concrete toward the abstract" (Artaud 1976, p 362).

---

19 According to DSM III-R, "the interviewer may observe that the person has spoken at some length but has not given adequate information to answer a question."

The preoccupation with ontological concerns, with issues pertaining to the nature of reality in general and to the general structure of self- world relations, is evident in this passage; and it has resulted in speech that is unlikely to seem meaningful to the person not attuned to such issues. Statements like these seem to be attempts to express things whose intrinsic nature renders them close to ineffable, experiences that are so total as to pervade the whole universe, yet so subtle as to seem at times like nothing at all—experiences of the being of Being, of the unreality of unreality, of existing both inside and outside one's own mind, or of feeling one's own epistemic centrality. If the sympathetic reader can grasp Artaud's meaning, this is a considerable tribute to Artaud's verbal skill (and it may also have something to do with the expectation of meaningfulness one typically brings to the work of a recognized literary artist). But the vast majority of schizophreniform patients are neither philosophers nor poets, without benefit either of a technical vocabulary or an exceptional metaphoric ability, and one should hardly expect their statements to be easy to follow; this may be one reason why they are so readily assumed to manifest poverty of content.

I would argue, in fact, that the famous obscurity of Heidegger's own highly abstract prose—which, it has been said, is "untranslatable, even into German" (Passmore 1968, p 603)—derives largely from the same source, for he was attempting to express the ontological without resorting to the distorting ontic metaphors or expressions of the philosophical tradition. Thus Heidegger could write such things as that "the world worlds" and that "the nothing itself nothings"; and, in a passage made famous when Rudolph Carnap quoted it as an example of the nonsensical nature of metaphysical philosophizing, he wrote that: "Nihilation is neither a nihila-tion of what is, nor does it spring from negation. ... Nothing annihilates itself" (Passmore 1968, p 477).[20] Heidegger believed, incidentally, that it was necessary to defend the philosophical concern with Being against common sense, since the latter reacts to the Being-question as an attack upon itself, and also from those forms of philosophy—Carnap's would doubtless be an example—that, in Heidegger's view, were essentially restatements of common sense in canonical form.[21] It would not be un-reasonable to compare the hostile or contemptuous responses to Heidegger of such empirically oriented analytic philosophers as Carnap, who claimed that most of Heidegger was devoid of cognitive significance, to the psychia-trist's dismissive assessment of "poverty of content" in some schizophrenic speech. There seems in both cases to be a similar impatience, verging sometimes on revulsion and contempt, for an attitude of mind that turns away from the noonday world of social and practical reality toward the

---

20 Heidegger's statements are, in fact, attempts to express some of the issues that have been central to this paper: e.g., the experience of an objectively existing and encompassing reality (this would be a world that "worlds"), and also the sense of the nothingness of the experiential subject or of its non-identity with its own objects of awareness (this is what is meant by "nihilation", a concept later taken up by Sartre).

21 Re. these issues, see W. Richardson (1974, pp 253, 251,229); also Olafson (1987, p 5).

elusive one of ontological speculation. But, anyone who has indulged in such musings, whether during adolescence or since, will know that anything said on such ultimate and totalistic topics can easily seem, even to the speaker, to waver between profundity and utter meaninglessness. Is this, perhaps, what is being alluded to in the following words spoken by yet another patient, a schizophrenic who had complained of feeling dead, of the world seeming unreal, and of being unable to express his thoughts?: "One talks and it seems one says nothing and then one finds one has been talking about the whole of one's existence and one can't remember what one said" (Rosser 1979, p 186).[22]

7. The Authenticity Question

The preoccupation with what seems to be the ontological dimension that is found in many schizophrenics raises the interesting question of whether such patients might be especially in touch with, or have a heightened awareness of, Being or the ontological difference. Could it be that the schizophrenic comes closer to the Heideggerian ideal of authenticity than does the normal human being? Actually, this question regarding authenticity, as I have just posed it, is far too blunt; and to explore it seriously we would have to consider some complicating factors that I only have time to mention: first, a couple of different reasons that Heidegger offers for the forgetting of the difference between ontic and ontological, and second, the different and, at least to some extent, inconsistent meanings of the term "Being".

In his later work, Heidegger explained the forgetting of the difference as a natural consequence of man's involvement in activities of everydayness, in the practical manipulations that focus attention on particular entities and goals while forcing one to presuppose and thus forget the encompassing horizon (see Heidegger 1930, pp 317-351; Olafson 1987, pp 162, 200). The fact that schizophrenics—persons who tend to be profoundly alienated from the pragmatic and social involvements of normal life—are particularly preoccupied with ontological issues is certainly consistent with this part of Heidegger's analysis. But, though there may be some evidence of the possibility of a *thinking* of the difference in schizophrenia, there seems to be less evidence of a naturally felt nearness to or embeddedness in Being, in the second sense of this term. Indeed, with its experiences of solipsism and world-catastrophe (and alienated objectivism, a phenomenon I have not had time to describe),[23]

---

22 Whether Carnap was right in saying that one should not even attempt to express such sentiments in other than artistic forms (he contemptuously defined metaphysicians as "musicians without musical ability") is not the issue here; I wish only to clarify some of the reasons for what is too readily dismissed as *mere* poverty of content.
23 The objectivist mode of experience in schizophrenia is described in the longer version of this paper that appears in *Philosophical Psychology*; Sass 1992a. There I also treat the authenticity question (and several other issues), in considerably more detail. Re. objectivism in schizophrenia, also see Sass 1990b, or Sass 1992b, Chapter 2.

schizophrenia would seem far closer to the mood of alarm that Heidegger associates with the end of philosophy than with the "wonder" so prominent at its beginning;[24] and it would be a mistake to assume that the schizophrenic's awareness of the difference is accompanied by the kind of heightened contact with Being that Heidegger believed to be characteristic of the preSocratic period. To understand this point, it will be useful to recall some of Heidegger's earlier thoughts regarding the sources of a forgetting of Being or the difference.

The tendency to be caught up in practical activity is not the only reason Heidegger gives for this forgetting. In his early work, including *Being and Time*, he emphasized what is almost an opposite one: the tendency for the stance of passive and detached visual contemplation, so natural to the philosophical or contemplative mind, to provide the basis for a misleading kind of ontological speculation, for certain illusions that thus tend, as he put it, to "settle down and nest with particular stubbornness precisely in philosophy" (Heidegger 1982, p 328). Given the passivity and detachment characteristic of schizophrenia, such patients might well be expected to manifest something akin to these "metaphysical" ways of obliviating Being and the difference which Heidegger concentrated on and criticized in his earlier work. And in fact, many of the schizophrenic experiences of the ontological dimension which I mentioned above may have more in common with these visions of reality that Heidegger disparages than with what he would consider a true understanding of *Dasein* or of Being.[25]

Summary

This paper offers a phenomenological or hermeneutic reading—employing Heidegger's notion of the "ontological difference"—of certain central aspects of schizophrenic experience. The main focus is on signs and symptoms that have traditionally been taken to indicate either "poor reality-testing" or else "poverty of content of speech" (defined in DSM III-R as: "speech that is adequate in amount but conveys little information because of vagueness, empty repetitions, or use of stereotyped or obscure phrases").

It is argued that, at least in some cases, the tendency to attribute these signs of illness to the schizophrenic patient results from a failure to

---

24 Incidentally, the later Heidegger no longer sees anxiety as a source of revelation, but instead as a sign of the "oblivion of Being" associated with modern nihilism (Heidegger 1956, p 211; also see Dreyfus 1991, chapter re. "attunement"). Heidegger claims, by the way, that Holderlin, a schizophrenic, did have the experience of the absolute presence of Being (in the second sense). Precisely this claim has, however, been disputed by Paul de Man. De Man acknowledges that Heidegger has accurately recognized the essential issue that preoccupied Holderlin in his late poetry (i.e., the issue of Being), but he thinks that what are actually statements of frustrated longing for Being are misread by Heidegger as being claims to have achieved a dwelling in Being (de Man 1983, pp 254-255).
25 A somewhat more elaborated version of this essay will appear in the journal *Philosophical Psychology* (Sass 1992a).

recognize that such patients—as part of a quasi-solipsistic orientation and alienation from more normal, pragmatic concerns—may be grappling with issues of what Heidegger would call an ontological rather than an ontic type, issues concerned not with entities but with Being (i.e., not with objects in the world but with the overall status of the world itself). An application of the Heideggerian concept of the ontological difference has the potential to alter one's sense of the lived-worlds of such patients, of what they may be attempting to communicate, and of why communication with them so often breaks down.

References

American Psychiatric Association: Diagnostic and Statistical Manual of Mental Disorders, Third Edition, Revised (DSM III-R). Washington, D.C., American Psychiatric Association, 1987

Andreasen N: Thought, language, and communication disorders, II, Diagnostic significance, Archives of General Psychiatry 36: 1325- 30, 1979

Andreasen N: Scale for the assessment of thought, language, and communication, Schizophrenia Bulletin 12: 473-482 1986

Artaud A: Selected Writings. New York, Farrar, Straus & Giroux, 1976.

Bleuler E: Dementia Praecox or the Group of Schizophrenias (1911), transl. J Zinkin, New York, International Universities Press, 1950

Bleuler M: The Schizophrenic Disorders. New Haven & London, Yale University Press, 1978

Boelen B: Martin Heidegger as a phenomenologist. In: Phenomenological Perspectives: Historical and Systematic Essays in Honor of Herbert Spiegelberg. The Hague, Martinus Nijhoff, pp 93-114, 1975

Coate M: Beyond All Reason. Philadelphia & New York, J B Lippincott Co., 1965

Cutting J: The Psychology of Schizophrenia. Edinburgh, Churchill Livingstone, 1985

de Man P: Heidegger's exegeses of Hölderlin. In: de Man P (ed) Blindness and Insight, pp 246-266, Minneapolis, University of Minnesota Press, 1983

Dreyfus H: Being in the World: A Commentary on Heidegger's Being and Time, Division I. Cambridge, Massachusetts, MIT Press, 1991

Gabrial TM: (1974, original article in Russian), cited in P Ostwald & V Zavarin Studies of language and schizophrenia in the USSR. In: Rieber RW (ed): Applied Psycholinguistics and Mental Health, pp 69-92 (see p 75), New York, Plenum, 1980

Heidegger M (1930) On the essence of truth. In: W Brock (ed) Existence and Being, pp 317-351, Chicago, Regnery, 1930

Heidegger M: The way back into the ground of metaphysics. In: W Kaufman (ed) Existentialism from Dostoevsky to Sartre, pp 206-221, New York, Meridian/New American Library, 1956

Heidegger M: An Introduction to Metaphysics. Garden City, New York, Doubleday, 1961

Heidegger M: Being and Time. New York, Harper & Row, 1962

Heidegger M: The Anaximander fragment, Early Greek Thinking. New York, Harper & Row, 1975

Heidegger M: The Question Concerning Technology and Other Essays. transl. W Lovitt, New York: Harper & Row, 1977

Jaspers K: General Psychopathology. Chicago, University of Chicago Press, 1963

Olafson F: Heidegger and the Philosophy of Mind. New Haven & London, Yale University Press, 1987

Passmore J: A Hundred Years of Philosophy. Harmondsworth, Middlesex, England, Penguin Books, 1968

Richardson W: Heidegger: Through Phenomenology to Thought. The Hague, M. Nijhoff, 1974

Rosser R: The psychopathology of feeling and thinking in a schizophrenic, International Journal of Psychoanalysis 60: 177-188, 1979

Sartre J: The Psychology of Imagination. New York, Washington Square Press, 1966

Sass LA: On delusions. Raritan 9: 120-141, 1990a

Sass LA: The truth-taking stare: a Heideggerian interpretation of a schizophrenic world. Journal of Phenomenological Psychology 21: 121-149, 1990b

Sass LA: Heidegger, schizophrenia, and the ontological difference. (to appear in) Philosophical Psychology, 1992a

Sass LA: Madness and Modernism: Insanity in the Light of Modern Art, Literature, and Thought. New York: Basic Books, (in press) 1992b

Schreber D: Denkwürdigkeiten eines Nervenkranken (1903). Frankfurt, Berlin, Wien, Ullstein, 1973

Schreber D: Memoirs of my Nervous Illness. transl. I. MacAlpine, RM Hunter, Cambridge, Harvard University Press, 1988

Sechehaye M (ed): Autobiography of a Schizophrenic Girl. New York, New American Library, 1970

Spitzer M: On defining delusions, Comprehensive Psychiatry 31: 377-397, 1990

Wallace C: Portrait of a Schizophrenic Nurse. London, Hammond and Co., 1965

Weiner I: Psychodiagnosis in Schizophrenia. New York, Wiley, 1966

Werner H: Comparative Psychology of Mental Development, revised edition. New York, International Universities Press, 1957

Language and Cognition

M. Spitzer, F.A. Uehlein
M.A. Schwartz, C. Mundt
(eds.): Phenomenology
Language & Schizophrenia.
Springer-Verlag, New York, 1992

Phenomenological Aspects on "Zerfahrenheit" and Incoherence

Henning Sass

1. Historical and Terminological Background

Since the time of Griesinger (1845) and Snell (1852), disturbances of thought and language have always been of special importance in descriptions and concepts of mental illness. This observation also applies to "dementia praecox" or "the group of schizophrenias" established by Emil Kraepelin (1899) and Eugen Bleuler (1911) at the beginning of our century. Kraepelin introduced the term "Zerfahrenheit" for special types of disturbances with very characteristic features, defined as "loss of internal or external connection of the chain of ideas," or as "loss of internal unity". His interpretation of these phenomena was similar to many contemporary concepts, e.g. that of Stransky (1914), who used the metaphor of "intrapsychic ataxia". Also, Eugen Bleuler's (1911) descriptions of schizophrenic thinking became of major influence. Bleuler gathered together—along with disturbances of affect, ambivalence and autism—the disorders of thought and language—especially "loosening of associations"—as characteristic fundamental symptoms which are always present in schizophrenia.

In concordance with Kraepelin and Bleuler, many German-speaking psychiatrists have regarded the phenomenon of "Zerfahrenheit" as one of the most typical signs of schizophrenia. But unfortunately, even in German-speaking psychopathological discussions, there is much inconsistency in the usage of Kraepelin's term "Zerfahrenheit". This is especially true regarding the ambiguous relationship of "Zerfahrenheit" to the similar term "Inkohärenz" or "incoherence", which can be traced back at least as far as to Griesinger (1845). Sometimes "Zerfahrenheit" is taken as a synonym for "Inkohärenz", but this is criticized by other authors. These authors point out that classical psychiatrists like Bleuler, Ewald, Mayer-Gross and Stransky stressed the distinction between the two terms, which is based mostly on nosological assumptions. Their intention was to distinguish "Zerfahrenheit" as a more or less typical form of schizophrenic thought and language disturbance from "incoherence" as a term for the somewhat different phenomena found in organic mental disorders. Other authors, for example Bash, Kleist and Leonhard, make no distinction between "Zerfahrenheit" and "incoherence" and use the terms as synonyms.

The situation has become even more complicated by difficulties in the translation of the texts of Bleuler (1911) and Kraepelin (1919) into English. Usually "Zerfahrenheit" is translated as "incoherence," and is conceptualized as similar to Bleuler's "loosening of associations" or to "derailment". The latter, a more precise term preferred by Andreasen (1979), is derived from the English version of Kraepelin's monograph on "Dementia praecox and paraphrenia" (1919). "Zerfahrenheit" itself has not been incorporated into the English-speaking psychopathological literature. A historical reason for this may be the incomplete translation of the early versions of Kraepelin's textbook into English, which left out some parts of his text, especially some general remarks on thought disorder and "Zerfahrenheit".

In recent years, "Zerfahrenheit" has lost its prominent role in schizophrenic symptomatology, and we find it explicitly neither in Kurt Schneider's (1959) "first rank symptoms," nor in the diagnostic criteria of DSM-III, DSM-III-R, and ICD-10. The German versions of these instruments, however, reintroduce the term "Zerfahrenheit" as equivalent to the English item "incoherence". This has been criticized by Peters (1991), who insists on the difference between "Zerfahrenheit" as schizophrenic and "Inkohärenz" as organic phenomena. To make matters even worse, the English usage of "incoherence" seems to be quite the opposite. Thus, Andreasen suggests that "incoherence" should be used only when an organic mental disorder has been ruled out as the cause of disturbed speech and language behavior.

Another aspect of the discussion regarding the meaning of the term "incoherence" comes from the modern linguistic concept of "Kohärenz" or "coherence", which refers to the internal consistency of a text. Several authors, such as Hoffman et al. (1982), Hoffman et al. (1986), and Tress et al. (1984), applied this concept in clinical studies. They found differences in the degree of "coherence" in schizophrenic speech when compared to other speech samples. These results seem to indicate a special significance for the concept of "coherence" in the analysis of schizophrenic thought disorder. Such research could support the translation of "Zerfahrenheit" as "incoherence", but we should keep in mind that the terms "coherence" or "incoherence" are nosologically neutral, whereas the term "Zerfahrenheit" for many psychiatrists implies a diagnostic (nosological) decision.

2. The Distortions of These Concepts in DSM–III

In an influential paper on thought, language and communication disorders, Andreasen (1979) prepared the concept of thought disorder for the chapter on schizophrenia in DSM–III. She explicitly referred to Bleuler, whose approach to the assessment of schizophrenia—which regarded thought disorder as a pathognomonic symptom—had been most influential in American psychiatry for many years. Nonetheless, Andreasen's theoretical and empirical analysis led to the conclusion that thought disorder is of little diagnostic significance. In particular, the concept of "loosening of associations" was regarded as having only little value for differential diagnosis between mania and schizophrenia. Additionally, Andreasen claimed that this concept was based upon outdated associationist psychology. This judgement does not seem to be completely justified. It might perhaps be true concerning older forms of associationist psychology, in which a general idea was decisive for the choice of the subordinated ideas. But, as Hoff (cf. this volume) pointed out, even Kraepelin's psychological teacher Wundt (1874) held quite different views. In contrast to the former associationist psychology, as represented by Herbart, Wundt stressed the special importance of consciousness and thinking for associations. He therefore spoke of apperceptions and emphasized that consciousness played an active role in the production of associations instead of passively responding to external stimuli. Thus we find a voluntaristic element in Wundt's theory, similar to the view accentuated by later authors that intentions lead the flow of ideas and associations.

Andreasen's (1979) reproach of an outdated associationist psychology is even less justified concerning the concepts of Bleuler, for he—in cooperation with his disciple Jung—had made a fruitful attempt to integrate psychoanalytical ideas about the role of unconscious elements into the analysis of associations. Bleuler's concept of "loosening of associations" mainly refers to Freud's theory, and on the other hand was inspired by Janet's (1903) views regarding the unconscious determination of the disturbed associations. Even before Bleuler's famous monograph *The Group of Schizophrenias* appeared in 1911, Bleuler and Jung (1908) had published a paper, entitled *Complexes and causes of illness in dementia praecox,* which introduced psychoanalytic concepts for the analysis of the symptomatology of schizophrenia. Nonetheless, Andreasen's (1979) critique that the term "loose associations" has been used so imprecisely until now as to be nearly meaningless, is appropriate. It will be the task of this paper to review some concepts of thought disorder in the German-speaking psychopathological tradition, in order to find out whether there is still a useful basis for the distinction between "loosening of associations" and "incoherence" on the one hand, and the special symptom of "Zerfahrenheit" on the other hand.

In DSM–III and DSM–III–R, "incoherence" (and "loosening of associations" as a milder form of it) are used as terms for formal thought disorders of schizophrenia which in the German-speaking literature are found under the heading of "Zerfahrenheit", in the sense of Kraepelin (1919), and under the heading of "loosening of associations", in the sense of Bleuler (1911). However, it does not represent the original ideas of Kraepelin and Bleuler if we merely put these forms together and distinguish them only on the basis of increasing severity. Kraepelin did not speak of "incoherence" nor of "loosening of associations". Instead, in the 5th edition of his textbook

(1896), he regarded "Zerfahrenheit" as symptom of a general type of confusion, to be found, for instance, in dementia or in mental deficiency. Kraepelin introduced "Zerfahrenheit" for the first time in his 6th edition (1899) as a specific thought disorder of dementia praecox.

What we call "loosening of associations" in the Bleulerian sense is viewed by Kraepelin as distinguishable from "Zerfahrenheit". He (1903/04, p. 199) compared two ways in which a loosening of the train of thought may occur—"flight of ideas" on the one hand and "Zerfahrenheit" on the other. In a similar way, Bleuler (1911) distinguished several forms of disturbances of associations and thought. One form was "flight of ideas", another and different one was the schizophrenic disturbance which Bleuler also called "Zerfahrenheit", with explicit reference to Kraepelin, in a special section of his chapter on associations.

In her recommendations for DSM–III, Andreasen (1979) criticized Bleuler's concept of "loose associations" and instead proposed Kraepelin's (1919) term of "derailment", characterizing the latter as "graphically descriptive". Nevertheless, in DSM–III, we find "incoherence or marked loosening of association" as the only item for thought or language disorder in the acute phase of schizophrenia. This seems to contradict the arguments of Andreasen (1979), who on the one hand did not agree with the term "loosening of association", and on the other hand found in empirical studies that incoherence is a relatively rare symptom.

3. Phenomenological Description of Schizophrenic Thought Disorder

To further investigate the question of a specific "Zerfahrenheit" as a typical schizophrenic thought disorder, we need to shift from terminological to phenomenological aspects. In a purely descriptive sense, a precursor of "Zerfahrenheit" is flight of ideas, which does not necessarily mean an acceleration (Aschaffenburg 1904), but often consists of excited thinking sustained by strong drive or enthusiastic affect. The flight and loosening of ideas can become so intense that a meaningful connection between the single associations can hardly be detected by the observer.

This also holds true for "Zerfahrenheit", but this form of thought disorder does not merely result from the loosening of associations by acceleration or retardation. "Zerfahrenheit" additionally means that the ideas go on to new areas, that the internal structure gets lost, that there is a derailment, and that associations or fragments of associations which stem from different chains of ideas are linked together. Especially these forms of disturbed associations represent the fundamental schizophrenic symptom which Bleuler and Kraepelin had in mind. Whereas in loosened thinking, or flight of ideas, the associative connections are in principle still present, although it may be difficult to follow them, thinking in the state of "Zerfahrenheit" has lost the rational ties between the associations. If the single elements are fragmented into very small units, "word salad" may even result.

Even more subtle than Bleuler and Kraepelin in the descriptive analysis of thinking and associations was Carl Schneider (1930), who published several detailed studies on schizophrenic thought disorder. One important issue was the similarities between these disturbances and the alterations of associations in thinking at the beginning of sleep or dream, a similarity which, among others, Kraepelin, Bleuler and Jung already had pointed out. According to Carl Schneider, there are three elements in the subjective experience of the patient which constitute the typical schizophrenic "Zerfahrenheit": Hastiness of thinking, loss of normal organization, and loss of connection which leads to separation and disjointed thinking. In accordance with these subjective experiences of altered thinking are the objectively noticeable disturbances of speech: (1) The objective disjointedness, the "Faseln", which means drivel or rambling, where the subunits of a complex train of thought are mixed up, (2) the derailments, where there is a shift from main thought to sidetracks which are not presented in parenthesis, but which are irregularly amalgamated with the main train, and (3) finally the substitutions and the building of gaps. Further formal characteristics of schizophrenic thinking include fusioning, where heterogeneous parts of speech are combined in a grammatically correct but senseless unit, and other phenomena as well. Besides these formal features, Carl Schneider (1930) described some organizing principles of schizophrenic thought and speech which take content into account as well as form, and which contribute to the impression of schizophrenic Zerfahrenheit: paralogies, neologisms, bizarreness, mannerisms, stereotypies, perseverations, iterations, verbigerations, viscosity.

4. Phenomenological Psychopathology of Schizophrenic Thought Disorder

In the following, we shall leave these early European conceptions, because they are relatively well-known in Anglo-American psychiatry through English translations of the classical textbooks, although, as we have seen, they sometimes have been misunderstood. In the years following Bleuler and Kraepelin, phenomenological psychopathology came into being. While there were various methodological influences, for example the early Husserl (1901) and Dilthey (1894), the introduction of phenomenological psychopathology into psychiatry was the contribution of Karl Jaspers (1913), who later held a chair in philosophy in Heidelberg. One of the main aspect of his analysis of abnormal psychic phenomena is intuition and empathy, which constitute the difference between a rational form and a sympathetic form of understanding. Jaspers tried to clarify whether sympathetic understanding of psychic phenomena could be achieved. By focusing upon the inner aspects of psychic experiences, the phenomenological method involved a deliberate extension of the merely descriptive intentions of Kraepelin. According to Jaspers (1913) and the phenomenological school inspired by him, psychic phenomena are psychotic when the subjective experience of the patient is not accessible to the sympathetic understanding of the examiner. Thus, disturbances of thinking are schizophrenic if a comprehending reconstruction of the reported experiences and of the observable language is not possible.

Gruhle (1922, 1929) and Berze (1929) emphasized Jaspers' phenomenological method in their studies of the psychology of schizophrenia. These investigators criticized Bleuler and Kraepelin for putting too much weight on objective disturbances of thinking, associations and language, whereas the inner life of the patient, his consciousness and his subjective experiences, were neglected. The phenomenological method had become very influential, and by 1929 Berze wrote that the internal way of psychopathological analysis seemed to prevail over external descriptions, and that perhaps this change might already have gone too far.

Obviously—concerning phenomenology in the sense of Jaspers, Gruhle and Berze—contemporary developments have been moving in the opposite direction once again. When preparing the concept of thought disorder for DSM–III, Andreasen wrote in 1979 that definitions should be clinical, empirical and atheoretical, and furthermore, that these definitions should emphasize observable verbal behavior as a way of evaluating thought disorder. The so-called atheoretical method and the preference for observable behavior are completely in line with the main principles of DSM–III, which aim at high reliability and therefore try to keep the degree of inference and interpretation very small. Such reverting to the beginning of the century in a neo-Kraepelinian approach tends to eliminate the achievements of phenomenological psychopathology, some of which could be valuable, as for example, the distinction of qualitatively different kinds of thought disorder.

First of all, it is questionable whether disorders of thought and language should be regarded as more or less of the same kind, as Andreasen (1979) advocated in the theoretical part of her paper. Berze and others before him had already argued that an idea in its conception contains all subunits simultaneously, whereas in speech the subunits follow each other successively. Even at the beginning of an idea there is an anticipated scheme—a preexisting order, which guides the production of the idea and the train of thought. Well-ordered thinking fills in the preexisting rule with adequate and correct contents. The importance of these anticipated schemes has been characterized by Beringer (1926) who used the metaphor of "the span of intentional arc".

When Berze (1929) analyzed the act of thinking which may result in speech, he distinguished between three elements. The first and most simple element involves focusing on the topic of the thinking; the second and more differentiated element represents the focusing on the task of thinking. The third element is the focusing on the special scheme or rule of thinking, which, when it is carried out, leads to the realization of the special task of thinking. Not until then do well ordered forms of speech come into being, and this finally results in a meaningful utterance of the idea, or the train of thought, respectively.

Berze's (1929) theory of schizophrenic thought disorder takes into account the content as well as formal elements of the disorder. Hence, he overcomes any strict distinction between disorders of the content and of the form of thought, as introduced by Griesinger (1845). Andreasen (1979), however, is in agreement with Griesinger, and even went further by restricting her usage of the term thought disorder to "formal thought disorder". However, Berze (1929) stresses that the analysis of formal disturbances of thought must also regard the content, because schizophrenic thinking, even if it is not delusional, often is characterized by a special peculiarity of associations. In particular, there are fluent transitions between abnormal phenomena of the form and of the content of thought. As we have seen, Jaspers (1913) and his followers regarded thought disorder as schizophrenic when in phenomenological examination the subjective experience is no longer accessible to sympathetic understanding. Therefore, phenomenological analysis examines the flow of associations and their content in addition to the formal elements. Thinking involves general aspects of the functioning of a person and is embedded in complex qualities such as will, intentions, drives, values, i.e. characteristics which cannot be analyzed under merely formal aspects.

An example of the interdependence of aspects of form and content is fusion, a phenomenon in which two or more ideas that seem to coincide more or less by chance combine in one thought. Berze (1929) noted that elements present in consciousness at the same time are not only linked associatively, but also that there is a tendency of the mind to relate them to each other. Only superior regulation can keep the newly founded relationship between the single elements of thought from being contradictory to the rules of thinking and to empirical knowledge. In schizophrenic thought disorder, this superior regulation is no longer effective. Furthermore, the tendency to establish new relationships in thinking which are illogical to normal judgement is enhanced by the coloring of thinking by emotions. Thus, it can happen that two ideas without a noticeable relationship—at least for the normal observer—are nevertheless connected to each other or even fusioned by a schizophrenic patient because there are relationships in some accompanying parts, e.g., in their emotional atmosphere.

It follows that in a phenomenological approach it is important to take the affective background of the situation into account. In contrast, Kraepelin's and Andreasen's concepts of thought disorder are almost exclusively based on aspects of cognitive functioning. To give an example: One of Gruhle's patients, in a specific affective state, noticed three marble tables in a café and was suddenly convinced that the end of the world was imminent. For Berze (1929), this experience represented an instance of fusioning of a perception (the three tables) with an idea (the forthcoming end of the world). The character of direct evidence, which originally is only justified for the perception (three tables), is now expanded and adapted to the totality of the idea. Therefore, the idea of the forthcoming end of the world gains the same quality that initially was connected to the perception only. The certainty of the idea stems from the certainty of the perception which was fused with it. Thus, the three tables can show the end of the world for the patient.

As result of such fusioning of thinking, which is influenced by emotional factors in addition to pure cognitive functioning, schizophrenic patients may have new experiences and poorly comprehensible strange ideas. If the failure to organize associations is even more severe, the formal rules are increasingly neglected, until a meaningful connection of the elements of thought can no longer be reconstructed. This is characteristic of the transition from strange ideas to typical schizophrenic "Zerfahrenheit". Some other criteria for the analysis of thinking are patterns of thought order, attentiveness, passive sticking to contents, quantitative increase with qualitative devaluation of thoughts, and actualization of peripheral contents.

The results of an "external" examination are not sufficient for a phenomenological approach to "Zerfahrenheit", because this method only permits the registration of observable disturbances of performance. Equally important is the "internal" examination, which, from the phenomenological viewpoint, considers both the subjective experience and the altered relationship of the ego to the experience. According to Berze (1929), the special symptom of "Zerfahrenheit" represents a primary schizophrenic thought disorder and results from a disbalance between affect and cognition. The organizing schemes of thinking, which lead to a meaningful relationship between contents, are weakened, so that affects and emotions reach a disturbing predominance over the sequence and order of thought.

5. The Positive/Negative Conception of Schizophrenic Thought Disorder

Berze's interpretation of "Zerfahrenheit" was based on his concepts of the causes, the psychology, and the course of schizophrenia, which cannot be described here in detail. Like most psychiatrists of his epoche and before, such as Kahlbaum, Kraepelin, Bleuler, Jaspers, Carl Schneider and Kurt Schneider, Berze assumed that dementia praecox is caused by a pathological process in the brain. He characterized a psychotic basic disturbance as essential for the specifically schizophrenic changes. This disturbance may be regarded as the psychopathological equivalent of the basic organic process. Berze characterized this psychopathological disturbance as a "primary insufficiency of mental activity" (1914), and some years later as a "hypotonia of consciousness" (1929). The so-called primary or process symptoms of schizophrenia directly stem from the psychotic basic disturbance. Moreover, the organic process can lead to lesions in the brain and, as a consequence, to defect symptoms which outlast the active process.

Therefore, in a longer lasting illness, the primary, specifically schizophrenic phenomena within the symptomatology mix with symptoms caused by organic changes. Over the course of a lifetime, these secondary features can prevail over the schizophrenic primary symptoms and even replace them; nonetheless, a new exacerbation of the organic process can always cause a reappearance of the primary symptoms.

For Berze, a clear distinction between process symptoms and defect symptoms was the necessary basis for a psychological theory of schizophrenia. Berze answered the decisive question of criteria for this distinction between primary and secondary—of active psychosis and defect—by a subtle psychopathological analysis. He emphasized the importance of the initial phase of the disease and—as a sign of the beginning psychotic process—he tried to find out whether a sympathetic understanding of the psychic experiences of the patient could be achieved by the phenomenological method.

Berze's concepts of an active process and a long lasting defect, as well as his distinction between primary and secondary symptoms, are of special interest for the concept of positive and negative forms of schizophrenia (Sass 1987, 1989). Especially since the appearance of Crow's (1980) paper on negative symptoms in schizophrenia, this concept has been widely accepted, although there are still important variations in their description and measurement. Negative symptoms are usually discussed in the context of the ideas of Jackson (1889) and Reynolds (1858), which have been revived by Wing and Brown (1970), Crow (1980) and Strauss (1985). However, despite its attractiveness, the positive-negative distinction contains several inconsistencies. Originally, Reynolds (1858) described positive and negative symptoms in patients with epilepsy. Negative symptoms were identified with "the negation of vital properties", whereas positive symptoms were thought to consist of "the excess or alterations of vital properties". Jackson (1989) used this distinction in his hierarchical model of the nervous system and of psychiatric disturbances. For Jackson, negative symptoms stem from paralysis affecting a level of functioning in the nervous system. Additionally, however, the paralysis of a higher center causes the functional release of a lower center. The uninhibited but healthy functioning of this lower center gives rise to new forms of behaviour that are defined by Jackson as positive symptoms. This concept implies that positive symptoms are a consequence of negative symptoms (Berrios, 1985). Neither Crow nor Andreasen use the term "negative symptoms" in the Jacksonian sense, because, according to this model, positive symptoms cannot occur without negative symptoms.

Following the discussion about positive and negative types of schizophrenic illness, there have also been efforts to distinguish positive and negative forms of thought and language disorders. Mayer-Gross (1955) and Fish (1962) had already described negative thought disorders which were characterized by a loss of the previous ability to think, whereas in positive thought disorders the patient produces false concepts by blending together incongruous elements. In a similar way Wing and Brown (1970) counted poverty of speech as a negative symptom and incoherence of thought and speech as a florid symptom. Strauss (1985) described thought disorder as a positive symptom in contrast to poverty of speech as a negative symptom. Andreasen (1982) considered negative symptoms as redefinitions of Bleuler's fundamental symptoms; however, based on empirical studies of frequency, she concluded that, as a whole, thought disorder was not pathognomonic for schizophrenia. Furthermore, "loosening of associations" had no empirical value for the task of differentiating between mania and schizophrenia. As a useful diagnostic distinction, however, Andreasen proposed that thought disorder be divided into positive and negative forms. She regarded incoherence as a positive form of thought disorder, whereas poverty of speech and poverty of the content of speech were regarded as negative forms.

There are interesting parallels of these modern Anglo-American opinions to former concepts in German psychopathological theories (see, for example, Gruhle 1922; cf. Sass 1989). Just as relevant are the ideas of Berze (1929), which I already introduced. Berze's distinction between "active process schizophrenia" and "inactive process schizophrenia", which sometimes can be reactivated, resembles Crow's concept of Type I and Type II syndromes, about which etiological and pathophysiological assumptions are also made. In the context of a distinction between positive and negative forms of thought disorder, Berze's differentiation between actual process-symptoms and secondary changes in the defect state is of special significance. For Berze, (1929) only schizophrenic "Zerfahrenheit" is based on the primary process of the illness, whereas other peculiar phenomena of schizophrenic thought and language are a product of secondary distortions in the personality. Examples are the typical peculiarities of post-acute, not completely remitted schizophrenics, summarized as "Verschrobenheit" ("eccentricity"), e.g., bizarreness, mannerisms, stereotypies, stilted speech, verbigerations, schizophasia. Referring to the common use of the term "schizophrenic incoherence", Berze critically commented that there is a false mixing up of schizophrenic "Verschrobenheit" or "eccentricity" of the defect state with schizophrenic "Zerfahrenheit" of the acute phase. In her definition of incoherence in 1979, Andreasen described a similar mixing up of disturbances which were thought to be due to different mechanisms.

Berze's (1929) distinction between acute and chronic schizophrenic symptoms is of special interest for treatment. For example, treatment with neuroleptics, which brings about a reduction of dynamics in drive and affect, seems to be effective especially for the primary process symptoms of the active phase and for those secondary negative phenomena, which can be understood as reactions to positive symptoms. Concerning the disturbances of thought and language, this would apply to "Zerfahrenheit". The true negative forms of thought disorder, however, including primary negative symptoms and "Verschrobenheit" (eccentricity) as a defect symptom in the sense of Berze (1929), can hardly be influenced by neuroleptics. Von Baeyer's (1951) observation that electroconvulsive therapy has no effect on pure defect symptoms can be interpreted in a similar way. True negative phenomena can be reached—if at all—by psychotherapy, behaviour therapy and social therapy, and possibly by activating psychopharmacological agents.For such therapeutic strategies, adequate definitions of symptoms are necessary in order to distinguish between the various types of thought disorder and prevent the mixing up of heterogeneous forms, as can be found even in DSM–III–R. However, the formulation of clear-cut new definitions is difficult, because the detection of thought disorders must be based on a complex clinical evaluation including a subtle personal assessment as well as self reports by the patient. I shall therefore conclude with some phenomenological proposals. Following the distinctions of Berze (1929), the special symptom of "Zerfahrenheit" as a primary schizophrenic thought disorder is registered by the patient in a subjective way, he feels disturbed and handicapped, sometimes helpless or perplexed, occasionally with delusional interpretations of the changed experiences. In addition, the psychiatrist fails to achieve a comprehending reconstruction of the reported experiences of the patient. So the initial process symptom of primary "Zerfahrenheit" has both an objective and a subjective aspect of disturbance. In contrast, "Verschrobenheit", or eccentricity, as a secondary defect symptom of schizophrenic thought disorder, is a phenomenon which in most cases can only be registered objectively. The patient himself considers his strange ideas, thoughts and bizarre language behaviour as the right result of his thinking. Self-confident certainty has replaced the perplexed uncertainty in the state of "Zerfahrenheit".

Summary

For DSM–III, Andreasen (1979) conceptualized an approach to thought, language and communication disorder, and developed a set of definitions which were incorporated into the glossary. These became, as Andreasen had expected, standard for American psychiatrists, and additionally, for all psychiatries influenced by the systematics, symptomatology and concepts of DSM–III. Andreasen equated formal thought disorder more or less with its observable phenomena, the disordered speech of the patient. Consequently, she proposed the use of the term "disordered speech" instead of thought disorder, and her definitions merely attempt to describe signs without aiming to characterize underlying cognitive and affective conditions. This so-called strictly empirical or observational approach results in broad categories of "loosening of associations" and "incoherence" which are derived from Bleuler and Kraepelin.

Phenomenological psychopathology, in contrast, employs methods of empathy and introspection to achieve a comprehending reconstruction of the experiences of the patient. This is done in order to subject the patient's motives, reflections and feelings to a—first of all—formal analysis, which, however, has also to regard the content. The distinction of primary and secondary, of acute process and of defect symptoms, is done by psychological means, and the way in which individual phenomena develop from one another with internal plausibility is heuristically valuable. Further research must show whether by such methods a clinically important distinction between primary "Zerfahrenheit" and secondary "eccentricity" can be achieved. This may be useful for the analysis of thought disorder in addition to, rather than as an alternative to, the approach of DSM–III–R. Divergent approaches are justified because behaviorally oriented researchers attempt to get information by neutral observation exclusively, whereas in the phenomenological tradition, listening to the patient in order to understand his subjective experiences through intuition and empathy is credited as a valid method.

References

Andreasen NC: Thought, language, and communication disorders. I. Clinical assessment, definition of terms, and evaluation of their reliability. II. Diagnostic significance. Archives of General Psychiatry 36: 1315–1321, 1325–1330, 1979

Andreasen NC: Affective and schizophrenic disorders. New York, Brunner/Mazel, 1982

Aschaffenburg G: Experimentelle Studien über Assoziationen. III. Theil: Die Ideenflucht. In : Kraepelin E (Ed): Psychologische Arbeiten, Vol. 4. Leipzig, Engelmann, pp. 235–373, 1904

Baeyer Wv: Die moderne psychiatrische Schockbehandlung. Stuttgart, Thieme, 1951

Berze J: Die primäre Insuffizienz der psychischen Aktivität. Leipzig, Wien, Deuticke, 1914

Berze J (1929) Psychologie der Schizophrenie. In: Berze H, Gruhle HW (Ed): Psychologie der Schizophrenie. Berlin Heidelberg New York, Springer, 1929

Beringer K: Denkstörungen und Sprache bei Schizophrenen. Zeitschrift für die gesamte Neurologie und Psychiatrie 103: 185–197, 1926

Berrios GE: Positive and negative symptoms and Jackson. Arch Gen Psychiatry 42: 95–97, 1985

Bleuler E: Dementia praecox oder die Gruppe der Schizophrenien. Leipzig, Wien, Deuticke, 1911

Bleuler E, Jung CG: Komplexe und Krankheitsursachen bei Dementia praecox. Zentralblatt für Psychiatrie und Nervenheilkunde 3: 220–227, 1908

Crow TJ: Molecular pathology of schizophrenia. More than one dimension of pathology? Brit Med Journal 280: 66–68, 1980

Crow TJ: The two-syndrome concept: Origins and current status. Schiz Bull 11: 471–485, 1985

Dilthey W: Ideen über eine beschreibende und zergliedernde Psychologie (1894). In: Misch G (Ed): Gesammelte Schriften, 4th ed, Vol. V, 139-237, Stuttgart, Teubner, 1974

Fish FJ: Schizophrenia. London, Wright, 1962

Griesinger W: Die Pathologie und Therapie der psychischen Krankheiten. Stuttgart, Krabbe, 1845

Gruhle HW: Die Psychologie der Dementia praecox. Z Neurol 78: 454–471, 1922

Gruhle HW: Psychologie der Schizophrenie. In: Berze J, Gruhle HW: Psychologie der Schizophrenie. Berlin, Springer, 1929

Hoffman RE, Kirstein L, Stopek S, Ciccetti DV: Apprehending schizophrenic discourse: A structural analysis of the listeners task. Brain and Language 15: 207–233, 1982

Hoffman RE, Stopek S, Andreasen NC: A comparative study of manic vs schizophrenic speech disorganisation. Archives of General Psychiatry 43: 831–838, 1986

Husserl E: Logische Untersuchungen. 2. Teil: Untersuchungen zur Phänomenologie und Theorie der Erkenntnis. Halle a.S., Niemeyer, 1901

Jackson H: On postepileptic states: A contribution to the comparative study of insanities. J Ment Science 34: 490–500, 1889

Janet P: Les obsessions et la psychasthénie. Paris, Alcan, 1903

Jaspers K: Allgemeine Psychopathologie (1st ed 1913). 9th ed, Berlin Heidelberg New York, Springer, 1973

Jung CG (Ed): Diagnostische Assoziationsstudien, 2 Vols. Leipzig, Barth, 1906/1910

Jung CG: Über die Psychologie der Dementia praecox. Halle, Marhold, 1907

Kraepelin E: Psychiatrie. 5th ed. Leipzig, Barth, 1896

Kraepelin E : Psychiatrie. 6th ed. Leipzig, Barth, 1899

Kraepelin E: Psychiatrie. 7th ed 2 Vols. Leipzig, Barth, 1903/04

Kraepelin E: Dementia praecox. Chicago, Chicago Med Book, 1919

Mayer-Gross W, Slater E, Roth U: Clinical Psychiatry. Baltimore, Williams and Wilkins, 1955

Peters UH: Die Verwerfungen im Sprach- und Textverhalten Schizophrener. In: Kraus, A, Mundt CH,(Hrsg.): Schizophrenie und Sprache, pp. 8–21. Thieme, Stuttgart, 1991

Reynolds JR: On the pathology of convulsions, with special reference to those of children. Liverpool Med. Chir. J. 2: 1–4, 1858

Sass H: The classification of schizophrenia in the different diagnostic systems. In: Häfner H, Gattaz, WF, Janzarik W (eds): Search for the causes of schizophrenia, pp. 19–28. Berlin Heidelberg New York Tokyo, Springer, 1987

Sass H: The historical evolution of the concept of negative symptoms in schizophrenia. Brit J Psychiatry 155 (suppl. 7): 26–31, 1989

Schneider C: Die Psychologie der Schizophrenen und ihre Bedeutung für die Klinik der Schizophrenie. Leipzig, Thieme, 1930

Schneider K: Clinical Psychopathology (transl. by Hamilton MW). New York, Grune & Stratton, 1959

Snell L: Über die veränderte Sprechweise und die Bildung neuer Worte und Ausdrücke im Wahnsinn. Allgemeine Zeitschrift für Psychiatrie 9: 11–24, 1852

Stransky E: Lehrbuch der allgemeinen und speziellen Psychiatrie. I. Allg. Teil. Leipzig, F.C. Vogel, 1914

Strauss JS: Negative symptoms: Future developments of the concept. Schiz Bull 11: 457–460, 1985

Tress W, Pfaffenberger U, Frommer, J: Zur Patholinguistik schizophrener Texte. Eine vergleichende Untersuchung an Schizophrenen, Depressiven, Hirnorganikern und Gesunden. Nervenarzt 55: 488–495, 1984

Wing JK, Brown GN: Institutionalism and schizophrenia. Cambridge, Cambridge University Press, 1970

Wundt W (1874) Grundzüge der physiologischen Psychologie. Leipzig, Engelmann, 1874

M. Spitzer, F.A. Uehlein
M.A. Schwartz, C. Mundt
(eds.): Phenomenology
Language & Schizophrenia.
Springer-Verlag, New York, 1992

Word-Associations in Experimental Psychiatry: A Historical Perspective

Manfred Spitzer

1. Introduction

The concept of association is one of the oldest and most fruitful in psychology. It has been used to describe and as well to explain various aspects of the experience and behavior of human beings. It also has been used to describe as well as to explain various aspects of psychopathology, especially pathological verbal behavior, in the field of psychiatry.

"We study associations in order to make inferences about the nature of human thought, and these associations are cast in the language which embodies the thought. [...] To the extent that verbal behavior is the mediator of thought, modern association theory is a theory of thought." (Deese 1965, p. 4).

This paper is focused on empirical (rather than conceptual) studies of associations in psychiatry, and therefore mainly deals with experimental work on the associations between words (rather than associations between concepts, ideas, or images).[1] A historical perspective is taken in order to show some of the conceptual as well as methodological roots of more recent approaches and findings.

1.1 How the Mind Works: Association Psychology

Aristotle, in a short manuscript on *Memory and Recollection,* discussed ways to hunt up memories by either reconstructing the temporal succession of events, or by thinking of things or events which are similar to, contrast with, or are in temporal or spatial continuity with the event or thing to be remembered. Associations can go "for instance from milk to white, from white to air, from air to damp" (p. 305), i.e., in various ways according to similarity, opposition, and contiguity.

Detailed accounts of associations and their workings were subsequently given by the English empiricists John Locke and David Hume. The physician David Hartley later established these ideas as a foundation for psychology. As Boring explained:

---

1 These studies have been supported by a grant (Sp364/1–1) from the *Deutsche Forschungsgemeinschaft.*

"He took Locke's little–used title for a chapter, 'the association of ideas,' made it the name of a fundamental law, reiterated it, wrote a psychology around it, and thus created a formal doctrine with a definite name, so that a school could repeat the phrase after him for a century and thus implicitly constitute him as its founder. [...] Whoever discovered 'association,' there is not the least doubt that Hartley prepared it for its ism" (Boring 1950, p. 194).

Various "laws of association" were formulated by Thomas Brown, James Mill, and John Stuart Mill. Brown contrasted the primary laws of association—similarity, contrast, and temporal and spatial contiguity—to the secondary laws which influence the establishment of association, viz., duration and vividness of a sensation, the frequency of its repetition, the lack of interfering material, the affective state, physical condition, habits, and personality of the person.

In his *Principles of Psychology*, William James devoted an entire chapter to *Associations*, where he summarized the findings of the by then well established school of thought called association psychology. Associations and the laws that connected them were meant to explain the succession of ideas and the flow of thought. In his *Psychology: Briefer Course*, James clearly laid out his thoughts on the order of ideas:

"But as a matter of fact, What determines a particular path? Why do we at a given time and place proceed to think of b if we have just thought of a, and at another time and place why do we think, not of b, but of c? Why do we spend years straining after a certain scientific or practical problem, but all in vain—our thought unable to evoke the solution we desire? And why, some day, walking in the street with our attention miles away from that quest, does the answer saunter into our minds as carelessly as if it had never been called for—suggested, possibly, by the flowers on the bonnet of the lady in front of us, or possibly by nothing that we can discover?

The truth must be admitted that thought works under strange conditions. Pure 'reason' is only one out of a thousand possibilities in the thinking of each of us. Who can count all the silly fancies, the grotesque suppositions, the utterly irrelevant reflections he makes in the course of a day? Who can swear that his prejudices and irrational opinions constitute a less bulky part of his mental furniture than his clarified beliefs? And yet, the mode of genesis of the worthy and the worthless in our thinking seems the same" (James 1892/1984, p. 224).

It is important to keep in mind that in association psychology up to the time of William James, associations were meant to be associations between *ideas*, i.e., between entities in the mental realm.

1.2 How the Brain Works: Associations in Speculative Neurophysiology

With the advent of physiology and neuroanatomy, the term "association" gained a new "biological" meaning: Not ideas, but brain parts—neurons—were thought to be associated, i.e., connected in a specific way. This stimulated several writers, including Sigmund Exner, Sigmund Freud, and William James, to engage in a sort of "speculative neurophysiology", which dealt with the associations and functioning of neurons.

The concept of neurons had just been introduced by Waldeyer in 1891, and it was energy (viz., electrical currents), rather than information that was thought to propagate through the paths in the nervous system.[2] Because of limited knowledge at the time, these early writers could only stipulate that there are associations between *brain* processes. As James put it: "... so far as association stands for a *cause*, it is between *processes in the brain* ..." (James 1892/1984, p. 225, italics in original). However, it is important to note that James avoided any reference to ideas: the flow of the ideas was what he wanted to explain. Therefore, he had to avoid referring to ideas in his explanation altogether, at least in principle.

In his review of the actual laws of associations, however, James had to use mentalistic terms, and here it becomes clear that his explicit "reductive" approach was merely a program and not a finding. The law of contiguity, for example, was introduced as follows:

"... objects once experienced together tend to become associated in the imagination, so that when any one of them is thought of, the others are likely to be thought of also... the most natural way to account for it [the law] is to conceive it as a result of the laws of habit in the nervous system; in other words, it is to ascribe it to a physiological cause" (James 1890/1981, p. 529).

As we can see, a mentalistic description of the association law is given first, and then, a physiological cause is stipulated. Along the same lines, the arguments in Exner's *Project of a Physiological Explanation of Mental Phenomena*[3] (1894) and in Freud's *Project for a Scientific Psychology*[4] (1895-1900) were constructed. All these approaches remained speculative. In the case of Freud, physiology was "officially abandoned" with the publication of *The Interpretation of Dreams* in 1900, and thereafter. Associations between ideas, and even between words, though in a less rigid sense than in association psychology, remained at the heart of the matter of psychoanalysis. The reader need only turn to one of Freud's most innovative and influential works, *The Psychopathology of Everyday Life*, in order to verify the importance of word–associations for Freud's thinking.

2. Word Associations: Francis Galton and Wilhelm Wundt

The technique of word–associations was introduced in 1879 by Francis Galton. In his *Inquiries into Human Faculty and its Development* (1883), Galton gave a detailed account of experiments he conducted on himself.

---

2 In addition to James, Sigmund Exner (1894) and Sigmund Freud (1895-1900, first published in 1950) wrote physiological associationist accounts of mental functioning. In these models, priming and inhibition play a crucial explanatory role for a great number of mental processes (Spitzer 1984).
3 Original German title: *Entwurf zu einer physiologischen Erklärung der psychischen Erscheinungen*.
4 These writings consisted of letters to his friend, Wilhelm Fliess. Freud abandoned such thinking with the publication of his Interpretation of Dreams (1900), however, the influence of such "physiological" though on his theory has been shown convincingly by several authors (cf. Hobson & McCarley 1977, Pribram & Gill 1976, Sulloway 1979). The letters to Fliess were finally published after Freud's death in 1950.

"When we attempt to trace the first steps in each operation of our minds, we are usually baulked by the difficulty of keeping watch, without embarrassing the freedom of its action. The difficulty is [...] especially due to the fact that the elementary operations of the mind are exceedingly faint and evanescent, and that it requires the utmost painstaking to watch them properly. It would seem impossible to give the required attention to the processes of thought, and yet to think as freely as if the mind had been in no way preoccupied. The peculiarity of the experiment I am about to describe is that I have succeeded in evading this difficulty. My method consists in allowing the mind to play freely for a very brief period, until a couple or so of ideas have passed through it, and then, while the traces or echoes of those ideas are still lingering in the brain, to turn the attention upon them with a sudden and complete awakening; to arrest, to scrutinize them, and to record their exact appearance" (Galton 1883, p. 185).

Galton first noted the ideas that came to his mind when he walked outside and watched various objects. Later he developed the technique of constructing a list, partly covered by a book, displaying only one word, to which he formed associations that he wrote down. He even measured the time it took him to do so.

"I held a small chronograph, which I started by pressing a spring the moment the word caught my eye, and which stopped of itself the instant I released the spring; and this I did so soon as about a couple of ideas in direct association with the word had arisen in my mind" (Galton 1883, p. 188).

From his work, Galton drew far–reaching consequences, especially if one looks at it from a psychiatric perspective.

"I have desired to show how whole strata of mental operations that have lapsed out of ordinary consciousness, admit of being dragged into light, recorded and treated statistically, and how the obscurity that attends the initial steps of our thoughts can thus be pierced and dissipated... Perhaps the strongest of the impressions left by these experiments regards the multifariousness of the work done by the mind in a state of half–unconsciousness, and the valid reason they afford for believing in the existence of still deeper strata of mental operations, sunk wholly below the level of consciousness, which may account for such mental phenomena as cannot otherwise be explained" (Galton 1879, p. 162; see also Galton 1883, pp. 202–203).[5]

In Germany, Wilhelm Wundt founded the world's first psychological laboratory in 1879, where a great deal of research on word associations would either be performed or at least stimulated. James McKeen Cattell, Wundt's first self–appointed assistant, developed an apparatus to measure reaction times, which was activated by movement of the lips. By means of this apparatus, the amount of time that word–associations take could be measured in the word-association task. Using these methods, Cattell found that when familiar words are used as stimuli, different people tend to give the same word as a response. Responses to concrete nouns were made

---

5 It is likely that Freud knew Galton's work on associations, although he does not mention Galton in this respect and claims to have developed the method of free associations by "following a dark presentiment" (cf. Jones 1978, p. 293). The similarities between Galton and Freud are, at any rate, striking. In an article full of antiscientific prejudices and unproven psychoanalytic claims, Zilboorg (1950) interpreted Freud's departure from the scientific method of Galton in the study of associations as a great advantage. In view of more recent developments, the opposite must rather be said.

faster than responses to abstract nouns (cf. Cattell & Bryant 1889). Emil Kraepelin worked in Wundt's laboratory, and was not only highly influenced by the empirical spirit of Wundt (see Hoff, this volume), but also was able to use some of the methods developed in Wundt's laboratory for purposes of experimental psychopathology.[6]

3. Experimental Psychopathology Using Word Associations: Emil Kraepelin and Gustav Aschaffenburg

Most psychiatrists regard the work of Emil Kraepelin on associations as theoretically uninteresting and practically irrelevant. After all, Kraepelin became famous for his clinical distinctions, his classification system introduced in several editions of a multi–volume textbook on (clinical) psychiatry. Kraepelin was not, and still is not, famous for his work in cognitive psychology and experimental psychopathology, although he himself was highly interested in these activities.

In 1892 Kraepelin published a monograph, *On the Modification of Primitive Mental Processes by some Drugs*[7], in which he used several experimental neuropsychological techniques. The first chapter of this book contains detailed discussions of methodological issues. For example, with respect to the measurement of word–associations, Kraepelin scrutinized Cattell's apparatus for measuring voice (i.e., lip–movement) activated reaction times in detail, evaluated the accuracy of the apparatus, and discussed statistical methods to calculate the results. He spent ten pages (pp. 22–32) to show that medians (he called them "possible means") are more appropriate than arithmetic means for the correct estimation of the "real" value of reaction times, because medians are less sensitive to outlyers.

Kraepelin also discussed the ways of classifying associations. Referring to Wundt (1893, vol. II, p. 455) and Wundt's disciple Trautscholdt (1883, p. 216), he classified word–associations as either internal (conceptual) or external (due to temporal and spatial contiguity)—a scheme derived from classical association laws. However, he introduced simplifications and additions to this scheme (see table 1) and discussed every type of association with great care. In general, he was not satisfied with the systems used in contemporary psychology, mainly because of their lack of reliability and their questionable validity.

---

6 This article is focused on psychopathology, i.e., on experiments with psychiatric patients and pathological phenomena, or on investigations with normal subjects, which were conducted by psychiatrists, and hence influential on their theories and thinking. It is beyond the scope of this paper to even summarize the enormous work on the associations of normal people done by psychologists in the two decades before and after 1900. To give just an example: The psychologist Hugo Münsterberg, who taught in Freiburg and later became professor of psychology at Harvard University, wrote four volumes (*Beiträge zur experimentellen Psychologie/Contributions to Experimental Psychology*) in which, among other things, he argued that there are three types of personalities which can be discerned by the way they react in word–association experiments (cf. Jung 1906a, p. 434).

7 *Über die Beeinflussung einfacher psychischer Vorgänge durch einige Arzneimittel.*

The results of word–association experiments conducted by Kraepelin and his successors are remarkable for several reasons: From a methodological point of view, these studies remain pertinent even in the light of currently used sophisticated standards. Great care was taken in the collection of data, large sets of data were obtained, and thoughtful analyses and interpretations were presented. Of course, what these authors lacked were inferential statistical methods. However, their detailed descriptions of results makes data re-analysis possible, using statistical procedures that were developed long after the original data had been gathered and published.[8]

In a "pilot study", using himself as the only subject, Kraepelin found a *decrease* in reaction time and an increase in external associations, notably in *clang* associations, under the influence of a moderate dose (30 g) of alcohol (cf. Kraepelin 1892, p. 52–53). From his results, the correlation between these two variables can be calculated. It turns out to be quite high, –.647, which means that 42% of the variability in the type of associations can be interpreted in terms of speed. Kraepelin further found that controlled thought processes, such as the logical subsumption of a stimulus word under a concept rather than free association, were disrupted by alcohol. Therefore, he demonstrated the "transition from associations that needed some mental effort to more simple or basic associations given by habit" (Kraepelin 1892, p. 54).

A repetition of the alcohol experiment with tea (pp. 107–125) did not yield any clear–cut results, but was at least suggestive of some opposite effects of tea on reaction time and type of association as compared to the effects of alcohol.

A large number of experiments on word–associations in normal subjects were carried out by Aschaffenburg (1896, 1899, 1904).[9] He used three methods: (1) free association to a word by writing down all the words which come to mind, (2) free association to a word by writing down the first word which comes to mind, and, (3) free verbal association to a word spoken by the experimenter, measuring reaction time with a voice key (Aschaffenburg used a modified version of Cattell's device). Among the many interesting results of Aschaffenburg's first study of normal subjects, the following findings seem to be of particular interest:

---

8 The correlation coefficient was introduced by Pearson in 1907. The concept of statistical significance had been developed by Fischer in 1925. The t-distribution and the respective method of testing for statistical significance had been described by Gosset in 1908 (cf. Bortz 1989).

9 At that time, Aschaffenburg worked together with Kraepelin, who among others served as a subject. Moreover, the results of that work were published in the first volume of a series named *Psychological Studies* which was edited by Kraepelin and devoted entirely to the experimental study of normal and pathological mental phenomena. All this work received little attention from the psychiatric community for reasons partly discussed later in the paper. Only the investigations on the work curve became known to some extent. In my view, the experimental work done by Kraepelin and his coworkers represents an example of how excellent work can be forgotten because it is too advanced for a given time. Moreover, little or nothing was known about the possible neuronal basis of the phenomena under experimental scrutiny, which meant that little or no inferences regarding underlying mechanisms could be drawn, and no "cross-fertilization" was possible. Nonetheless, the general spirit of the work, the striving for methodological improvement, the great care taken regarding measurements, and the thoughtful discussions of results certainly put Kraepelin and his group among the ranks of sophisticated cognitive neuropsychologists.

Table 1: Classification schemes of word–association types

Source	Scheme		
Association psychology	the 4 "laws" of association	(internal)	similarity opposition
		(external)	temporal contiguity spatial contiguity
Trautscholdt/ Wundt	internal	coordination	similarity opposition
		sub– / superordination	superordination subordination
		dependency	cause–effect means–ends
	external	part / whole	part to whole whole to part
		independently coexisting ideas	
		succession, sound	right order changed order
		succession, vision	right order changed order
Kraepelin	internal	coordination/ subordination	
		predicate relations	
	external	temporal and spatial coexistence	
		speech reminiscences	
		similarity by clang	
Aschaffenburg	"semantic"	internal	coordination/subordination predicate relations cause–effect
		external	temporal and spatial coexistence identity speech reminiscences

	"non–semantic"	effects of sound	word complementations
			clang and rhyme
			      making sense
			      not making sense

		effect of mere stimulation	repetition repetition of a not directly preceding association association to a previous word reactions without any noticeable relation

The first method produced the largest inter-individual variety of responses. With respect to the second and third method, the following can be said: Clang–associations increased under the influence of fatigue and alcohol. Absolute reaction times varied considerably in normal subjects. When two–syllable words were used, there was less intra-individual variation in absolute reaction times in normal subjects compared to one-syllable words. Indirect associations were rare (about 4%) and took longer than direct associations. External associations, as defined above (cf. Aschaffenburg in table 1) were more frequent than internal associations, and there was a tendency for them to be given faster. Monosyllable words produced faster reaction times (900–1200 ms), when compared to two–syllable words (1100–1400ms). However, reaction times were more reliable using two–syllable words. Most individuals tended to give nouns as associations (85–92% nouns, 1–9% verbs) although a smaller number of individuals responds with fewer nouns (59–68% nouns and 22–31% verbs).

In a second study, Aschaffenburg (1899) investigated the effects of fatigue on word associations (see figure 1). He used his colleagues as subjects and gave them lists of words regarding which they were instructed to note word associations at about 9 p.m., midnight, 3 a.m. and 6 a.m. Aschaffenburg analyzed the data according to the scheme of association-types as used in the previous study. He also obtained reaction times from some of his subjects. The effects of fatigue were summarized as follows:

"The general finding of the experiments at nighttime is a decrease in the quality of associations. Conceptual relations are replaced by loose associations to the clang of the stimulus word, whose meaning seems to have no influence upon the reaction. We did not find any exception to this rule, although the effect size of the phenomenon varied to a considerable extent..." (Aschaffenburg 1899, p. 48, transl. by the author).

Aschaffenburg noticed that the clang relation was not restricted to rhyming words but could further extend to meaningless rhyming syllables. Moreover, in some cases, he noticed not so much rhyming associations but completions of words according to clang characteristics.

In general, focused conceptual relations (Aschaffenburg: "high-quality associations") gave way to relations which relied on more "material" or "sensual" aspects of the words ("low-quality associations"), especially to sound-characteristics.[10] The latter was furthermore found to be the case in mentally ill patients (see below) and, to a degree, in one subject who was investigated while suffering from a severe flu. Aschaffenburg noted that increasing fatigue did not lead to an increase in totally unrelated associations nor to an increase in simple repetition, as one might have expected.[11]

---

10 Aschaffenburg was eager not to give the impression that he was "pathologizing" poetry: "The tendency to rhyme has to be unquestionably interpreted as a worsening of the association process. This view may provoke fewer contradictory voices, however, if we emphasize that there is a sharp distinction between 'rhyme' and 'poetry'" (Aschaffenburg 1899, p. 50).

11 In fact, from the data on one subject diagnosed as suffering from some form of "neurasthenia", Aschaffenburg concluded that simple fatigue and neurasthenia are quite different. This subject had an unusually high number of stereotype repetitions, and no clang associations (except when he was very tired; cf. Aschaffenburg 1899, pp. 54–55).

Figure 1: Effect of increasing fatigue on the frequency (means and standard errors) of clang–related associations, defined as rhyming words, meaningless rhyming syllables, and completions of words according to clang–characteristics. Word–associations were obtained from 9 subjects. 5 subjects were given 4 blocks (at the 4 specified times of night) of 50 monosyllable words each, in 4 subjects, 4 blocks of 100 two–syllable words were used. At 3 a.m., the difference to 9 p.m. is significant (two–tailed t–test; p = .0471); at 6 a.m., this difference is highly significant (two–tailed t–test; p = .0018). Data from Aschaffenburg 1899, tables III, V, VII, IX, XI, XIII, XV, XVII, and XIX, re-analyzed.

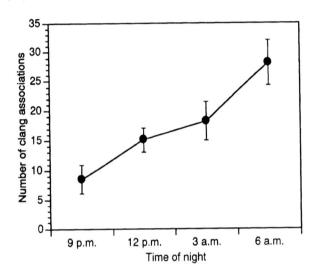

"Put into a scheme, the process of association displays the following changes under the influence of fatigue: Tight connections between the stimulus word and the reaction are loosened and increasingly replaced by types of associations which come into existence because of long standing habits. In particular, relations of language [as opposed to conceptual relations] prevail. However, even these tend to become increasingly superficial. The stimulus concept, as well as the spontaneous associations to it, are no longer apprehended as such, but produces its effects merely by its sound, pitch and rhythm. If fatigue is increased, the tendency increases to string one clang to another clang, until the new association similar in clang ceases to be a word, and all that remains is the pure clang, the syllable which sounds similar" (Aschaffenburg 1899, pp. 49-50, transl. by the author).

Aschaffenburg discussed his findings on clang associations in terms of everyday observations. For example, he stated that jokes which involve rhyming are more likely to make people laugh if they are tired or drunk or both (cf. Kraepelin's findings on clang associations and alcohol). From the apparently parallel course of measurements of simple reaction time and clang associations, Aschaffenburg drew the conclusion that the latter are caused predominantly by somatic fatigue, which was thought to increase motor activity, to decrease conceptual performance, and for these reasons increase clang associations. His comments are worth quoting at some length:

"A direct confirmation of the tight connection between rhyme and—though almost entirely somatic—fatigue can be obtained from a look at any visitors book on mountain tops and in mountain huts. Of course, I disregard those products which obviously had been written under the influence of alcohol. It seems as though everyone has to admit that a poem which really is rich in content only rarely ornates the visitors books of mountain huts. This is true and not all of these cases are instances of uneducated people having authored these poems. Rather, in the quietness of their studies, these authors would be ashamed of having written such thoughtless rhymes" (Aschaffenburg 1899, pp. 51-52, transl. by the author).

The hypothesis of a simple "correlation" (the mathematical concept of a correlation coefficient had not yet been established in scientific practice) between somatic fatigue and clang associations was questioned later on by Hahn (1910) and by Jung (see below) on the grounds of further detailed empirical investigations.

In his third paper on associations, Aschaffenburg (1904) described the associations of 11 patients (who would most likely be classified as suffering from bipolar disorder by present day standards) in great detail. His material consisted of 12,900 associations, and in 6150 of these he measured reaction times. Some of the patients were examined several times in different stages (manic and depressed) of their disorder. Aschaffenburg discussed the findings of every single patient in great detail so that it is difficult to draw general conclusions. However, as in his other papers, he provided a detailed report of the results so that it is possible to re–analyze them. In general, he found a higher degree of distractibility, no increased attention, and an increase in clang associations in manic patients. Clang associations were also noticed in some catatonic patients. Reaction time data did *not* confirm the clinical impression that the associations in manic patients were more rapid.

4. Carl Gustav Jung: Methodological Refinements and More Results

Working under the supervision of Eugen Bleuler in the famous Burghölzli psychiatric hospital, from the year 1902 on Carl Gustav Jung conducted a number of studies on associations in normal people and in patients. Just as in many of the above–mentioned studies, a word was spoken to a person who then had to say aloud, as quickly as possible, whatever came to his or her mind upon hearing the word. For example, if the word "white" was spoken by the experimenter, most people responded by saying the word "black". In his first lecture (Antrittsvorlesung), entitled *On the Psychopathological Significance of the Association–Experiment*[12], Jung commented on this method as follows:

"The experiment is similar to any experiment conducted on physiology... By means of a stimulus word, we bring a mental stimulus to the mental organ. We introduce an idea into the consciousness of the subject, and then let us notice what further

12 *Die Psychopathologische Bedeutung des Assoziationsexperiments.*

idea has thereby been produced in the brain of the subject. This way we can obtain a large number of relations between ideas, or associations, respectively, within a relatively short period of time. From this material, and by comparisons between subjects, we are able to state that a given stimulus in most cases leads to a particular reaction. Hence, we possess a means to study the 'laws of the associations of ideas'" (Jung 1906b/1979a, p. 431).

Jung already attempted to established tentative norms for "correct" associations (i.e., those that are given by most people). Such norms had to be established if the method of word-associations was to become clinically relevant. The enthusiasm of Jung for the method of word-associations is clearly visible in the following statement:

"You associate just in the way you are. The psychiatrist Weygand recently stated most appropriately: 'Tell me how you associate, and I tell you who you are.' This is not an empty statement" (Jung 1906b/1979a, p. 438)

Using a stop watch[13], Jung further carried out studies on reaction times, which were also published in 1906 (*On reaction time in the association experiment*).

A detailed paper, entitled *Experimental study on the associations of healthy people*[14], which Jung published together with Franz Riklin in 1904 and 1906, contains data on about 35,000 associations from about 150 subjects (cf. Jung 1906a/1979a) and is worth a closer look.

Jung introduced new independent variables, gender and educational level, in order to clarify the reasons for the considerable variation in the data on word-associations. He also used a rather modern technique to study the influence of attention: He had his subjects perform the word association test under normal conditions and then under one of two conditions that were thought to divert attention: Subjects had either to visually imagine the object denoted by the stimulus word, or had to make strokes on a piece of paper with a pencil according to the rhythm of a metronome. With both methods for the diversion of attention, the frequency of conceptually-driven ("internal") associations decreased while clang associations increased (see figure 2). Jung concluded that the increase of clang associations is not a result of a general somatic fatigue, as hypothesized by Aschaffenburg, but rather represents an attentional phenomenon.

"Whenever we have been successful in diverting attention during the experiment, i.e., in those cases in which the conditions of the experiments have been accomplished, we found the same phenomenon, viz., an increase in external and clang associations and a decrease of the internal associations. That is to say, we saw a shift in the direction of the habitual and of what is already primed, i.e., mechanical visual or speech relations" (Jung 1906a/1979a, p. 149-150, transl. by the author).
If attention decreases, associations become increasingly superficial, i.e., their value decreases (Jung 1906a/1979a, pp. 58-59).

---

13 Jung thought that a more sophisticated method of measuring reaction time was not indicated because of its possible influences on attentional factors, especially in mentally ill patients (cf. Jung 1906c/1979, p. 241).
14 *Experimentelle Untersuchungen über die Assoziationen Gesunder.*

Figure 2: Frequency of 3 types of word-associations in 3 normal subjects under 2 conditions: Attention was either not influenced ("normal" condition) or diverted by an imagery or motor task, respectively. A decrease in "conceptually driven" internal associations and an increase in associations due to clang is clearly visible (inferential statistics were not performed due to the small number of subjects). Data from Jung (1903/1978, pp. 180-181), re-analyzed.

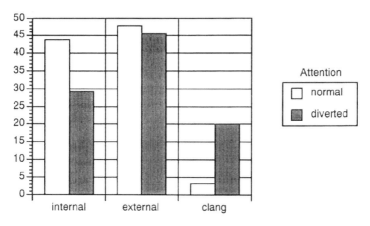

Like Aschaffenburg, Jung found a decrease in internal and an increase in external associations under diverted attention in addition to the increase in clang associations. When Jung analyzed the data for subjects with high versus low educational level separately, he found a considerably larger effect size, i.e., a larger increase in clang associations under diverted attention conditions in the high educational level group (see figure 3, for further discussion, see section 9.4).

Jung's discussion of his findings was rather advanced. He thought that attention serves the purpose of maintaining a particular idea within consciousness and stabilizing its direction or goal. Such a goal directed idea ("Richtungsvorstellung") facilitates associations which are related to the idea and the goal and inhibits non-related associations.

"Now, if the attentional tone of a non-related idea is increased, the goal-directed idea is repressed from the focus [of attention], i.e., it loses its [attentional] tone. Accordingly, the intensity of its effects decreases, and thereby the differences of the thresholds of all the other associations decrease. The selection of the goal-directed association becomes increasingly difficult and subject to the law of frequency. That is to say, those associations which constitute the most frequent content of consciousness by practice and habit and therefore have low thresholds, will push forward. The law of frequency now takes over the role which was played by the goal-directed idea" (Jung 1906a/1979a, p. 150).

Jung's comments on clang associations are also worth detailed consideration. In the first place, he clearly saw the need to assume that these associations are inhibited during normal thought:

"Normally, clang-associations are inhibited, because they are usually extremely inappropriate for the process of thinking, and therefore are switched off. Hence, there will always be a tendency to suppress clang-associations. It will be the stronger, the smaller the disturbance of attention is, and vice versa" (Jung 1906a/1979a, p. 188).

Jung also observed a negative relationship between clang-associations and mediated associations (i.e., associations between two ideas which are related only by a third one) which he interestingly interpreted as follows: Mediated associations are produced by a disturbance of attention which is not large enough to produce clang associations but suffices to divert the focus from the conceptually driven goal-directed idea to a weakly related one (cf. Jung 1906a/1979a, pp. 188-189).

Figure 3: Percentage of clang associations in subjects with high and low educational level, with and without distraction of attention (data from Jung 1906a/1979a, re-analyzed). While the increase of clang association due to attentional distraction is highly significant in both groups, the effect is much larger in subjects with high educational level .

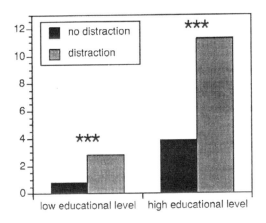

Jung definitely found mediated associations and was strongly opposed to those researchers, Münsterberg, for example, who doubted their existence. He blamed methodological drawbacks in their investigations for the fact that they were not able to find any.

"Münsterberg boldly states 'there are no mediated associations by unconscious links'; however, he just did not find any" (Jung 1906a/1979a, p. 191).

In sum, Jung found that word-associations are influenced by attention, educational level, and individual differences. He did not observe major differences between men and women. Individual differences were thought to be due to various factors, such as the tendency of some people to respond with verbs rather than nouns (this tendency was even found to run in families (cf. Jung 1906b/1979a, p. 438), and several "types" of responders (the objective type and the egocentric type). An exhaustive review of Jung's findings is far beyond the scope of this paper.

5. C.G. Jung and E. Bleuler: Associations and Schizophrenia

Jung strongly believed in the clinical applicability and usefulness of the method of word-associations:

"... the association experiment, more or less as we have conducted it in our clinic for several years now, will play an important role in the future diagnosis of mental disorders ..." (Jung 1906c/1979, p. 243)

He published several papers in which he gave detailed accounts of single patients whom he investigated with this method. In these, he commented on the peculiar way in which the associations were changed in individuals with epilepsy, factitious disorder, hysteria, and finally in a subject who was a thief (Jung 1905/1979a, 1906a/1979a, 1906b/1979a, 1906c/1979a)

Most noteworthy in this context, however, are Jung's investigations of patients with dementia praecox. Given the fact that Jung worked under the supervision of Eugen Bleuler, the influence of Jung's work on Bleuler's concept of schizophrenia as it developed during that period of time can hardly be underestimated.

Jung even explained single symptoms in terms of word-associations, as can be seen from the following example from his article *The Psychology of Dementia Praecox* written in 1906. According to Jung, negativism is a symptom of a rather "mild" disturbance of associations, because the negatively associated word is strongly associated to the original word (as, for example, "black" to "white").

"... Why are contrast associations so frequent? They are closest to one another. In ordinary language, we can observe a similar thing: words which represent ordinary contrasts are strongly associated and therefore belong to well-established relationships in language (black-white, etc.). In some primitive languages there is sometimes even only *one single* word for two opposite (contrasting) ideas. Hence, in order to produce the phenomenon of negativism, ... we need only a slight disturbance of mind" (Jung 1906/1979, p. 19, transl. by the author).

Sommer (1899) had found an increase of the frequency in clang associations and of mere repetitions in catatonic patients, which was interpreted as a sign of somewhat more disturbed associational processes in these patients.

Although Jung thought that the processes of association were somewhat different from normal in dementia praecox, he opposed the view that thought processes of such patients are totally different from normal. Such a view had been proposed by the Austrian psychiatrist Erwin Stransky on the grounds on his empirical investigations of thought disorder. Stransky had coined the term "intrapsychic ataxia" to literally denote the way in which the associations behave in patients suffering from dementia praecox. However, from the experiments conducted by Kraepelin, Aschaffenburg and Jung, it seemed obvious that associational processes could gradually shift, and that minor changes in activation or inhibition of associations or in the allocation of selective attention could lead to pronounced behavioral changes. Therefore, Jung commented on the position held by Stransky:

"Generally speaking, I think that it is always a daring undertaking in the natural sciences to suppose something totally (toto coelo) new and absolutely unfamiliar. In dementia praecox, where in fact innumerable normal associations exist, we have to expect that the laws of normal mental life are in place, until we learn to know the faint processes which are [different from normal and] truly specific [to schizophrenia]. However, our knowledge of the normal psyche is restricted to a primitive level. This is detrimental for psychopathology, where the only thing we can agree upon is the vagueness of the concepts that we use" (Jung 1906/1979, p. 8).

One has to be parsimonious with new principles to explain phenomena: Therefore, I reject the clear and witty hypothesis of Stransky (Jung 1906/1979, p. 23).

It is not entirely clear what position Bleuler took in his famous monograph on schizophrenia, first published in 1911, because he oscillated between the *descriptive* and the *explanatory* use of "association" in his writings. A few quotes from Bleuler's book on schizophrenia may illustrate this point:

"In this malady the associations lose their continuity. Of the thousands of associative threads which guide our thinking, this disease seems to interrupt, quite haphazardly, sometimes such single threads, sometimes a whole group, and sometimes even large segments of them. In this way, thinking becomes illogical and often bizarre. Furthermore, the associations tend to proceed along new lines, of which so far the following are known to us: two ideas, fortuitously encountered, are combined into one thought, the logical form being determined by incidental circumstances. Clang-associations receive unusual significance, as do indirect associations" (Bleuler 1911/1950, p. 14).

This is the second paragraph of chapter 1, entitled *The Fundamental Symptoms*, and Bleuler clearly meant to *describe* the clinical picture of schizophrenia, using the term "association" in a descriptive sense. This is not the case in the following quotes, where "association" in meant to have explanatory significance:

"Of course, the association disturbances are responsible for most of the confusion in logical thinking. Logical thinking is a reproduction of associations which are equivalent or analogous to those which experience has taught us. Through the loosening of the customary connections between concepts, thinking becomes detached from experience and takes a turn into deviant pathways" (Bleuler 1911/1950, p. 80)

Note that in this quote, associations represent an explanatory concept for overt psychopathology. In this passage, it is not false associations that are being described, and deviant pathways of thought are explained by association-mechanisms. The explanatory function of the concept of association is even more obvious in the following passage:

"The association disturbances were conceived of as being primary; from these we can derive the majority of secondary symptoms: Although this cannot be done with absolute certainty, they can still be understood in terms of this uniform viewpoint" (Bleuler 1911/1950, p. 355).

A disorder of associational processes is seen as the primary event, from which other symptoms can be derived.

To conclude: Jung had carried out his experiments in the famous Burghölzli Hospital, chaired by Eugen Bleuler, who drew heavily upon Jung's experiments as well as upon a background in association psychology when he formed his concept of schizophrenia. In Bleuler's view, schizophrenia is a disorder of the associations. Because of the indeterminateness of the term "association", and, in particular, because the term has to serve a descriptive and explanatory function, it is not entirely clear what his theory really meant. However, it is quite possible that this very fact has made Bleuler's theory so appealing , because many aspects could be subsumed under the heading "disordered association". Bleuler himself engaged in some "speculative neurophysiology", writing about hypothesized weakened nervous activity (Schaltschwäche) in schizophrenic patients.

Historically, only the descriptive aspect of Bleuler's theory became famous and influential; his neurophysiological speculations as well as his explanations (in which associations were meant to flow along more normal lines as compared to the disrupted surface) were largely forgotten. Hence, when Bleuler's association psychology account of the clinical symptoms of schizophrenic patients is mentioned nowadays, only the descriptive aspect is remembered: Schizophrenic patients suffer from *weaker*, as well as from *"false"*, associations.

6. The Search for Empirical Norms and Further Results

In 1910, Kent and Rosanoff published a large scale study on associations in normal subjects and insane patients. With respect to methodology, they were dissatisfied with the somewhat unreliable Aschaffenburgian classification of associations and introduced an empirical way of classifying associations. Kent and Rosanoff established *norms* against which the associations of mentally ill patients could be checked.

> "Many attempts have been made to modify and amplify the classical grouping of associations according to similarity, contrast, contiguity, and sequence, so as to make it serviceable in differentiating between normal and abnormal associations. In this study, we attempted to apply Aschaffenburg's classification of reactions, but without success... The criterion of values which is used in this study is an empirical one... With the aid of our method the difficulty of classifying the reactions quoted above is obviated, as it is necessary only to refer to the table to find their proper values" (Kent & Rosanoff 1910, p. 45).

The essential feature of their method, which had already been developed by Sommer in his book on *Diagnosis of Mental Disorders*, was the "statistical treatment of results obtained by uniform technique from a large number of cases" (Kent & Rosanoff 1910, p. 37). Kent and Rosanoff carefully compiled a list of 100 words and collected data on word associations from one thousand (!) normal subjects, "in order to establish a standard which should fairly represent at least all the common types of association and which should show the extent of such variation as might be due to differences in sex, temperament, education, and environment... From the records obtained from these normal subjects, including in all 100,000 reactions, we have compiled a series of tables, one for each stimulus word, showing all the different reactions ... and the frequency with which each reaction has occurred" (Kent & Rosanoff 1910, pp. 38-39).

In particular, the method used to analyze the data was as follows:

"... the reactions contained in [the frequency tables] will fall into two classes: the *common* reactions, those which are to be found in the tables, and the *individual* reactions, those which are not to be found in the tables. For the sake of accuracy, any reaction word which was not found in the table in its identical form, but which is a grammatical variant of a word found there, may be classified as *doubtful*.
The value of any reaction may be expressed by the figure representing the percentage of subjects who gave it. Thus the reaction, *table—chair*, which was given by two hundred and sixty-seven out of the total of our one thousand subjects, possesses a value of 26.7 per cent" (Kent & Rosanoff 1910, p. 40, italics in original).

The most striking finding of this investigation of normal subjects consisted of the fact that their reactions mainly (91.7%) were of the common and rarely (6.8%) of the individual type (1.5% were classified as doubtful). No major differences were found with respect to gender, age, and educational level.

Kent and Rosanoff comment on the advantage of obtaining empirical values for the classifications of associations as opposed to Aschaffenburg's method of judgment as follows:

"Logically the combination *health—wealth* may be placed in any one of four classes, as follows:

$$
\text{health—wealth} \left\{
\begin{array}{l}
\text{intrinsic} \left\{ \begin{array}{l} \text{causal dependence} \\ \text{coordination} \end{array} \right. \\
\text{extrinsic} \left\{ \begin{array}{l} \text{speech reminiscence} \\ \text{sound similarity} \end{array} \right.
\end{array}
\right.
$$

But since our table shows this association to have an empirical value of 7.6 per cent, it becomes immaterial which of its logical relations is to be considered the strongest. It is mainly important, from our point of view, to separate reactions possessing an empirical value from those whose value is zero" (Kent & Rosanoff 1910, p. 46).

In the second part of their paper, Kent and Rosanoff report the results of the same word association test, carried out with 247 mentally ill patients. The most general finding was that of a weakening of the normal tendency to respond by common reactions. In order to analyze these individual reactions and their relationship to various clinical forms of mental disorder, the authors had to introduce their own classificatory system, despite their criticism of such systems as presented above.[15]

---

15 Kent and Rosanoff basically sacrificed validity for reliability in their system, which largely eliminated personal judgment, but allowed for about one third of all words to be classified as "unclassified" (cf. Kent & Rosanoff 1910, p. 318).

With respect to specific diagnostic groups, several findings seem worth reporting them here. In the 108 cases of dementia praecox the average number of individual reactions (34.4%) not only exceeded the normal range to a marked degree but also exceeded the number of individual associations found in any of the other mental disorders (to give an example: 21.5% individual associations were found in manic-depressive disorder). A detailed analysis of the associations of these patients revealed their clinically known pathology:

"A further examination of the individual test records shows that there is no uniformity of associational tendencies in this clinical group, but that several tendencies are more or less frequently met with either alone or in various combinations. Yet some of these tendencies, when appearing at all prominently, are so highly characteristics of dementia praecox as to be almost pathognomonic. Among these may be mentioned: (1) the tendency to give *neologisms*, particularly those of the senseless type; (2) the tendency to give unclassified reactions largely of the *incoherent* type; and (3) the tendency toward *stereotypy* manifested chiefly by abnormally frequent repetitions of the same reaction. Fairly characteristic also is the occasional tendency to give sound reactions" (Kent & Rosanoff 1910, p. 331, italics in original).

Once norms for the frequency of associations were established, their commonness and uniqueness could be assessed.[16] The findings of Bleuler and Kent & Rosanoff have subsequently been refined by using such norms. They can be summarized as follows (cf. Cramer 1968): Compared to normal controls, schizophrenic patients give fewer responses which are ordinarily given (fewer primary responses, less response commonality), they give more different responses (larger associative-response domain), which are less stable on retest. Moreover, schizophrenic patients give more clang responses and more "distant" responses. These findings are generally related to chronicity and seem to be specific in so far as they have not been obtained in neurotic depressed or alcoholic patients. According to Cramer, these results indicate a disinhibition or increased activation of associative pathways.

"The problem of the schizophrenic is that he is unable voluntarily to restrict his associations, and as a consequence is flooded with competing responses, many of which fall outside the usual—i.e., normal—associative domain" (Cramer 1968, p. 216).

Even the prolonged reaction time of schizophrenic patients in the word association test can be interpreted as a result of activation or disinhibition (rather than general slowing or decreased activation):

"... this increased reaction time appears to be a function of the schizophrenic's inability to restrict his associative domain. That is, the greater number of response alternatives results in greater response competition, and it is this competition among

---

16 According to Cramer, the most popular quantitative measure of association-response strength is the *Primary*, defined as "that response which occurs with the greatest frequency to any one stimulus" (Cramer 1968, p. 26). A related measure of response strength—*response commonality*—has been defined as the frequency of the Primary in a selected set of stimuli. In addition to these measures of associative strength, the *associative-response domain*, i.e., the number of different responses to a stimulus word, has turned out to be of interest in schizophrenia research.

potential responses which is responsible for the delay. Unlike the depressive or alco-holic, the schizophrenic' delayed reaction time does not result from searching for an acceptable response, but rather represents his inability to choose *a* response from among too many. This hypothesis is supported also by the finding that the reaction time of schizophrenics to multiple-, as opposed to single-, meaning stimuli is signifi-cantly longer, while for normal subjects the reverse is true. That is, *schizophrenics have difficulty in restricting the activation of associative pathways*, and this difficulty is increased when the stimulus itself is connected with several different associative domains" (Cramer 1968, p. 214, italics added).

Before further evidence for the activation or disinhibition of association pathways in schizophrenia will be discussed in section 9, the question of why research on association declined during the first half of this century and the problem of an adequate integrative framework for association research will be discussed.

7. Loss of Interest in Word-Associations: Possible Reasons

Given the amount of activity spent on the problem of associations in the fields of psychology and psychiatry, and the additional theoretical impact of the concept on these two fields, it is hard to understand why people seem to have lost interest in the problem for almost half a century in Europe as well as in The United States. Some tentative speculations may be offered.

First, researchers might have been discouraged by the idea that the results of Aschaffenburg and Jung, the findings of Kent and Rosanoff (1910), and the insights of Freudian interpretations left nothing more to be done. Furthermore, as individual differences seemed so striking, a hermeneutic approach might have appeared to be more applicable to word-association data.[17] As recently as in 1979, the editors of the second volume of Jung's collected works (Gesammelte Werke) claimed that Jung saved the method of word-associations from "scientific pedantry" by using a more interpretational approach (cf. Jung 1979a, p. 9). In short, even quite recently, the scientific vigor of the method—with its tables, means, graphs and numbers, was seen as a drawback!

The fact that Kraepelin, Aschaffenburg and Jung had to deal with numbers while methods of deriving adequate computational parameters had not yet been developed, was certainly a major obstacle to further development of their line of research. Inferential statistics did not exist, and—given the considerable variability of the raw data—, there was no way to find out whether the difference between two means was statistically significant.

Secondly, Gestalt psychology, one of the main movements in psychology of the first half of this century, had associationism as its

---

17 In fact, the very use of interpretation to classify associations according to various schemes may have contributed to the loss of interest in empirical association research. As Cramer (1968, p. 4) noted: "Part of this decline in popularity may well be the result of the ineffectiveness of the old a priori classificatory system to make meaningful discriminations."

declared intellectual antipode. With the predominance of gestalt-oriented approaches in psychiatric thinking, and, in particular, with experimentally oriented psychiatrists turning to gestalt psychology, research on word-associations almost naturally died out. As Lange noted in an experimental paper on the effects of cocaine, scopolamine and morphine, published in the last volume of Kraepelin's *Psychological Studies*:

> "Shortly after experimental psychology was founded it flourished to an extraordinary extent. However, by now the number of followers has decreased, and there is silence in the field... Yet, at any rate, we are still convinced of the value of such 'experimental trivialities'..." (Lange 1922, p. 354, transl. by the author).

Thirdly, psychoanalysis, though conceptually resting on associationist models of the mind, turned increasingly "hermeneutic" and decreasingly "scientific". As a consequence, we have already seen that the "scientific" study of associations was disregarded as being the fundamentally wrong one. Moreover, from a clinical point of view the rise of the use of projective techniques—notably the Rorschach and the Thematic Apperception Test—gradually pre-empted the Word Association Test as a diagnostic instrument. The new projective techniques were believed to provide a much better window into unconscious processes of the patient, and it was felt that they permitted inferences about the patients' motives and intentions more directly than word-association methods could. This made them more amenable to psychoanalytic interpretation.

Fourthly, behaviorism may have contributed to the lack of interest in associationist models of the mind and research, especially in the United States. After all, in the "black box", nothing needed to be modeled! Although learning paradigms made considerable use of word-pairs to be learned, associations due to the specific organization of the mind could only count as error variance. Learned word-associations were also unlikely to become a major paradigm for psychiatric research since learning itself suffers from a major impairment in the mentally ill. Hence, all that could be stated along these lines is the hardly interesting finding that learning words is merely another paradigm in which patients did worse than normals.

In summary, the lack of links to other fields, the lack of adequate statistical methods, and the growing influence of gestalt psychology and behaviorism in psychology and of psychoanalysis in psychiatry brought about decreasing research interest in the rather "basic" phenomenon of word associations.

8. Bridging the Gap Between Associations on Neurons and Associations of Words

Several findings, discoveries, and innovative ideas have led to a revival of work on associations in physiology as well as in psychology.

8.1 Neurobiology: Neurons and Synapses

The problem of linkage of the association of concepts to the association of nerve cells has been a major motivational force for the development of neuroscience in this century. James, as we have already seen, could merely stipulate such links.

The first attempt to link mind and matter on a neuronal basis was made by McCulloch and Pitts (1943). Although the particular assumptions about the functioning of neurons made in their famous paper, *A logical calculus of the ideas immanent to nervous activity,* later turned out to be wrong, the authors were able to show that neurons could be conceived of as computing devices capable of performing propositional logic. Interestingly, McCulloch and Pitts drew some conclusions about psychiatry. Referring to "tinnitus paraesthesias, hallucinations, delusions, confusions and disorientations" (p. 25), they claim that their account of the functioning of neuronal assemblies allows for a physiological account of the phenomena:

> "Certainly for the psychiatrist, it is more to the point that in such systems 'Mind' no longer 'goes more ghostly than a ghost.' Instead, diseased mentality can be understood without loss of scope or rigor, in the scientific terms of neurophysiology" (McCulloch & Pitts 1943/1989).

Some years later the Canadian psychologist Hebb (1949/1989) for the first time proposed a mechanism by means of which associations of neurons could actually be influenced through experience, i.e., a mechanism which makes learning possible. In other words, Hebb outlined the operating principles of the "association" of single nerve cells, the synapse, and how such associations could be influenced by "meaningful" associations, i.e., something to be learnt. Only seven years later, the first successful simulation of such synaptic activity was reported (Rochester et al. 1956/1989), using a device that was to revolutionize research on associations in the years to follow—a computer. After some modifications were introduced to Hebb's model, patterns appeared in the activity of the simulated "cells". Although the precise biological mechanisms regarding how changes in synaptic strength can provide a basis for memory are still largely unknown, considerable progress has been made over the last two decades. Not only did Kandel show how learning and synaptic modification occur parallel in the marine snail *Aplysia californica* (see Kandel 1991, for a review), but also mechanisms of synaptic modification in the human brain, most notably in the hippocampus, have been proposed (see, for example, Brown et al. 1988).

Although many details are still well beyond scientific understanding, neurobiology has come a long way from the assumption that there must be something in the head (doing the various kinds of processing) to working hypotheses about the underlying mechanisms of thought. Such hypotheses provide valuable constraints for any model developed by scientists who are more interested in "pure" function than in the details of implementation.

8.2 Computer Science and Artificial Intelligence:
Serial and Parallel Computers

In the 1950s, digital computers became accessible, not only as tools for research, but also as models for "thinking machines". Named after the person whose brainchild they were, the von–Neumann–machine was the model for all computers. Most of the computers of the present day still work like the machines designed forty years ago. Information is processed serially, i.e., a central processing unit (CPU) handles a single "chunk" of information at a time. To compensate for this limitation, such processing happens very quickly. Compared to the switching devices on silicon computer chips, neurons are terribly slow: For example, the computer used to type this paper contains memory chips with a switching speed of less than a tenth of a microsecond (< .0000001 s), whereas neurons take a few milliseconds (> .0001 s) to respond to input, i.e., to switch. If we take reaction time data from the experiments reported above and below as examples, i.e., reaction times as low as 500 milliseconds, we can conclude that the neural algorithm which performs, for example, lexical decisions cannot consist of more than about a hundred consecutive steps (cf. Rumelhart 1989, p. 135). However, everyone who has some experience with computer programming knows that a hundred step program is far too limited to accomplish even quite simple tasks.

This line of reasoning directly implies that the task of a lexical decision (see below) cannot be performed by neurons working in the same manner as my personal computer. It is quite obvious that the rather slow neurons must work massively in parallel to perform the many computations necessary for word-associations.

In addition to the argument from considerations of speed, a similar argument in favor of a parallel design for the associations-handling device called "brain" can be made from considerations of precision. In a classic monograph, *The Computer and the Brain*, John von Neumann (1958) had already pointed out that the level of precision which can be accomplished by neurons is several orders of magnitude less than the level of precision that computers can achieve. This implies that long programs relying on many steps cannot possibly be handled by such systems because an error occurring within one such step will be easily propagated and multiplied in subsequent steps.

For these reasons, the idea that associations form some sort of a network[18] is so plausible that it is rarely doubted or even discussed. But how is this network organized? Psychologists working on the structure of semantic memory answered this question in the 1970s by postulating

---

18 It must be mentioned that the term "network" is as ambiguous as the term "association": Associationist psychology has shown that meanings of words are associated according to various "laws", i.e., that on a conceptual or semantic level, associations play an organizing role. On the level of neurons, microanatomy has demonstrated that neurons are associated via distinctive fibers. There are "networks" of meaning and "networks" of cells and fibers. Of course, the identity of the name—network—does not provide any insight about similarities.

highly structured networks of concepts. According to these investigators, language consists of rules which operate on a set of distinctly stored representations. More recently, "loose" types of networks have been proposed to account for a variety of aspects of the human faculty of language. In these networks, idealized neurons, i.e., computing devices, are supposed to be in a certain state of activity (represented by a number), and are connected to other neurons with *connections of varying strength* (also represented by a number). Hence the name *connectionism* for the whole approach to the architecture of ideal neurons. Because these neurons work in parallel, and because the work is done in different location (rather than in only a single CPU), the term *parallel distributed processing* (PDP) has been used to characterize these models.[19] As David Rumelhart, a major proponent of the connectionist approach, has put it:

"The basic strategy of the connectionist approach is to take as its fundamental processing unit something close to an abstract neuron. We imagine that computation is carried out through simple interactions among such processing units. Essentially the idea is that these processing elements communicate by sending numbers along the lines that connect the processing elements... The operations in our models then can best be characterized as 'neurally inspired.' ... all the knowledge is in the connections. From conventional programmable computers we are used to thinking of knowledge as being stored in the state of certain units in the system... This is a profound difference between out approach and other more conventional approaches, for it means that almost all knowledge is implicit in the structure of the device that carries out the task rather than explicit in the states of the units themselves" (Rumelhart 1989, pp. 135-136).

8.3 Network Models of Semantic Memory

Network models of semantic memory had already been proposed in the 1960s and 1970s as a result of research which attempted to unravel the nature of the representational code in which information is stored. However, these networks were highly structured and technically rather than psychologically inspired. In other words, although they consisted of nodes and connections, they did *not* have the connectionist model architecture:

"In associative networks, lexical concepts are represented by nodes. The properties of a concept are stored at its node; its relations to other concepts are given by labeled links between nodes... The meaning of any word is given by its node and by the relations made explicit in the network" (Miller & Glucksberg 1988, p. 436).

A small part of such a network is shown in figure 4. Such networks can explain some experimental data. For example, it has been proposed that memory search consists of activation spreading from node to node along links in such a network. It has been further proposed that

"people store lexical information in the form of a strict hierarchy. Information about subordinates and superordinate relations among concepts is explicitly represented in the hierarchy by means of labeled links between concepts. Information

---

19 For brief introductions , see Anderson 1988, Bechtel & Abrahamson 1991, and Rumelhart 1989.

about properties is stored at concept nodes, and is stored non-redundantly. If the property *has skin* is stored at the node for the concept *animal*, then it is not stored at any hyponymic nodes in the network, but applies to all of them... consider these statements:

1. Canaries are yellow.
2. Canaries can fly.
3. Canaries have skin.

According to the model, such statements are evaluated by a memory search that is accomplished by the spread of activation from the relevant concept node—from canary in this case. Under this model certain predictions could be made: Statement (1) would take the least time to evaluate, since it can be evaluated from information stored at the canary node itself; statement (2) requires that activation spread from one node to another, so evaluation would take somewhat longer; and statement (3) requires a search two links deep, and so would take the longest time" (Miller & Glucksberg 1988, pp. 436-437).

Although it turned out that reaction times in a respective experiment were consistent with these assumptions, the model has been challenged for several reasons which are beyond the scope of this paper (cf. Miller & Glucksberg 1988, pp. 437-439). It is important to note, however, that references to networks, nodes, activation and its spreading have become commonplace in psycholinguistics. Instead of the old "memory traces", "connected nodes" are now supposed to carry and to pass on, information.

Figure 4: Hierarchical Associative Semantic Network (modified from Miller & Glucksberg 1988, p. 436).

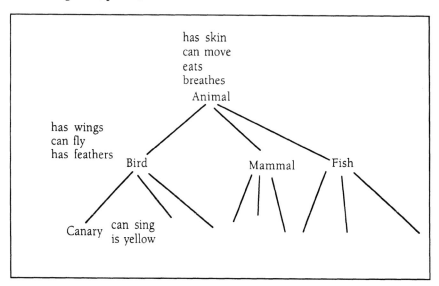

8.4   Network Models and Semantic Associations

The structure of semantic memory has been investigated using tasks in which word-associations play a major role. For example, from the above-mentioned fact that familiar stimulus words tend to produce the same response word in many subjects, it has been concluded that the organization of semantic memory is quite uniform across individuals. Moreover, from the fact that word-associations are produced faster when common words are given as stimuli, it has been concluded that the organization of semantic memory—also referred to as the *mental lexicon*—somehow takes into account frequency. In other words, the relationship between word frequency (as measured in a large corpus of various texts[20]) and accessibility (as measured by the time it takes to produce an associated word) is taken to reflect, at least in part, the structure of the mental lexicon. Since the time of Kraepelin, the frequency as well as conceptual and syntactic features of words have been known to serve as organizing principles regarding the way in which these words are stored in our minds.

If one wants to study specific types of word-associations, the method of free associations, as described above, has the drawback that the analysis of the type of association can only be post hoc; i.e., the experimenter cannot specify a certain association and then test it, he rather has to wait until it occurs spontaneously. Moreover, the experimenter may want to test the associations between concepts without referring to particular words, or he may be interested in the special role of reading and pronunciation. Several methods have been developed to give more specific answers to these kind of questions. For example, words can be read to subjects or they can be presented visually. Moreover, pictures may be presented to bypass a particular word (for example, its phonetic characteristics) in the process of presenting a concept. Furthermore, the technique of lexical decision, in which the subject has to decide whether a given string of characters is a word or not, has been widely employed. To test specific types of associations, word pairs can be presented either simultaneously or one after the other. Then, the effect of the relation between the words on the specific task involved (such as reading the words or deciding whether both of them are in fact words) can be measured in terms of the time it takes to perform the task.

The technique of lexical decision has now become one of the most widely used in experimental psychology. A robust phenomenon that has been discovered using this technique is *semantic priming*. If a word is shown first and then a string of characters is shown,[21] and the subject is asked to press a key labeled "yes" if the second string is a word, and a key labeled "no" if it is not a word, the response is faster if both words are related. To give an example: "black" is recognized faster as a word if it is presented after "white" as compared to being presented after a non-related word, such as "soft".

The numerous studies which have been conducted using this methodology are suggestive of a representation of semantic information

---

20 The best and most widely used example of such a "frequency-table" is Francis and Kucera and 1982
21 When this effect was demonstrated for the first time by Meyer and Schvanaveldt (1971), the two strings of characters were presented at the same time.

which is not totally unstructured, but which is also not as hierarchically ordered (by only one principle) as the model outlined above. In other words, we have to assume that concepts are represented in a network of links which in turn represent various kinds of relationships. As a first approximation, these may be conceived of as similar to the old association laws. *Black* may be linked to *white*, to *color*, and to *ivory black*, also to *night*, *shadow*, *darkness*, *devil*, *ink*, *coal*, *pitch*, *coffee*, and, even further, to *blackout*, *blackball*, *black eagle*, *blackjack*, *black letter*, *blackout*, *blacksmith* etc. We know some of the more obvious relations, but others may still await discovery.[22] A sketch of what semantic networks may look like according to what we just have said is depicted in figure 5.

Figure 5: Structure of the semantic network as suggested by research on word-associations.

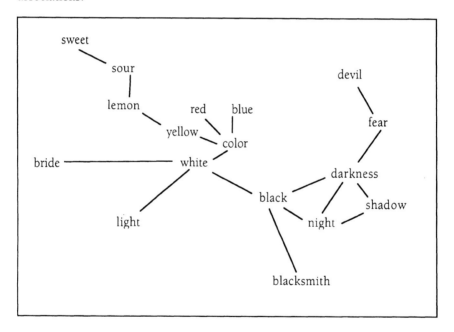

Although the technique of lexical decision seems to involve some arbitrary features when compared to the simple free word-association test, it has a major advantage in that word-associations can be specified in advance and then be subjected to measurement. Various types of word-associations as well as some examples are shown in table 2. The stimulus-word usually is presented first and is called the *prime*, the string of characters that has to be detected as being a word or a non-word usually comes later and is called the *target*. The interval between the onset of the

22 In particular, it is interesting to note and contrast the large effect sizes which Jung found for affectively laden word-associations, and the little attention which the problem of affect has attracted so far from contemporary experimental psychologists In my view, it is not unlikely that the study of semantic networks can produce valuable insights into the nature of affect .

prime and the onset of the target is called *Stimulus Onset Asynchrony* (SOA) whereas the interval between the end of the prime and the onset of the target is called *Inter Stimulus Interval* (ISI). It follows that the SOA equals the duration of the prime plus the ISI. Both the SOA and the ISI are used in the literature.

Table 2: Types of word-associations as used in lexical decision studies.

Type of association	Examples
	prime—target
word—non-related word	cloud—tree
word—semantically related word	table—chair
word—indirectly related word	lion—(tiger)—stripes
word—clang related word	house—mouse
word—non-word	frame—brun

9. Word–Association Research in Schizophrenia: Data and Theory

It is beyond the scope of this paper to summarize all the work on word associations in the field of clinical psychology and psychopathology. Even with respect to only a single disorder, schizophrenia, an exhaustive review cannot be given here. Instead, sketches of the work of some groups presently working in this area, including my own, are given.

9.1 Semantic Associations

Only recently, the method of semantic priming in lexical decision tasks has been applied to the study of psychopathological processes, in particular, to aspects of cognitive malfunctioning in schizophrenic patients (Chapin et al. 1989, Fisher & Weinman 1989, Maher et al. 1987, Manschreck et al. 1988). Using this technique, Manschreck et al. (1988) discovered an increased semantic priming effect in schizophrenic patients who suffered from formal thought disorder, as compared to non-thought disordered schizophrenic patients and normal control subjects. The authors interpret their results as evidence for an activated semantic network, which is visible clinically as disordered thought but which also allows word associations to spread faster, and hence, produces a larger priming effect.

The finding of a larger semantic priming effect in thought disordered schizophrenic patients was confirmed by Kwapil et al. (1990) using a different method. After the prime word, visually degraded words were presented and the degree of degradation at which it was correctly identified was taken as the dependent variable. The difficulty of the task was adjusted in such a way that performance of patients and subjects was generally equal, and differences between the experimental conditions within each group were largest. It is important to note that while this task did not measure reaction times, i.e., the speed of a decision, it yielded the same result of a larger semantic priming effect in thought disordered schizophrenic patients.

Taken together, the studies on semantic associations suggest that the argument between Jung and Stransky can be settled in favor of Jung's position. In other words, it seems as though we do not have to call for specific aberrant associations in schizophrenic thought, or for specific laws of associations in schizophrenia. Instead, association-networks in thought disordered schizophrenic patients are essentially the same as those of normal subjects. Minor changes in the speed of processing and the failure of proper timing of processes involved in certain tasks of reasoning can account for the clinical phenomena. In particular, inhibitory processes by which irrelevant associations are normally excluded from consciousness are defective in schizophrenic patients. As the maintenance of an organized sequence of thought and of an organized language utterance requires the operation of a goal-directed organization of thoughts—as pointed out by Bleuler—, it can only be accomplished by the active inhibition (exclusion) of associations that are irrelevant to the intended utterance. This means that the intrusions of associations into schizophrenic utterances create the end-result of disrupted utterances. It should be mentioned that inhibitory processes are assumed by researchers on attentional processes, and that a failure of such inhibitory processes has been taken to explain aspects of the performance of schizophrenic patients in selective attention tasks.

From a historical point of view, it is interesting to note that observations about formal thought disorder and faster reaction times are not new. In a footnote in his chapter on associations, William James had already referred to experiments on the reaction times of mentally ill patients.

"The only measurements of association-time which so far seem likely to have much theoretic importance are a few made on insane patients by von Tschisch [...]. The simple reaction time was found about normal in three patients, one with progressive paralysis, one with inveterate mania of persecution, one recovering from ordinary mania. In the convalescent maniac and the paralytic, however, the association-time was hardly half as much as Wundt's normal figure [...] whilst in the sufferer from delusions of persecution and hallucinations it was twice as great as normal (1.39" instead of 0.7 "). [...] Herr von Tschisch remarks on the connection of the short times with diminished power for clear and consistent processes of thought, and on that of the long times with the persistent fixation of the attention upon monotonous objects (delusions)" (James, *Principles*, p. 528).

Tschisch had published his paper in 1885. His data on simple reaction time and the time of word association are presented in table 3. He commented on his results as follows:

188   M. Spitzer

"The duration of the associations certainly is influenced by the nature of the disease process: In K. the decrease of mental powers produces a decrease in the capability to form decisive and clear thoughts; in P. the decrease of mental energy is related to the abnormal predominance of some ideas (delusions) in consciousness. — In the third patient S. there is strictly speaking no weakness of mental power, but the capability for clear and precise thoughts is reduced because of the past stage of agitated incoherence and the currently present exhaustion. Hence, the time of association is similar to that of K. [...] We have to conclude that a decrease of mental powers leads to a pronounced decrease in the time of association, but only so, if the decrease of mental powers is not related to fixation of attention by single thoughts (delusions), which leads to a delay of the association processes" (Tschisch 1885, p. 219).

From this quote it is quite obvious that, more than a hundred years ago (even before Bleuler's account of schizophrenia) it was hypothesized that there might be a *connection between formal thought disorder and faster word associations*.

Table 3: Simple reaction time (150 measures per patient) and time of word association (300 measures per patient) in milliseconds (ms) in normal controls and three patients (adapted from Tschisch 1885).

subject	measure		
	clinical description	simple reaction time (ms)	rt in word association test (ms)
patient K.	36 year old physician suffering from general palsy with manic like symptoms and formal thought disorder for about one year	80	230
patient P.	36 year old veterinarian suffering from hallucinations and persecutory delusions for several years	120	1390
patient S.	student, suffering from mania for 8 months, in remission; at the time of the investigation slightly exhausted	70	280
control subjects	(number and age not specified)	100	700

9.2 Semantic Associations and Context

Eugen Bleuler already noted that schizophrenic patients are unable to focus on the relevant meaning of a word as suggested by the context. With respect to a concept which has several meanings depending upon the context, he noted:

"... in the normal mind only those part concepts dominate the picture that belong to a given frame of reference. The others exist only potentially, or at least retreat into the background so that we cannot even demonstrate their influence... [However] ... patients may lose themselves in the most irrelevant side-associations ..." (pp. 17-18).

Since the classic work of Chapman (cf. Chapman et al. 1964) on differences in responses to words with two or more different meanings (polysemous words, homonyms) in schizophrenic patients compared to normal controls, homonyms have been used in several studies to investigate the context dependency of associative processes. Swiney (1984), for example, was able to demonstrate contextual insensitivity in chronic schizophrenic patients using a cross–modal lexical priming technique. The patients were auditorily presented with sentences and were required to make visual lexical decisions at specified points in time: while the sentence which contained the priming word was being presented, and following the priming word in the sentence. He found that shortly after the presentation of the polysemous word, all of its meanings are activated (context–insensitive lexical access), i.e., produce a semantic priming effect. About a second later in time, however, only the contextually constrained meaning is selected in normal subjects, whereas in thought disordered schizophrenic patients such a constraining process does not occur and both meanings remain activated.

Contextually relevant information seems to be processed by specific neural assemblies in the frontal lobe. Recently, neural network models have been developed to account for the difficulties schizophrenic patients experience in processing context information (cf. Cohen and Servan–Schreiber 1992). Such models may guide the search for more specific and sensitive experimental procedures which in turn may provide new insights into the nature of the schizophrenic defect.

9.3 Indirect Semantic Associations

Bleuler already commented on empirical studies of indirect associations:

"In experimental investigations of association, we find a notable frequency of 'mediate associations.' I suspect that only the lack of sufficient observation has been responsible for our inability to demonstrate them more frequently in the thought-processes of our patients. The above mentioned example, the association 'wood (wood-coffin)—dead cousin,' may be considered as a mediate association. Certainly to this group belong such examples as 'tea—spirit' by way of the mediate concept of soul; cook—pole by way of 'Cook—Northpole'" (Bleuler 1911/1950, p. 26).

Bleuler even claimed indirect associations to be significant in the differential diagnosis of mania and schizophrenia:

"Truly indirect associations hardly ever play a particularly striking role in the mania of manic-depressives whereas they are quite common in schizophrenia" (Bleuler 1911/1950, p. 308).

To my knowledge, there is no study of indirect, or mediated, associations in schizophrenic patients employing methods such as naming, reading, or lexical decision. Only recently, our group began a series of semantic priming investigations words which are indirectly associated to the target word, as for example, lemon—(sour)—sweet (see table 2). The few studies that have been conducted on normal subjects using indirect semantic priming revealed mainly negative findings, i.e., the word "lemon" does not facilitate the detection of the word "sweet". When such word pairs are presented using a short SOA, however, a priming effect can be found in schizophrenic patients (cf. Spitzer 1992). Hence it seems as though associations in schizophrenic patients are in fact propagating faster through associational networks than is the case for normal subjects.

9.4 Associations by Clang or Rhyme

As I have already pointed out in previous sections, associations by clang or rhyme were extensively studied by psychologists and psychiatrists almost a hundred years ago. Moreover, clang associations are mentioned by Bleuler as an integral part of schizophrenic symptomatology:

> "Furthermore, clang associations are very frequent. Head-bed; frog-bog; sad-mad-bad; beaten-betrayed-beloved-bedecked. ... the identity or even the similarity of one single sound suffices to give the direction of the association. Thus, the clang association very often has the schizophrenic mark of the bizarre" (Bleuler 1911/1950, pp. 24-25).

Given this interest in clang associations, their clinical significance, and the findings of the past, it is surprising that no experimental work on clang-associations can be found in the more recent psychopathological literature. Even more so, it is striking that there are no well-established data regarding the effect of clang relations between words on tasks such as lexical decision or picture naming carried out by *normal* subjects. In fact, the results of the few studies on this issue are conflicting, and facilitatory as well as inhibitory effects have been reported.

In light of these conflicting reports, we carried out several clang-association experiments with normal control subjects and schizophrenic patients using the lexical decision paradigm. The results may be summarized as follows:

(1) Whether a prime related by clang facilitates or inhibits the recognition of a target is dependent on the interval between the two words. Short intervals inhibit and longer intervals facilitate lexical decisions on clang-related targets.

(2) The experiments were not designed to investigate the effects of fatigue. However, a post hoc analysis was carried out in order to determine whether tiredness caused by the experimental procedure may have had an effect on clang associations (assuming that the combination of boredom and exhaustion produced some variability in the data). The results nicely paralleled those obtained by C.G. Jung: In subjects with high educational level fatigue tends to facilitate clang associations.

(3) In schizophrenic patients, clang related primes have a facilitatory effect on target processing, even if the interval between prime and target is

short: There is a positive clang or phonological priming effect in schizophrenia.

(4) When the clinical picture improves, this phonological priming effect reverts to zero, i.e., schizophrenic patients go back to normal on this measure.

Interestingly, the time course of decreasing clang associations in patients remitting from a psychotic episode had already been described by Sommer in 1899 in his *Textbook of Research Methods in Psychopathology*. Sommer commented on his findings as follows:

"Accordingly, this method enables us not only to state the presence or absence of certain psychopathological symptoms, but rather allows for their fixation *in the form of a number*, in some sense to *measure* them. This should be the aim of an *exact symptomatology*" (Sommer 1899, p. 388).

10. Conclusions

Of course, the findings presented in the previous section have to be replicated before any major conclusions can be drawn. In particular, studies in patients with other diagnoses have to be undertaken, as well as investigations of the effects (if there are any) of treatment on the reported phenomena. Additionally, their long-term stability and their presence in relatives have to be investigated. Some experimentally induced phenomena may turn out to be state-dependent whereas others may be more like traits. In spite of the scarcity of data, however, some speculative thoughts may be allowed.

From a *theoretical* point of view, the fine-grained experimental study of thought processes in schizophrenia as well as in other mental disorders should enhance our understanding of these disorders. We need to know more about what goes wrong in the minds/brains of patients in order to improve our efforts to treat, rehabilitate, or even simply to talk to them. Cognitive science approaches to psychopathology are, on the one hand, "biological" enough to mesh with findings from the "hard-sciences" (such as studies on neurotransmitters and receptors). On the other hand, they serve a greatly needed bridging function for results from "soft-science" approaches to psychopathology.

From a *methodological* point of view, the following remark has to be made. It is a generally accepted strategy to correlate the results of experiments such as the ones described above with psychopathological measures. Fundamentally, these measures consist of ratings of gross pathology. However, since overt symptoms are the result of a complex and poorly understood interplay of impaired mental functioning, possibly impaired reactions and (possibly impaired) adaptive strategies, and interpretations by the patient, such correlations will almost never reach high values. A better strategy might involve the correlation of various experimental measures, and the use of these, along with the symptoms, as independent descriptions of clinical syndromes.

From a *clinical practical* point of view, the possibility of measuring some aspects of the psychotic state seems within reach. Because of the large variation which is characteristic of almost all data collected from mentally ill, and especially from schizophrenic patients, a single measure is not likely to be successful. However, a combination of several measures testing various aspects of mental functioning may provide us with a profile or an index which has clinical significance. If we were able, to give just one example, to determine the course of illness of a chronic schizophrenic by monitoring some "profile of activity" each month, we might successfully predict relapse. If we could do so, we could reduce prophylactic medication with neuroleptics or possibly even do without them, thereby reducing the risk of tardive dyskinesia.

A final word must be said to the skeptic who might be inclined to make the following argument at this point: Kraepelin devoted great efforts to experimental psychopathology but became famous for having accomplished something else. Jung completed major experiments on various aspects of word–associations, but his findings were later regarded as little more than an ill conceived empiricist's attempt to validate Freud's psychodynamic speculations. Even the more recent approaches of clinical psychologists are literally unknown to most psychiatrists and have not had any major theoretical, let alone clinical-practical, impact on the field. So why should the psychiatrist be concerned with association psychology and experimental psychopathology at all?

In my view, although this argument seems rather convincing, it is nonetheless wrong. We have already discussed the reasons why the findings of early experimental psychopathologists did not gain major recognition: Early studies not only became old fashioned with the advent of Gestalt psychology and behaviorism, they also were too advanced and hence could not be linked to anything else that was known in the field. Even in the 1960s, the gap between psychology and neurophysiology was huge, and hence, little cross-fertilization could occur. Today, this situation has changed: The functioning of neurons has been described down to a mathematical level and neurobiological findings can provide constraints to such mathematical models of neuronal assemblies up to the human cortex. Experimental psychopathology will certainly profit from these developments. Just as there is computational neuroscience, there might be computational psychopathology at some time in the future. In short, Kraepelin, Jung and others could not connect to connectionism. Their findings could not be interpreted by any other theory, and in particular, could not be linked to neuroscience, as known at that time. However, the general spirit in which Kraepelin and his group worked on word-associations—most clearly visible in a programmatic paper entitled *The psychological experiment in psychiatry*[23]—may still serve as a strategy. In this first article in the first volume of what became a multi–volume effort in experimental psychiatry, Kraepelin's enthusiasm for experimentation, as well as his discontent with

---

23 *Der psychologische Versuch in der Psychiatrie.*

speculation—as popular in psychiatry then as it has been in the recent past—is clearly outspoken.

"Even though industrious optimism may be sometimes diminished by obstacles and disappointments, and even though some of the far reaching tasks of the present may turn out not to be solvable, experience at this point already confirms that psychological experiments represent fully justified and irreplaceable elements in the array of our methods of scientific research. This is all the more important, since in psychiatry, to a much larger extent than in any other branch of medicine, interpretation and systematization rather than observation is the rule. In particular, in our psychological accounts, we habitually suffer from an abundance of spirit and idiosyncrasy. Their bold arbitrariness finds free room to play, until finally the slow progress of real knowledge will narrow the field. Without doubt, almost every professor of psychiatry feels justified—one is even inclined to say, feels compelled to—construct [to timber] his own edifice of psychological theory, built either upon some rough observations of patients and animals or upon literary studies. However, which textbook of internal medicine would dare, for example, announce a new system of physiology which was not already tiresomely worked out in the laboratory?

It is timely that we start to replace witty claims and deep inventions by sound and conscientious single experiments. We do not proceed with claims that cannot be proven or rejected. We need facts, not theories. Of course, no science can completely do without summarizing views and preliminary assumptions. However, we must not forget that these are not of any intrinsic value. They are nothing but means to certain ends. They can only be justified by the fact that they lead to certain questions, and hence, to new investigations. I think that we do have enough questions. We intend to start to answer them, not in the armchair [original: at the green table], but in the laboratory, not with brilliant ideas, but with measurements and observations" (Kraepelin 1896, pp. 90–91, transl. by the author).

Summary

In the general framework of association psychology, word associations were first introduced as a tool for psychological research in the 1880s by Francis Galton. Soon thereafter and stimulated by Wilhelm Wundt, research on word–associations in psychiatry began, headed by Emil Kraepelin. Under the supervision of Eugen Bleuler, Jung introduced methodological refinements and produced data which heavily influenced Bleuler's concept of schizophrenia. For several reasons which are tentatively discussed, research on word-associations almost ended in the 1920s, and the empirical findings gathered at the turn of the century were almost completely forgotten. Advances in the fields of neurophysiology, neuropsychology, and artificial intelligence research, i.e., the advent of a whole new field—cognitive science—brought about a revival of interest in associations. For about three decades, word–associations have once again been studied by clinical psychologists and psychiatrists. With emphasis upon my own work, recent findings on word–associations in schizophrenic patients are discussed in the light of what was already known at the turn of the century.[24]

---

24 I am indepted to Brendan A. Maher, Michael A. Schwartz, and Friedrich A. Uehlein for comments on an earlier version of this paper.

References

Anderson JA: General Introduction. In: Anderson JA, Rosenfeld E (eds): Neurocomputing. Foundations of Research, pp. xiii-xxi. Cambridge, MA, London, England, MIT Press, 1988

Anderson JA, Rosenfeld E (eds): Neurocomputing. Foundations of Research. Cambridge, MA, London, England, MIT Press, 1988

Aristotle: On Memory and Recollection. Loeb Classical Library, Aristotle VIII, On the soul, parva naturalia, on breath, transl. by WS Hett, Cambridge MA, Harvard University Press, 1975

Aschaffenburg G: Experimentelle Studien über Associationen I. In: Kraepelin E (ed): Psychologische Arbeiten I, pp. 209–299, Leipzig, Engelmann, 1896

Aschaffenburg G: Experimentelle Studien über Associationen II. In: Kraepelin E (ed): Psychologische Arbeiten II, pp. 1–83, Leipzig, Engelmann, 1899

Aschaffenburg G: Experimentelle Studien über Associationen III. In: Kraepelin E (ed): Psychologische Arbeiten IV, pp. 235–373, Leipzig, Engelmann, 1904

Bleuler E: Dementia Praecox or the Group of Schizophrenias (1911), transl. by Ziskin J, Lewis ND; New York, International Universities Press, 1950

Bechtel W, Abrahamnson A: Connectionism and the Mind. An Introduction to Parallel Processing in Networks. Cambridge MA, Basil Blackwell, 1991

Boring EG: A history of experimental psychology, 2nd ed. New York, Appleton–Century– Crofts, 1950

Borz J: Statistik. Berlin, Heidelberg, New York, London, Paris, Tokyo, Springer, 1989

Brown TH, Chapman PF, Kairiss EW, Keenan CL: Long-term synaptic potentiation. Science 242, 724-728, 1988

Cattell JMcK, Bryant S: Mental association investigated by experiment. Mind 14: 230-250, 1889

Chapin K, Vann LE, Lycaki H, Josef N, Meyendorff E: Investigation of the associative network in schizophrenia using the semantic priming paradigm. Schizophrenia Research 2: 355-360, 1989

Chapman LJ, Chapman JP, Miller GA: A theory of verbal behavior in schizophrenia. In Progress in Experimental Personality Research, Vol. I. B.A. Maher (Ed.). New York & London: Academic Press. Pp.49-77, 1964

Cohen J, Servan–Schreiber D: Context, cortex and dopamine: A connectionist approach to behavior and biology in schizophrenia. Psychological Review 99: 45-77, 1992

Cramer P: Word association. New York and London, Academic Press, 1968

Deese J: The structure of associations in language and thought. Baltimore MD, Johns Hopkins Press, 1965

Exner S: Entwurf zu einer physiologischen Erklärung der psychischen Erscheinungen. Leipzug, Wien, Deuticke, 1894

Fisher M, Weinman J: Priming, word recognition and psychotic tendencies. Personality and Individual Differences, 10(2), 185–189, 1989

Francis WN, Kucera H: Frequency Analysis of English usage. Lexicon and Grammar. Boston, Houghton Mifflin 1982

Freud S: Project for a scientific psychology (1895). The Standard Edition of the Comlete Psychological Works of Sigmund Freud, vol. 1, pp. 283–397. London, Hogarth Press, 1978

Freud S: Die Traumdeutung (The Interpretation of Dreams). Gesammelte Werke II/III. Frankfurt, S. Fischer, 1976

Freud S: Zur Psychopathologie des Alltagslebens (On the Psychopathology of Everyday Life). Gesammelte Werke IV. Frankfurt, S. Fischer, 1978

Galton F: Psychometric experiments. Brain 2: 149–162, 1879

Galton F: Inquiries into Human Faculty and Its Development. London, MacMillan, 1883

Hahn R: Über die Beziehungen zwischen Fehlreaktionen und Klangassoziationen. In: Kraepelin E (ed): Psychologische Arbeiten V, pp. 163–208, Leipzig, Engelmann, 1910

Hebb DO: The organization of behavior (1949). Quoted from: Anderson JA, Rosenfeld E (eds): Neurocomputing. Foundations of Research, pp. 45–56. Cambridge, MA, London, England, MIT Press, 1988

Hobson JA, McCarley RW: The brain as a dream state generator: An activation-synthesis hypothesis of the dream process. American Journal of Psychiatry 134: 1335–1348, 1977

James W: Principles of Psychology. Cambridge Mass., London, Harvard University Press, 1983

James W: Psychology: Briefer Course. Cambridge Mass., London, Harvard University Press, 1984

Jones E: Das Leben und Werk von Sigmund Freud, vols. 1-3. Bern, Huber, 1978

Jung CG: Über Simulation von Geistesstörung (1903). Gesammelte Werke 1 (Psychiatrische Studien), 2nd ed., pp. 169-201. Olten, Freiburg, Walter, 1978

Jung CG: Experimentelle Beonachtungen über das Erinnerungsvermögen (Experimental Obervations on the Faculty of Memory, 1905). Gesammelte Werke 2 (Experimentelle Untersuchungen), pp. 289-307. Olten, Freiburg, Walter, 1979a

Jung CG: Experimentelle Untersuchungen über Assoziationen Gesunder (1906a) Gesammelte Werke 2 (Experimentelle Untersuchungen), pp. 15-213. Olten, Freiburg, Walter, 1979a

Jung CG: Die Psychopathologische Bedeutung des Assoziationsexperiments (1906b). Gesammelte Werke 2 (Experimentelle Untersuchungen), pp. 429–446. Olten, Freiburg, Walter, 1979a

Jung CG: Über das Verhalten der Reaktionszeit beim Assoziationsexperimente (1906c). Gesammelte Werke 2 (Experimentelle Untersuchungen), pp. 239-288. Olten, Freiburg, Walter, 1979a

Jung CG: Analyse der Assoziationen eines Epileptikers (Analysis of the Associations of an Epileptic Patient, 1906d). Gesammelte Werke 2 (Experimentelle Untersuchungen), pp. 214-238. Olten, Freiburg, Walter, 1979a

Jung CG: Über die Psychologie der Dementia Praecox (1906). Gesammelte Werke 3 (Psychogenese der Geisteskrankheiten), 2nd ed., pp. 3-170. Olten, Freiburg, Walter, 1979b

Kandel ER: Cellular Mechanisms of Learning and the Biological Basis of Individuality. In: Kandel ER, Schwartz JH, Jessell TM (eds): Principles of Neuroscience, 3rd ed, pp. 1009-1031 (ch. 65).New York, Amsterdam, London, Tokyo, Elsevier, 1991

Kent GH, Rosanoff AJ: A study of associations in insanity. American Journal of Insanity 66/67: 37-47 (part I), 317-390 (part II), 1910

Kraepelin E: Über die Beeinflussung einfacher psychischer Vorgänge durch einige Arzneimittel. Jena, G. Fischer, 1892

Kraepelin E: Der psychologische Versuch in der Psychiatrie. In: Kraepelin E (ed): Psychologische Arbeiten I, pp. 1–91, Leipzig, Engelmann, 1896

Kwapil TR, Hegley DC, Chapman LJ, Chapman JP: Facilitation of word recognition by semantic priming in schizophrenia. Journal of Abnormal Psychology 99: 215-221, 1990

Lange J: Psychologische Untersuchungen über die Wirkungen von Kokain, Skopolamin und Morphin (Experimental studies of the effects of cocain, scopolamine, and morphine). In: Kraepelin E (ed): Psychologische Arbeiten VII, pp. 354-412, Berlin, Springer, 1922

Maher BA, Manschreck TC, Hoover TM, Weisstein CC: Thought disorder and measured features of language production in schizophrenia. In: Harvey P, Walker E (eds): Positive and negative symptoms in psychosis: Description, research and future directions. Hillsdale, NJ, Erlbaum, 1987

Manschreck T, Maher BA, Milavetz JJ, Ames D, Weisspeim C, Schneier ML: Semantic priming in thought disordered schizophrenic patients. Schizophrenia Research 1: 661–666, 1988

McCulloch WS, Pitts W: A logical calculus of the ideas immanent in nervous activity (1943). In: Anderson JA, Rosenfeld E (eds): Neurocomputing. Foundations of Research, pp. 18–27. Cambridge, MA, London, England, MIT Press, 1988

Meyer DE, Schvaneveldt RW: Facilitation in recognizing pairs of words: Evidence of a dependence between retrieval operations. Journal of Experimental Psychology 90: 227-234, 1971

Miller GA, Glucksberg S: Psycholinguistic aspects pragmatics and semantics. In: Atkinson RC, Herrnstein RJ, Lindzey G, Luce RD (eds): Steven's Handbook of Experimental Psychology (ch. 6), pp. 417-472. New York, Wiley, 1988

Neumann Jv: The computer and the brain. New Haven, Yale University Press, 1958

Pribram KH, Gill MM: Freud's 'project' re-assessed. New York, Basic Books, 1976

Rochester N, Holland JH, Haibt LH, Duda WL: Tests on a cell assembly theory of the action of the brain, using a large digital computer (1956). In: Anderson JA, Rosenfeld E (eds): Neurocomputing. Foundations of Research, pp. 68-79. Cambridge, MA, London, England, MIT Press, 1988

Rumelhart DE: The architecture of mind: A connectionist approach. In: Posner MI (ed): Foundations of cognitive science, pp. 133–159. Cambridge, MA, London, England, MIT Press, 1989

Sommer R: Lehrbuch der Psychopathologischen Untersuchungsmethoden. Berlin, Wien, Urban & Schwarzenberg, 1899

Spitzer M: Freuds Traumtheorie vor dem Hintergrund des Standes der physiologischen Forschung von damals und heute (Freud's theory of dreams and the state of physiological research then and now). unpublished Diploma Thesis, Freiburg, 1984

Spitzer M: Assoziative Netzwerke, formale Denkstörungen und Schizophrenie. Zur experimentellen Psychopathologie sprachabhängiger Denkprozesse (paper submitted) 1992

Sulloway FJ: Freud, Biologist of the Mind. New York, Basic Books, 1979

Swinney D: Theoretical and methodological issues in cognitive science: A psycholinguistic perspective. In: Kintsch W, Miller JR, Polson PG (eds): Method and Tactics in Cognitive Science. Hillsdale, NJ, Erlbaum, 1984

Trautscholdt: Experimentelle Untersuchungen über die Association der Vorstellungen. Wund's Philosophische Studien 1: 213–250, 1881

Tschisch Wv: Ueber die Zeitdauer der einfachen psychischen Vorgänge bei Geisteskranken (On the duration of mental processes in mentally ill patients). Neurologisches Centralblatt 3: 217–219, 1885

Wundt W: Grundzüge der Physiologischen Psychologie, 4th ed., vols I &II. Leipzig, Engelmann, 1893

Zilboorg G: Some sidelights on free associations. The International Journal of Psychoanalysis 33: 489-495, 1952

M. Spitzer, F.A. Uehlein
M.A. Schwartz, C. Mundt
(eds.): Phenomenology
Language & Schizophrenia.
Springer-Verlag, New York, 1992

Language Planning and Alterations in the Experience of Will

Ralph E. Hoffman

Many of the bizarre symptoms of schizophrenia correspond to alterations in the experience of the will (Bleuler 1911/1950). Typical examples are those patients who complain that nonself forces (such as a famous individual or some more insidious force like the CIA) control their actions, thoughts or speech. The experience of an alien will has its mirror opposite—those patients who believe that they possess special abilities to influence the thoughts and actions of others. These bizarre misattributions of willfulness are all the more puzzling given experimental data indicating that the reasoning abilities of schizophrenics, in general, are intact (Maher 1974).

1. Alterations in the Schizophrenic Patient's Experience of Will

What then causes the schizophrenic to draw false conclusions regarding the limits of his own will and/or the will of others? I will argue in this paper that an examination of language phenomena in schizophrenia sheds some light on this problem.

But the first point I want to make is that once one tries to look at "will" phenomenologically, it is very hard to pin down.

Consider for a moment what the psychotic person is expressing when he reports that his thoughts are controlled by an outside force. A first and necessary condition, I think, is that such thoughts be experienced as involuntary. This is very simple—if the ideation is experienced as being willed by the self, then the likelihood of that ideation being attributed to a nonself agency is small. Yet this doesn't get us very far since most of our thoughts are involuntary—mostly we don't decide to have them. They just pop into our heads. Yet somehow we are not bothered by them. It might perhaps be simpler to consider our actions. Most of the things we do, we don't intend to do in the sense of making a conscious decision about doing it and then doing it. Rather we just do it. For example, when I go to work in the morning, there is a whole range of actions—locking my apartment, walking to my car, driving down the freeway—that I do more or less (depending on the day) automatically. Yet I do not question who is in control. It all seems according to some plan, my own plan, whose goal is to get me to work; this plan seems to unfold regardless of whether I'm attending to its substance or not.

What about an involuntary scratching of the forehead or an irrelevant thought about a movie that I saw last night *which just popped into my head* as I drive to work. These events ordinarily just aren't alarming in the least. We all have unedited thoughts and actions. We can free-associate. Irrelevant material can enter our consciousness. Yet we ordinarily do not conclude that that these unedited thoughts and actions derive from a nonself origin. We glide along, conscious of a constant spectacle of images, affects and actions, and are not concerned about whether we are "in control." What in the schizophrenic patient's mind then raises the question of being "in control" given the apparent disorder of moment–to–moment consciousness for all of us?

Consider a small mental exercise: Suppose you were on the highway driving in your car and you had a flat tire. You get out of the car and begin to change the tire. Now suppose while you are changing the tire, you developed an involuntary nervous twitch in your shoulder. This may be alarming, but certainly would not constitute an experience that would make one feel possessed by an alien force.

But now instead suppose that as you reached for the tire, your right hand involuntarily shot up in the air and started waving at the cars. My prediction is that this experience would be quite a bit more alarming—as if an alien, nonself force had taken possession of your arm. *It would be as if the arm had its own plan of action.*

This prediction is supported by a very interesting stroke syndrome studied by Goldberg (1985). These patients suffer from lesions of the supplementary motor area of the frontal lobes; this cortical area has been identified as being central to the initiation of purposeful motoric actions (Goldberg 1985). These patients develop "alien hands" which undertake a sequence of actions that seem planned to accomplish a particular goal. For instance, the hand may attempt to unbutton one's shirt when the subject has no intention of doing so. This rare form of stroke can produce a kind of psychosis. Some of these patients, none of whom have prior histories of prior psychiatric disturbance, have come to believe that their arms have been possessed by alien, nonself forces (G. Goldberg, personal communication).

Thus I propose that the alien ideation of schizophrenics reflects some coherent sequence of thoughts or images which seem "planful," and whose "planfulness" is somehow experienced as unfolding autonomously with respect to the individual. Scratching one's head or having idle thoughts about a recent movie do not present a threat because they are merely unplanned—they do not represent an alternative plan which competes with one's current goals and actions.

What does all of this have to do with schizophrenic language?

2. Language Production Processes in Schizophrenia

The connecting link is that spoken language has an inner counterpart—the speech that we use to "talk" to ourselves. "Inner speech" was best described by Vygotsky who presenting convincing evidence the words that we all use to talk to ourselves derive developmentally from outward directed social speech (Vygotsky 1978). Thus a study of the organization of outward speech may shed light on inner speech, the language of thought. Moreover, the production of speech reflects a hierarchy of cognitive planning par excellence: words are organized into sentences, and sentences are organized into discourse with an organizational plan expressing the communicative intention of the speaker.

It has long been appreciated that some—though not all—schizophrenic persons produce irregular utterances which are difficult for listeners to follow and understand (Bleuler 1911/1950). These speech difficulties are diverse in nature. For instance, some schizophrenics seem to have difficulties in generating acceptable words. The results, in neurolinguistic terms, are paraphasias; for example:

(1) he is a *grassical* person (Hoffman & Sledge 1984).

(2) ... you have to have a *plausity* of amendments to go through for the children's code, and it's no mental disturbance of *puterience*, it is an *amorition* law... (Chaika 1974).

Other schizophrenics produce paragrammatical sentences, e.g.,

(3) After John Black has recovered in special neutral form of life the honest bring back to doctors agents... (Chaika 1982)

On the basis of examples such as these, it has been argued that schizophrenics can demonstrate a kind of intermittent aphasia Chaika (1974, 1977, 1982). In my experience most schizophrenics do not often produce language deviance with the density of an organic aphasic patient, particularly in this age of aggressive use of neuroleptic medication. However, a careful study of transcriptions of their spontaneous speech do reveal certain types of more subtle and frequent syntactic difficulties which seem out of the ordinary.

Consider a schizophrenic speaker who produced the following (from Hoffman & Sledge 1984):

(4) the communists who have a class–struggle creation

and a few seconds later

(5) a creation class-struggles.

Examples (4) and (5) both seem to reflect difficulties in generating the noun phrase, "creation of (a) class-struggle(s)".

In order to analyze these grammatical errors, a preliminary word on nomenclature. Ordinarily, the lexicon of languages like English and German can be broken down into two classes. The first class is referred to as "open class" elements. This term refers to the nouns, verbs, adjectives and adverbs of the language; these are the words through which the language expands and evolves. On the other hand, "closed class" elements are those words that do not change—they are grammatical words such as prepositions, conjunctions, articles, etc. Consider then the following speech errors made by normal speakers (Garrett 1975):

(6) Although *murder* is a form of *suicide* (intended: suicide is a form of murder)
(7) McGovern favored *pushing busters* (intended: busting pushers)

Here it can be appreciated that different open class lexical items have exchanged places. Studies of speech errors such as these suggest that at a preliminary stage of preconscious sentence planning, the open class items relevant to the speech intention are clustered together in an unordered fashion. At a later stage, these words are slotted into a syntactic "frame" constructed from the closed class elements and other grammatical morphemes such as "ing" and "er" that attach themselves to open class elements. Open class items are sometimes misfiled in the syntactic frame when they resemble another item that is slotted for that place in the syntactic frame. Thus "murder" is exchanged with "suicide" since they both deal with death, and "push" is exchanged with "bust" since they are phonetically similar. For the second case, the syntactic frame looks like:

$$\text{Subject—verb—Slot}_1\text{–ing—Slot}_2\text{–ers.}$$

where "push" and "bust" are missorted into the two slots.

It should be clear that these speech errors are quite different than the speech errors produced by the schizophrenic speaker. A re-examination of the these examples suggests that there was a successful grouping together of two open class elements, "creation" and "class-struggle" *prior* to being slotted into a syntactic frame. However, a syntactic frame such as

$$\text{Slot}_1 \text{ of (a/the) Slot}_2$$

necessary for a syntactic realization of a phrase combining "creation" and "class struggle" seems lacking.

This case prompted us to undertook a systematic study which compared grammatical deviance generated by two groups of speakers (Hoffman et al. 1988). One group consisted of eleven schizophrenics with acute illnesses requiring short-term hospitalization. A second comparison group consisted in nine patients with psychiatric disorders other than schizophrenia also in need of acute hospitalization. Both groups were well matched in terms of age, gender and educational level. Each patient in the study was requested to respond to a series of neutral queries such as, "Tell me about your experiences in school" or "Tell me about where you grew up." Two of the responses were randomly selected for careful transcription and analysis of grammatical deviance. For the purposes of this study, grammatical deviance was defined as words that did not belong to the English lexicon, or combinations of words that violated syntax. Slang and variations due to local dialect were not scored as deviant. Of note is the fact that we did not choose normal subjects as a control group but rather other psychiatric patients; it was hoped that "nonspecific" factors tending to produce speech errors—anxiety, stress, fatigue, etc.—would be present in both groups, and therefore would be at least partially controlled for.

Two types of scores were generated for each patient. The first was the number of grammatically deviant segments produced relative to the total number of clauses produced. The second was an assessment, for each instance of deviance, as to the ambiguity of corresponding speech intention. All analyses were conducted blind to diagnosis.

The major finding was that the mean number of instances of deviance per clause was 0.11 for the schizophrenic group and 0.045 for the nonschizophrenic comparison group, a difference that was statistically significant at the 0.02 level.

This finding was consistent with other recent studies demonstrating that schizophrenics showed an increased frequency of language deviance (Morice & Ingram 1982; Fraser et al. 1986); these earlier studies, however, did not analyze the type and severity of deviance. Our study attempted to address these issues. In terms of the type of error, there was a roughly equal number of inappropriate or poorly formed open-class words (nouns, verbs, adjectives, adverbs) among the two subject groups. Here are two examples:

(8) Fish *school* in their communities... ("school" inappropriately used as a verb; example from a schizophrenic patient)

(9) The Israelis and the Arabs need to know that they are part of a strategic area and are *located* to world peace (possible target is important/critical; example from a manic patient)

There was only two cases of paraphasia (more commonly referred to in the psychiatric world as neologism): "edumacating" substituted for "educating" in a speech segment produced by a schizophrenic, and "wirth," apparently a condensation of "with" and "where" when viewed in context (Hoffman & Sledge 1988, p. 98).

However, there were many more errors involving grammatical morphemes (prepositions, conjunctions, suffixes, etc.) among the schizophrenic patients compared to nonschizophrenics. The following are two typical examples:

(10) That was a decent things to do
(11) We could be wheelchairs (intended: we could be in wheelchairs)

The second category used to score grammatical errors was the degree of ambiguity of what the speaker seemed to want to say, the speech intention. The speech intentions for (10) and (11) are quite unambiguous. However, in analyzing all the speech segments that we had, there was a strong trend in the direction of more ambiguous deviance within the schizophrenic corpus. Included among this group of errors was a relatively large number of syntactic "blends," consisting in the inappropriate combination of distinct syntactic structures. Here are two representative examples:

(12) I'm very sad to see it in some of the patients aren't really that rotten you see

This segment combines two alternative syntactic structures:

I'm very sad to seem it in some of the patients

and

Some of the patients aren't really that rotten you see

A more complex example is the following:

(13) I don't know where I'm going or wherever I'll go, but I'll let you know.

This seems to reflect a combination of two competing structures

I don't know where I'm going, but wherever I go I'll let you know

and

I don't know where I'm going or where I'll go, but I'll let you know (when I go)

These data suggest that schizophrenics produce two kinds of speech errors during the preconscious process of sentence planning. First, they have sporadic difficulties in elaborating the syntactic frame itself. Second, alternative syntactic frames seem at times to compete for expression. These two types of errors may reveal two distinct stages of language production that can be disrupted in schizophrenia, the former being the elaboration of any syntactic frame, with the latter corresponding to the selection of one of more than one alternative syntactic frames. These two types of errors of course do not account for the production of deviant words—paraphasias and other neologistic constructions—but such lexical problems did not seem to be excessive in the corpus of errors produced by schizophrenics.

Besides disruptions in sentence production there are other stages of language production commonly disrupted in schizophrenic patients that direct the juxtaposition of sentences in extended, coherent discourse. Of interest is that a similar pattern of disturbance can be observed.

3. Discourse Organization in Schizophrenia

Discourse planning requires the sequence of clauses, sentences or statements so that a specific communicative intention is expressed. This discourse plan is transformed into lower level representations such as syntactic units which form the basis of sentences and phonetic strings (Garrett 1975; Arbib 1982; Hoffman & Sledge 1984). As in the case of sentence planning, discourse planning processes generally occur outside the conscious awareness of the individual, although, at times, the speaker may be consciously aware prior to speaking of two or three key words that will figure into the discourse product.

James Deese (1978) has discussed a particular model of discourse planning whereby abstractly represented propositions which compose a communicative intention are arranged into a hierarchically organized data set. Topical propositions occupy high nodal positions in the tree. Structural subordination within the tree occurs if the truth of one proposition is presupposed in order to discern pragmatic sense of a second (dependent) proposition. A well-organized multi-sentence discourse structure or "frame" can be illustrated with a speech segment that was produced by a fifty-four year old woman hospitalized for depression (also discussed in Hoffman et al. 1986):

> (14) Interviewer: Can you describe where you live?
> Patient: Yes, I live in Connecticut. We live in a fifty year old Tudor house. It's a house that's very much a home...ah...I live there with my husband and son. It's a home where people are drawn to feel comfortable, walk in, let's see...a home that is furnished comfortably—not expensive—a home that shows very much my personality.

The overall message of the above segment is fairly obvious—the woman is extolling the virtues of her house in terms of how it reflects on herself as a person. This resulting discourse structure is illustrated in figure 1.

It can be demonstrated that a segment of discourse is experienced as coherent, as expressing well-planned communicative intention, if the statements in the text can be organized into a strong hierarchy. This roughly means a strict tree form with no loops or unusual branchings. Using Deese's approach, I and colleagues were able to devise a metric of textual deviance that reflects the degree with which the propositional structure of discourse departs from a strict tree form (Hoffman et al. 1982). The simple presence/absence of nonhierachical discourse structure, blindly determined, differentiated schizophrenic versus non-schizophrenic speakers with 80% accuracy.

Figure 1: Discourse structure of example (14). Lower level statements presuppose higher level statements. Each pair of statements is textually linked: either one statement presupposes the other, or they both presuppose a third statement. This allows the text as a whole to be experienced as coherent by the listener/reader (Hoffman et al. 1986). © 1986 American Medical Association. Reprinted with permission of the publisher.

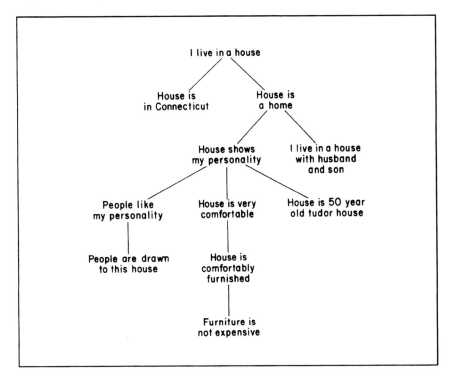

Though a full description of the analysis is beyond the scope of this presentation, textual deviance can be illustrated with the following three schizophrenic speech segments:

(15) Interviewer: Have you ever been out of New York?
Patient: No, I've never been no where—no where.....If I could go I would go...I feel like cashing in my welfare check now and just leaving...and I was gonna keep my-my two checks and save them and get an apartment. I wanna save them and just leave.
(16) Interviewer: Did you ever try to hurt yourself? (patient being asked about her suicidality after being admitted to a psychiatric hospital)
Patient: I cut myself once when I was in the kitchen trying to please David. I was scared for (sic) life because David didn't want me and if David didn't want me then no man would.
(17) Interviewer: Tell me about school?

Patient: School? Well there are schools of play and schools of fish, mostly you see fish school, people edumacating (sic) themselves, you see, sea is one thing and education is another. Fish is school in their community, that's why the community of man stands in the way of the community of the sea, and once they see the light of sunny sunshine then they will let it be...

For segment (15), the incoherence is due to the fact that "saving/keeping checks" has two different senses imposed by a shifting context—in the first case to provide money to leave NYC and in the second case to provide money to stay. This corresponds to the deviant tree structure represented in figure 2. Here the two separate chains of dependencies converge upon the single saving/keeping money statement. As can be seen, presupposed statements corresponding to staying and leaving NYC do not, in themselves, presuppose any third statement; hence this "upward branching" of presuppositional chains violates axiom (I) defining partial ordering.

Figure 2: Discourse structure of example (15). Two alternative hierarchical structures converge on the "I want to keep/save my two checks" statement, thereby lending two different interpretations to this segment. This structure is not a "strong hierarchy" because the discourse structure laws a superordinate statement that is presupposed by all other statements; in other words, there is no central "trunk" from which all the different statements branch out. (Hoffman 1986). © 1986 Cambridge University Press. Reprinted with permission of the publisher.

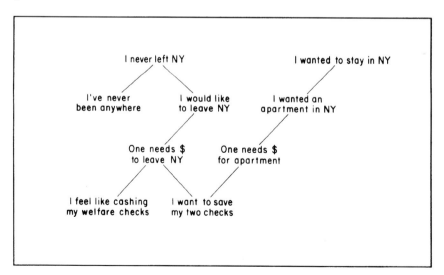

Segment (16) also suggests a condensation of two disjoint messages. This is illustrated in figure 3. The right hand chain of statements describes a state of high stress of the type that might lead to suicidal behavior. This description substantiates the paragrammatical statement, "I was scared for life," which could be interpreted as "I was scared *of* life," or "I feared that my life was over." The left-hand hierarchy seemingly refers to an incident where the speaker accidently cuts herself. In this context, "I was scared for life " seems to refer to her reaction to seeing that she had accidentally cut herself. The result is a departure from a strict hierarchical ordering of statements since statements such as "no man wants me" and "David doesn't want me" presuppose the "I was scared for life" statement and are referable to the suicide theme, but not the "I (accidentally) cut myself" statement.

Fig. 3 Discourse structure of example (16). The jagged line represents a break in transitivity of the presupposition relationship: "I was scared (for/of?) my life" seems to presuppose the "I cut myself in the kitchen statement, and forms the basis for talking about suicide (reflected in the chain of statements on the right hand side of the figure). On the other hand, "I cut myself in the kitchen" does not seem to be related to the suicide theme (unless we assume the unlikely interpretation that she tried to commit suicide to please her boyfriend David). This is another type of departure from a "strong hierarchy" discourse structure. (Hoffman 1986). © 1986 Cambridge University Press. Reprinted with permission of the publisher.

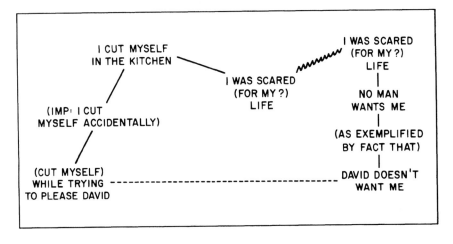

Segments (15) and (16), as mild discourse deviations, yield planning structures which condense disjoint messages corresponding to multiple statement hierarchies that deviate from any single communicative goal. On the other hand, segment (17) represents a rather total loss of hierarchical structure such that statements are juxtaposed primarily on the basis of word play and phonetic similarity.

Thus we can see a parallel when one compares problems in sentence construction among schizophrenics with their problems in generating multi-sentence discourse structure. In certain instances there seems to be a breakdown in syntactic planning; this was most clearly illustrated in the "creation of class struggle" examples. On the other hand schizophrenics also produced many more instances where different syntactic plans compete for expression. At a textual level segments such as (17) reflect a general breakdown of hierarchical planning, whereas segments (15) and (16) suggest, again, competition of alternative plans.

This heuristic view of language planning deviance in schizophrenia has a certain intuitive appeal. It is likely that the creation of structure (at either the sentence and discourse level) occurs somehow prior to that stage of language planning where structures compete for expression. Thus it may be possible that different types of language deviance may point to these different levels of language planning. Second, it suggests that the same types of cognitive pathology may be active in different parts of the schizophrenic's brain. Discourse planning—insofar as it involves "intentional" cognitive processes—probably occurs in prefrontal cortical areas closely associated with the supplementary motor area (Goldberg 1985), whereas syntax has classically been associated with the Broca's area.

4. Language Planning and the Will

I have argued that schizophrenics demonstrate two types of language planning disturbances. The first produces deficient structure, while the second yields simultaneous well-formed structures that compete for expression. This pattern of deviance was noted to occur both at the level of sentence construction, as well as when the speaker is attempting to combine multiple sentences into larger discourse structures. The latter corresponds to the formation of conversational intentions, i.e., the crystallization of the "gist" of what the speaker has in mind to say.

Recall that the bulk of these language planning processes occur outside of the awareness of the speaker. We can choose, when speaking, to be aware of syntactic rules of sentence construction or, in a rough fashion, the interweaving of topics and subtopics of what we are preparing to say. Yet, in general, we are not consciously attending to these processes. By and large we merely speak as we rely on our preconscious selection, combinatorial, and monitoring operations to yield acceptable utterances.

Try now to imagine what it is like to have one thing in mind to say, and instead, produce discourse that says something quite different. The closest most of us have come to this experience is when we generate slips of the tongue and other speech errors of the sort discussed earlier in the chapter. These errors generally seem motivated primarily by fatigue, phonetic similarity of exchanged elements, etc. The error itself doesn't often express it own "message," unless, of course, one is undergoing a Freudian psychoanalysis and has received special training in interpreting the "meaning" of slips in terms of, for instance, Oedipal wishes. You may be surprised, irritated, or amused by the slip, but ordinarily it doesn't clearly say to you something that is distinct from what you had mind to say. Now suppose that, instead of a slip involving a word or two, the speech product included one or more sentences that not only were were inconsistent with what you had in mind (as in the case of ordinary speech errors), but have sufficient structure to express a own fully elaborated, coherent "message," a message that you did not have any awareness of.

This is precisely the experience that is predicted by if the schizophrenic suffers from the *second* type of microgenetic language disturbance, i.e., a failure in (unconsciously) sorting out of competing discourse plans. This in turn produces a potential disparity between the "message" that is consciously registered in the mind as the intended speech act, and the intrusion of a competing discourse plan. It is similar to the "alien hands" described earlier, *except a string of linguistic elements (rather than a set of motoric actions) are produced seeming to have their own purpose.* Consequently the patient may also draw the conclusion that these manifestations derive from nonself forces. In short, the schizophrenic is thrust into a realm of experience where the origin of speech intentions is thrown into question; it may be that the only confirmation that he is the one who is originator of the speech act is the proprioceptive experience of his own vocal musculature while he is speaking. Thus he is likely to happen upon a variety of misconstrued beliefs (which to us seem bizarre, but to him quite reasonable) about the effectiveness of his own will and the willfulness of others.

These propensities may not simply apply to overt speech production, but to covert, "inner" speech as well. If schizophrenics suffered from failure is sorting out competing discourse plans, this failure would also be expressed in one's own inner speech. Under these conditions, the experience of inner speech, in essence, of one's own thought, could be extremely disconcerting if one experienced the intention behind the thought as alien. Once again this would reinforce certain misconstrued beliefs as to the effects of an "alien will" which is operating on the self.

A particularly vivid manifestation of this type of language pathology are the verbal hallucinations or "voices" of schizophrenics—these patients often report hearing the voice of another individual who is either not present or if he is present isn't actually speaking to him. These experiences are highly prevalent among schizophrenics. I have hypothesized that these experiences derive from competing, discordant discourse plans operating on inner speech.

The evidence for this claim is the following:

First, verbal hallucinations, like ordinary inner speech, seem to be accompanied by subtle activation of vocal musculature that is electromyographically detectable (Gould 1948, Junginger & Rauscher 1987). This strongly suggests that verbal hallucinations involves ordinary language production processes.

Second, a positron emission tomography study of chronic schizophrenics with and without verbal hallucinations suggests functional coupling of areas of the brain ordinarily involved in speech production in the former group (Cleghorn et al. 1990).

Third, the presence of verbal hallucinations is a strong predictor of the presence of disruption of language production processes reflected as defects in multisentence discourse planning (Hoffman 1986). Based on a metric of discourse planning deviance, mean scores among hallucinators were more than double that of nonhallucinators, a difference that was statistically significant at a very robust level.

Fourth, recent attempts to enhance the discourse planning abilities of schizophrenics with severe verbal hallucinations have resulted in significant improvement the intensity of their hallucinatory experiences (see also Hoffman, in press). This has been observed in three of four cases: a novel type of speech therapy has been attempted by myself where patients practice combining words into sentences, combining sentences into discourse, and completing brief stories. Moreover, I gave them a number of conversational exercises to practice at home, including reading aloud and talking to relatives. The one patient who failed to respond to this treatment was someone one had a very dense deficit in verbal memory—she could not remember what she had said from one sentence to the next—and therefore could not be trained to produced any kind of coherent discourse.

To conclude, I have argued that studying language planning disturbances, besides being of interest in its own right, may shed light on other components of the phenomenology of schizophrenia. In particular, these structural difficulties, if mirrored in the inner speech—or "language of thought"—could produce message structures possessing their own discordant intentionality which in turn could produce certain disturbances in the experience of willfulness of ideational processes so often reported by these patients. Focusing on verbal hallucinations, there is empirical evidence to support the hypothesis that language planning disturbance are etiologically related to alien/nonself aspects of their experience.

Summary

Schizophrenic patients often report ideation experienced as deriving from an alien, nonself force. A phenomenological analysis of involuntary actions suggests that such ideation reflects internally coherent cognitive plans. It is hypothesized that these cognitive plans unfold independent of, and are in conflict with, the conscious goals and actions of the individual. An examination of speech disturbances produced by schizophrenics may provide clues as the mechanism leading to these symptoms. At both syntactic and discourse levels of speech production, it is often the case that different planning structures simultaneously compete for expression. Outward speech provides the basis of "inner speech," the language of thought. If multiple, alternative planning structures also were elaborated during the production of inner speech, certain language plans may be fully elaborated but remain more or less out of consciousness. If these preconscious language plans were expressed as verbal images, the resulting mentation would be experienced as having an alien, nonself origin. It is hypothesized that verbal/auditory hallucinations derive from this form of language pathology.

210   R.E. Hoffman

References

Arbib MA: From artificial intelligence to neurolinguistics. In: Arbib MA, Caplan D, Marshall JC (eds): Neural models of language. New York, Academic Press, 1982

Bleuler E: Dementia praecox or the group of schizophrenias. New York, International Universities Press, 1911/1950

Chaika E: A linguist looks at "schizophrenic" language. Brain und Language 1: 257-76, 1974

Chaika E: Schizophrenic speech, slips of the tongue, and jargonaphasia: a reply to Fromkin and to Lecours and Vanier-Clement. Brian and Language 4: 464-75, 1977

Chaika E: A unified explanation for the diverse structural deviations reported for adult schizophrenics with disrupted speech. Journal of Communication Disoreders 15: 167-89, 1982

Cleghorn JM, Garnett ES, Nahmias C, Brown GM, Kaplan RD, Szechtmann H, Szechtman B, Franco S, Dermer SW, Cook P: Regional brain metabolism during auditory hallucinations in chronic schizophrenia. British Journal of Psychiatry 157: 562-570, 1990

Deese J: Thought into speech. American Scientist 66: 314-21, 1978

Fraser WI, King KM, Thomas P, Kendell RE: The diagnosis of schizophrenia by language analysis. British Journal of Psychiatry 148: 275-278, 1986

Garrett M: The analysis of sentence production. In: Bower G (ed): The psychology of learning and motivation, Volume 9. New York, Academic Press, 1975

Goldberg G: Supplementary motor area structure and function: Review and hypotheses. Behavioral and Brain Sciences 8: 189-230, 1985

Gould LN: Verbal hallucinations and the activity of vocal musculature: an electromyographic study. American Journal of Psychiatry 105: 367-73, 1948

Hoffman RE: Verbal hallucinations and language production processes in schizophrenia. Behavioral and Brain Sciences, 9: 503-548, 1986

Hoffman RE: The Duphar Lecture: On alien, nonself attributes of schizophrenic hallucinations. Psychopathology (in press)

Hoffman RE, Kirstein L, Stopek S Cicchetti D: Apprehending schizophrenic discourse: a structural analysis of the listener's task. Brain and Language 15: 207-33, 1982

Hoffman RE, Sledge W: A microgenetic model of paragrammatisms produced by a schizophrenic speaker. Brain and Language 21: 147-73, 1984

Hoffman RE, Sledge W: An analysis of grammatical deviance occurring in spontaneous schizophrenic speech. Journal of Neurolinguistics 3: 89-101, 1988

Hoffman RE, Stopek S, Andreasen NC: A comparative study of manic versus schizophrenic speech disorganization. Archives of General Psychiatry 43: 831-838, 1986

Junginger J, Rauscher FP: Vocal activity in verbal hallucinations. Psychiatry Research 21: 101-109, 1987

Maher BA: Delusional thinking and perceptual disorder. Journal of Individual Psychology 30: 98-113, 1974

Morice RD, Ingram JC: Language analysis in schizophrenia: diagnostic implications. Australian and New Zealand Journal of Psychiatry 16: 11-21, 1982

Vygotsky LS: Mind in society: the development of higher psychological processes. Cambridge, Mass., Harvard University Press, 1978

M. Spitzer, F.A. Uehlein
M.A. Schwartz, C. Mundt
(eds.): Phenomenology
Language & Schizophrenia.
Springer-Verlag, New York, 1992

The Structure of Schizophrenic Incoherence

Jörg Frommer & Wolfgang Tress

1. Introduction

Speech in acute and chronic mental disorders was characterized well over one hundred years ago by Wilhelm Griesinger as temporally incoherent (Griesinger 1861). Later on, under the influence of Kraepelin (1913) and Bleuler (1911), the expression "Zerfahrenheit" (distractedness), currently used in German psychiatry, became dominant for speech disorders of patients suffering from "dementia praecox". In English speaking countries as well as in France the expression incoherence continues to be prevalent. At the present time the German translation of the DSM–III (1980) is reimporting this older expression.

Many authors feel that speech disorder is a pathognomic symptom of schizophrenia (Pavy 1968, Mundt & Lang 1987). However, the evaluation of speech disorder is difficult because of the lack of a clear and universally accepted definition (Andreasen 1979). The long history of investigating this symptom shows that dominant research paradigms in other sciences such as psychology and sociology have always exerted great influence. In the beginning, descriptive-clinical psychiatry and neuropathology were the starting point, but association psychology, differential psychology, phenomenology, cognitive psychology, developmental psychology, and psychoanalysis became increasingly important from about the early 1900's on. Later, expressional psychology, communication sciences, systems theory and finally experimental psychology became relevant (Frommer 1991).

Modern research, interested in quantitative results, has used linguistic approaches for orientation. Here, a trend was apparent in recent years which Dawson et al. described as follows:

"A modern, functional approach to the study of the use of language ... moves from the study of single sentence to the study of text (larger semantic units), and from there to the study of interpersonal and social context" (Dawson et al. 1980).

As a part of this trend, the Czechoslovakian school of structuralism as well as the Parisian school of structuralism were applied in investigations of speech disorders. These approaches permitted the qualitative examination of pathological phenomena and their contexts in individual cases, such as, for example, the phenomena of "Zeichenfeldstörung" (Peters 1973) or "Symbolisationsstörung" (Lang 1982). However, the quantitative analysis of larger numbers of cases is problematic using these methods.

It is easier to quantitatively examine disturbances in the language of schizophrenic texts with the "cohesive ties" theory as developed by Halliday and Hasan. These ties are defined as "the means whereby elements that are structurally unrelated in the text are linked together" (Halliday & Hasan 1976). They represent syntactic interdependences of the individual elements in a text. Rochester and colleagues were the first investigators to examine thought disordered schizophrenics with this method and to compare them with non-thought disordered schizophrenics and with normal controls. Their subjects were asked to tell a story and the resulting texts were then judged for the appearance of the following types of cohesive ties: pronominal, demonstrative, and comparative reference; nominal, verbal, and clausal substitution; nominal, verbal, and clausal ellipsis; additive, adversative, clausal, temporal, and continuative conjunction; lexical cohesive ties as same root, synonym, superordinative, and general item. The authors found fewer cohesive ties in schizophrenic experimental subjects than in the normal controls. Thought disordered schizophrenics could be differentiated from non-thought disordered schizophrenics because the former group relied more on lexical ties. The authors also found that schizophrenics characterized as thought disordered were forming syntactically correct sentences and using the same lexical fundus as healthy subjects in the control group (Rochester 1978, Rochester & Martin 1979). Later Wykes and Leff demonstrated that the texts of manic patients contained significantly more cohesive ties than those of schizophrenics (Wykes 1981, Wykes & Leff 1982). Schonauer and Buchkremer used the same method to evaluate therapy for schizophrenics (Schonauer & Buchkremer 1986). Contrary to reported results, studies published by Allen and Allen (1985) and Rutter (1985) did not confirm the finding of a lower rate of cohesive ties in the texts of schizophrenic patients.

Other authors assumed that the typical characteristics of schizophrenic speech disorders could be understood more precisely by investigating semantic aspects. In this context it is useful to recall that speech utterances can always be classified into two categories: first something given, regarding which something is being said, and second something new, telling about the given (Halliday & Hasan 1976). This iterating basic structure of linguistic texts results in a "thematic progression" (Hellwig 1984) or a meaningful netting together of individual sentences. This connecting to a whole is termed "coherence".

In Chomsky's (1965) generative grammar, a concept which has dominated for many years, the context of a sentence is defined as a hierarchical pyramid of metalinguistic deep structures underlying the actual text. The actual text itself is called the surface structure (Chomsky 1965). This model, developed at first for sentences, was expanded later to include larger semantic units. Nöth was one of the first to use it to examine schizophrenic texts. According to Nöth (1976), schizophrenic incoherence results from the lack of coherence within the various hierarchical levels of the deep structure of a text. Similar models were applied by Hoffman et al. (1982), and Hoffman, Stopek, and Andreasen (1986), who found a higher rate of coherence in the texts of manics than in the texts of schizophrenics.

2. Empirical Studies

2.1 First Study

Our own studies are primarily influenced by the computer linguist Peter Hellwig, who defines coherence as "a matter of communicatively meaningful speech sequences" (Hellwig 1984). Hellwig assumes that all texts, including monologs, have an underlying implicit dialog structure. The basic pattern of this structure is a continually repetitive question-answergame. In most cases, however, the author of the text only says aloud the answer, whereas the question remains unspoken. In other words: speakers structure their texts so that each sentence can be understood as an acceptable answer to a question generated by the listener as a reaction to the portion of the text mentioned up to that point. Each coherent sentence must therefore pick up a theme of the already mentioned part of the text and add a meaningful statement to it. Hellwig describes the process of deciding whether a sentence is coherent in relationship to the rest of the text as follows:

"As reading normally progresses from the first to the last sentence, one tries to formulate a question to each statement in such a way that (1) the question is answered—at least partially—by the specific statement, and (2) posing the question is an involuntarily response to one of the earlier statements, or in case of the first sentence, to the external situation." (Hellwig 1984, translation by V.F. Sherbow).

We would like to explain this process utilizing the beginning of a famous American novel as a sample text:

1. "He was an old man who fished alone in a skiff in the Gulf Stream."
2. "And he had gone eighty-four days now without taking a fish."
3. "In the first forty days without a fish the boy's parents had told him, that the old man was now definitely and finally salao, which is the worst form of unlucky."
4. "And the boy had gone at their orders in another boat which caught three good fish the first week" (Hemingway 1952).

Let us judge this text with regard to its coherence and fill in questions between the individual sentences according to the approach of Hellwig :

1. "He was an old man who fished alone in a skiff in the Gulf Stream." *How successful was he?*
2. "And he had gone eighty-four days now without taking a fish." *Which reactions did this provoke?*

3. "In the first forty days without a fish the boy's parents had told him, that the old man was now definitely and finally salao, which is the worst form of unlucky."
    What did the boy do after that? ...

Each individual sentence can be judged by how well the criteria for text coherence are being fulfilled; that is to say, whether the sentence contributes to the thematic progression of a specific communication situation in a meaningful way.

In our own empirical studies we first utilized the story "Die Fabel vom Salzesel" (The story of the salt carrying donkey), a story often used in German clinical psychiatry, which was to be re-narrated by the experimental subjects.

Fourteen acutely ill, thought-disordered schizophrenics were included in this study (ICD 9: 295.1, 295.3). Further selection included organic psychosis (N = 14), major depressive disorders (N = 14), and healthy subjects (N = 14). All patients had been newly admitted to the psychiatric clinic of the University of Heidelberg within a defined time period. The control group consisted of staff members of the medical department. All subjects were similar in their educational background. They were diagnosed by their physicians according to the ICD–9 independent of the research team (for further details, see Tress et al. 1984).

The texts narrated by experimental subjects and recorded on casette tape were transcribed and broken down into individual sentences. Then, as a measure of cohesion, the number of co-references (words or phrases which re-addressed topics appearing in the text in a direct or modified way) was determined. This procedure was carried out for all topics which occurred in the text. The total number of co-references was then correlated with the number of sentences in the text. The computed rate of cohesion showed the lowest values in the group of schizophrenics (mean: 148%). Texts of patients with organic psychosis had values slightly higher than average (mean: 183%), whereas depressed subjects (mean: 177%) and healthy subjects (mean: 175%) did not differ substantially. However, the differences which were obtained were not statistically significant.

The coherence of each text was investigated by individuals unaware of the diagnosis of the narrator. Investigators were asked to formulate a coherent question for each sentence in the narration and examine whether the sentence can related to the rest of the text and situation in a meaningful way. If the above mentioned conditions for coherence were not fulfilled by a sentence; that is to say, if it could not be appreciated how the sentence was connected to the rest of the text, then the sentence received a straight line instead of a question. In the end straight lines of missing coherence questions were added up and the sum correlated with the number of sentences in the text. In this way a measure of incoherence was developed which is independent of the absolute length of the text.

The results significantly separated schizophrenics from other experimental subjects. Schizophrenics showed an average rate of incoherence of 31%, while incoherence in depressed subjects and healthy subjects was 0%. Finally, although patients with organic psychoses did demonstrate incoherence, the prevalence rate was extremely low. (4%) (Tress, Pfaffenberger, and Frommer 1984).

2.2 Second Study

In a second study we investigated how lay subjects describe a videotaped interview with a schizophrenic person in comparison to an interview with a patient suffering from dementia.

Eighteen subjects, all healthy volunteers, were presented with two interviews. The first was with an acutely ill schizophrenic patient who expressed numerous delusional ideas in disordered speech. The second interview was with a patient suffering from Alzheimer's disease who had completely lost orientation to time and space and who had become incapable of performing simple mathematical calculations. Subjects were instructed to describe each interview through the device of a letter to an imaginary person. Letters were to be as detailed as possible without using qualifying expressions such as "craziness", "stupidity", etc.

The evaluation of the "letters" yielded completely normal cohesion values as expected from mentally healthy people. However, while the conversation with the patient with Alzheimer's disease was described in a mostly coherent fashion, incoherences were often present in the descriptions of the interview with the schizophrenic patient. In descriptions of the schizophrenic's interview, passages kept reappearing in which subjects indicated that they had something to report which could not be meaningfully connected to what had occurred previously. Nevertheless, the writer had to put the unintelligible down on paper. The following example from a subject's letter illustrates this incoherence:

1. "The conversation revolved about the second person."
2. "It wasn't really a conversation."

2.3 Third Study

In the third study, we decided to examine naturally occurring dialogs instead of artificially constructed monologs. We also included thought disturbed manic patients in the study in order to examine the difference between manic and schizophrenic language. This topic has been the subject of ongoing controversy (Andreasen 1979, Hoffman, Stopek & Andreasen 1986).

Subjects for this study were 15 thought disordered schizophrenics (ICD 9: 295.1, 295.2, 295.7, 295.9, 292.1), 15 thought disordered manics, 15 patients with severe senile and presenile organic psychosis, and 15 patients with major depressive disorders. All subjects were involved in two dialogs.

Dialog I: Subjects were shown the picture "Die bestrafte Unschuld" ("An innocent is punished", introduced initially to the psychiatric examination by Bobertag). The picture shows two young boys and a man in front of a house with a broken window. The man is spanking one of the boys. However, at a closer look, one can see that the other boy, hidden behind a stack of firewood, is holding several snowballs in his hands. After viewing this picture, subjects were asked to tell its story, and to put into words its scenic plot. Interviewers added several standardized contributions to the resulting dialog.

Dialog II: Subjects were asked to describe the circumstances of their admission to the clinic. When the interviewer could not understand the progression of the resulting narrative, he/she contributed to the dialog with questions aimed at increasing his/her comprehension of the subject's story (e.g "what do you mean by that?").

Through the use of such standardized interviewer comments, investigators could explore how schizophrenics react in a dialog when they are supposed to follow a request, respond to a question or a comment, or clarify an unintelligibly uttered passage. Once again, as in the monolog study, the rate of cohesion was lowest among schizophrenics, although the result did not reach statistical significance. Detailed information on the average coherence values for both types of interviews are presented elsewhere (Frommer and Tress 1989). To summarize, incoherences appeared almost exclusively among schizophrenic patients (Dialog I: 10%, Dialog II: 15%), whereas they were very rare among patients with organic psychoses (Dialog I: 1%, Dialog II: 1%), and were missing altogether in the depressed group. Additionally, incoherences were not found in manic patients even when considerable thought disorder was present. One exceptional manic case should be mentioned in which a single incoherence did appear. This case, however, involved a manic syndrome in a patient with schizoaffective psychosis.

In Dialog II, interviewer questions were mainly asked to clarify understanding in conversations with schizophrenics These questions failed to achieve their purpose most of the time. In most cases, patients could not come up with a satisfactory explanation of the misunderstanding, but instead made statements which included further incoherences and caused more misunderstandings. In contrast, even though it was occasionally necessary to ask questions in order to improve understanding in conversations with patients suffering from organic psychoses, these questions generally led to clarification by the patient of the preceding incoherence and were not followed by new incoherences. In the dialogs with depressed and manic subjects, questions by the interviewer of this particular type were not necessary.

The following excerpt of one of the interviews with a schizophrenic patient will illustrate these results (coherence questions are printed in italics):

1. "Well, there is this: I'm sitting in my room or we could ride the trolley sometime."
   ------
2. "And then the conductor has, oh, someone is here, and he makes it possible, that something can happen on the train."
   ------
3. "When someone says: Yes we will do something with him."
   What does one think about it?
4. "Well, what will we do with him now."
   What else does one think?
5. "What should happen today?"
   What meaning does this have for the concrete situation?
6. "Or what will happen now."
   What does that mean for the people who are involved in this situation?
7. "What are you doing, what are you doing, what are you doing?"
   ------
8. "It is such a woman's game, I guess, or life also."
   How does the partner react to a statement which he did not understand?
9. Interviewer: "What do you mean?"
   ------
10. "Ha, one can do so many things with the brain."
    What things can one do with the brain?
11. "One can give feelings there and so how one thinks that."
    How does the partner react to a statement he did not understand?
12. Interviewer: "I don't quite understand that."
    ------
13. "Are you married?"
    What does one experience when one is married?

3. Discussion

Our investigations confirmed that linguistic incoherence is a typical schizophrenic symptom. We did not usually find linguistic incoherence in manics or in patients with senile dementia. While spatiality and temporality are disturbed within this last group, situational adequacy remains, although with distorted memories. With schizophrenic patients, however, memory is preserved although situational adequacy is weakened and even destroyed. As a result, subjects which are immediately relevant to the patient and are the topic of his/her statements cannot be elicited consistently and cannot be described in a uniform text. Even though the patient remains a spatial and temporal object for us, he/she is no longer at the center of a subjective coordinating system.Taking on an expression created by Karl Bühler (1934), one of us, Wolfgang Tress, named this condition of semantic disorganization "Dissolution der Deixis" (dissolution of textual reference; cf. Tress 1987).

Our dialog study also indicates that the disruptions that appear in conversations with schizophrenics cannot be eliminated communicatively. Normally, a dialog partner takes a questionable statement back or gives additional information. This affords us a different context to look at what initially seemed unintelligible, so that it can become more understandable. In most cases, however, schizophrenics do not contribute to the clarification of misunderstandings. Misunderstandings and disruptions occur because, at crucial moments, dialog statements of schizophrenics lacking an implicit question-answer-structure. A sentence appears suddenly in a text for which the listener is unable to find a question which would indicate that the sentence has a meaningful connection to what has already been said. On a practical level, according to our study, schizophrenic speakers suffer from a deficit in their capacity to put themselves into the role of the listener and then formulate their statements according to the listener's needs. Similar conclusions were drawn by Rochester (1978) and by Harrow and Quinlan (1985).

George Herbert Mead (1934) already emphasized the prominence of "taking the role of the other" in the formation of personal identity. Herein is a connecting link between schizophrenic speech disorder and the schizophrenic disturbance of the experience of the self, which has been appreciated as a central component of schizophrenic pathology since Bleuler (1911).

We would like to conclude, therefore, with a look at the internal structure of the disturbance in subjectivity characteristic of schizophrenics. Here we find old conceptual problems, already known in philosophic discussions of German idealism at the turn of the 19th century. As recently emphasized by Spitzer (1988), these issues are also relevant for the modern discussions of psychopathology. Part of the problem can be bypassed by focusing on the use of the word "I" in ordinary language instead of on the subject or the "ego". Everyone uses the word "I" to describe him/herself. Following the arguments of philosopher Dieter Henrich, what is meant by that "I" has a double structure. When "I" is correlated with the personal pronouns "he"/"she" or "you", it describes the speaker as one person among others. But when "I" is correlated with the neutral third person "it", the speaker becomes a subject apart from and over against all other entities (Henrich 1982). Therefore we understand ourselves (the bearers of the personal pronoun of the first person) in two ways: 1. As person we are part of the objective world, creatures identifyable in space and time, defined by our bodies. 2. As subject we are at the same time everything else who defines him/herself in the context of the history of his/her private experiences without reference to any identification in the social process. Neither one of these two perspectives can be omitted or reduced to the other. Conscious living and personal identity involve the development of self descriptions and of norms guiding ones actions which respect and nurture both tendencies (Henrich 1987).

In schizophrenic patients, a disturbance of conscious self-reference corresponds to the semantic destruction of sentence subjects (Tress 1987). Schizophrenics fail when attempting to overcome the tension between being a person and being a subject in their interpretation of the world and themselves. The split between being a person and being a subject is evident in the extremes of megalomanic delusion ("I am purely subject") and schizophrenic defenselessness ("I am defenselessly object") (Blankenburg 1971). The disturbance of the dynamic of being a person and being a subject, which Frommer (1990) describes as "Grund-verhältnisstörung" (a basic-proportions disturbance), results in the inability of schizophrenics to see themselves in a stable and consistent way as both an object (i.e., a person) and also a subject (i.e., a self). Linguistic capability, however, requires our taking on the role of the social other as a precondition for producing communicative texts. Those who cannot take on the perspective of others in a stable way cannot play the constitutive game with its unspoken questions that connect the individual statements of a text. Schizophrenics miss the oscillation between the perspective of the speaker and the perspective of the listener which is indispensable for the production of monologs and dialogs. This is the reason why we perceive their texts as unintelligible and incoherent. When this experience occurs repeatedly and our attempts to clarify resulting misunderstandings fail continually, we discontinue our efforts and describe the speech and the speakers as "schizophrenic".[1]

Summary

Texts of schizophrenic patients show significantly more incoherence than those of patients with non–schizophrenic syndromes (manics, depressives, and patients with organic psychosis) and normals. In our theory, incoherence means a disorder in the implicit dialog structure of texts. It is based on deficits in the capacity of taking the role of the other person in social communication. These deficits can be conceived as a common structure of schizophrenic speech disorders and the symptoms of ego–dissociation typically found in schizophrenia. The disturbances in the process of role-taking in social interaction are caused by fundamental disturbances in the

---

1 We wish to acknowledge our indebtedness to Ute F. Sherbow and Michael A. Schwartz who helped in the translation of our text.

self–awareness and self–consciousness of schizophrenic patients, because they are unable to see themselves in a stable and consistent way as both an object and a subject. In our paper results of three empirical studies are presented, which evaluate and confirm our theoretical approach. They show that out text linguistic approach can greatly contribute to a better understanding of central characteristics in schizophrenic speech disorder.

References

Allen HA, DS Allen: Positive symptoms and the organization within and between ideas in schizophrenic speech. Psychological medicine 15: 71-80, 1985

American Psychiatric Association: Diagnostic and statistical manual of mental disorders. 3rd ed. Washington, 1980

Andreasen NC: Thought, language, and communication disorders. I. Clinical assessment, definition of terms, and evaluation of their reliability. II. Diagnostic significance. Archives of General Psychiatry 36: 1315-1321, 1325-1330, 1979

Blankenburg W: Der Verlust der natürlichen Selbstverständlichkeit. Stuttgart, Thieme, 1971

Bleuler E: Dementia praecox oder Gruppe der Schizophrenien. Leipzig Wien, Deuticke, 1911

Bühler K: Sprachtheorie. Jena, Fischer, 1934

Chomsky N: Aspects of the theory of syntax. Cambridge Mass., MIT Press, 1965

Dawson DFL, Bertolucci G, Blum HM: Language and schizophrenia: Toward a synthesis. Comprehensive Psychiatry 21: 81-90, 1980

Frommer J: Über den Zusammenhang von Sprachstörungen und Störungen des Ich-Erlebens bei Schizophrenen. Unpublished paper, 1990.

Frommer J: Sprachauffälligkeiten Schizophrener: Historische Wurzeln moderner Forschungsperspektiven. In: Kraus A, Mundt Ch (eds) Schizophrenie und Sprache, Thieme, Stuttgart New York, pp 117-139, 1991

Frommer J, Tress W: Merkmale schizophrener Rede. Eine vergleichende patholin-guistische Untersuchung von Dialogen mit Schizophrenen, Manikern, Depres-siven und Hirnorganikern. Fortschr. der Neurologie Psychiatrie 57: 85-93, 1989

Griesinger W: Die Pathologie und Therapie der psychischen Krankheiten für Aerzte und Studirende. 2nd ed. Krabbe, Stuttgart, 1861

Halliday M, Hasan R: Cohesion in English. Longman, London, 1976

Harrow M, Quinlan DM: Disordered thinking and schizophrenic psychopathology. Gardner, New York London, 1985

Hellwig P: Grundzüge einer Theorie des Textzusammenhangs. In: Rothkegel A, Sandig B (eds) Text - Textsorten - Semantik, Buske, Hamburg, pp 51-79, 1984

Hemingway EM: The old man and the sea. Cape, London, 1952

Henrich D: Fluchtlinien. Philosophische Essays. Suhrkamp, Frankfurt, 1982

Henrich D: Philosophy and the conflict between tendencies of life. In: Henrich D, Konzepte, Suhrkamp, Frankfurt, pp 117-127, 1987

Hoffman RE, Kirstein L, Stopek S, Cicchetti DV: Apprehending schizophrenic discourse: A structural analysis of the listeners task. Brain and Language 15: 207-233, 1982

Hoffman RE, Stopek S, Andreasen NC: A comparative study of manic vs schizo-phrenic speech disorganization. Arch. of General Psychiatry 43: 831-838, 1986

Kraepelin E: Psychiatrie. 8. ed, Vol III. Barth, Leipzig, 1913

Lang H: Struktural-analytische Gesichtspunkte zum Verständnis der schizophrenen Psychosen. In: Janzarik W (ed) Psychopathologische Konzepte der Gegenwart. Enke, Stuttgart, pp 150-157, 1982

Mead GH: Mind, Self, and Society. Chicago University Press, Chicago, 1934

Mundt Ch, Lang H: Die Psychopathologie der Schizophrenien. In: Kisker K P, Lauter H, Meyer J-E, Müller Ch, Strömgren E (eds) Psychiatrie der Gegenwart. Vol IV. Springer, Berlin Heidelberg New York, pp 39-70, 1987

Nöth W: Textkohärenz und Schizophrenie. Zeitschrift für Literaturwissenschaft und Linguistik 6: 175-194, 1976

Pavy D: Verbal behavior in schizophrenia. Psychological Bulletin 70: 164-178, 1968

Peters UH: Wortfeld-Störung und Satzfeld-Störung. Interpretation eines schizophrenen Sprachphänomens mit strukturalistischen Mitteln. Archiv für Psychiatrie und Nervenkrankheiten 217: 1-10, 1973

Rochester SR: Are language disorders in acute schizophrenia actually information processing problems? Journal of Psychiatric Research 14: 275-283, 1978

Rochester SR, Martin J R: Crazy talk. A study of the discourse of schizophrenic speakers. Plenum Press, New York, 1979

Rutter DR: Language in schizophrenia. The structure of monologs and conversations. British Journal of Psychiatry 146: 399-404, 1985

Schonauer K, Buchkremer G: Zur sprachlichen Manifestation schizophrenen Denkens außerhalb akuter Krankheitsepisoden. European Archives of Psychiatry and Neurological Sciences 236: 179-186, 1986

Spitzer M: Ichstörungen. In search of a theory. In: Spitzer M (ed) Psychopathology and Philosophy, Springer, Berlin Heidelberg New York, pp 167-183, 1988

Tress W: Sprache Person Krankheit. Springer, Berlin Heidelberg New York, 1987

Tress W, Pfaffenberger U, Frommer J: Zur Patholinguistik schizophrener Texte. Eine vergleichende Untersuchung an Schizophrenen, Depressiven, Hirnorganikern und Gesunden. Nervenarzt 55: 488-495, 1984

Wykes T: Language and schizophrenia. Psychological Medicine 10: 403-406, 1980

Wykes T, Leff J: Disordered speech: Differences between manics and schizophrenics. Brain and Language 15: 117-124, 1982

M. Spitzer, F.A. Uehlein
M.A. Schwartz, C. Mundt
(eds.): Phenomenology
Language & Schizophrenia.
Springer-Verlag, New York, 1992

Cognitive Abnormalities and the Symptoms of Schizophrenia

David R. Hemsley

1. Introduction

There is increasing awareness of the need to construct a model of schizophrenic dysfunction which is able to integrate both its neural and perceptual/cognitive aspects. Although information processing models appear useful as a means of linking biological and social factors relevant to the disorder, Anscombe (1987) has noted that "there remains a gap between the computer terminology in which attentional theories are couched, and the patient's experience of schizophrenia" (p. 291). It is clearly important that disturbances of information processing be shown to be related to more complex forms of psychopathology in schizophrenia, as a means for validating the deficit and demonstrating that it is not trivial.

The present paper will begin by considering briefly some possible relationships between experiential phenomena and traditional experimental studies of schizophrenics' disturbances of perception and cognition. Emphasis will be placed on abnormalities of selective attention, although the vagueness of this term, and the variety of theoretical models which have been drawn upon, will be noted. The present author's earlier model of schizophrenic symptomatology will be summarized (Hemsley 1987), together with recent experimental studies which have been carried out to test the model. The data are broadly supportive of the 1987 formulation but some modifications have proved necessary. In particular, the original discussion concerning the formation and maintenance of delusions has required considerable elaboration. The modified cognitive model outlined has been one of the bases upon which Gray et al. (1991a,b) have attempted a detailed neuropsychological theory of schizophrenia. A final section will summarize some of its main points.

2. Perceptual Disturbances and Information Processing

It is clearly important to relate "the concepts and objects of clinical observation to the concepts and experimental data from general psychology"

(Cohen and Borst 1987, p.189). The most ambitious aim of psychological research in this area is to specify a single cognitive dysfunction, or pattern of dysfunction from which the various abnormalities resulting in a diagnosis of schizophrenia might be derived. Influential in this endeavor has been the concept of selective attention, and the reports by schizophrenics about their functioning during the early stages of their condition led McGhie and Chapman (1961) to suggest that the primary disorder is that of a decrease in the selective and inhibitory functions of attention.

Although this approach has continued to provide the impetus for much research, it has become apparent that there are numerous difficulties associated with it. First, there is no agreed model of normal cognitive functioning, and in particular the concept of selective attention is often ill-defined. Models are frequently designed to explain performance on a small range of tasks, and each uses a somewhat different conceptual framework. Their more general applicability (or ecological validity?) has yet to be demonstrated. As Shallice (1988) notes "large scale information processing theories are very loosely characterized; adding a connection, a constraint, or another subsystem to a model is unfortunately only too easy" (p. 321). Second, schizophrenics perform poorly on most tasks. Third, it is difficult to relate such work to biological models.

My own early research derived considerably from that of Broadbent (e.g. 1971) and led to the suggestion that schizophrenics fail to establish appropriate response biases, and hence do not make use of temporal and spatial redundancy to reduce information processing demands (Hemsley 1985). It is generally accepted that perception is dependent on an interaction between the presented stimulus and stored memories of regularities of previous input. The latter result in 'expectancies' or 'response biases' and serve to reduce information processing demands. Norman and Bobrow (1976) therefore make a distinction between 'conceptually driven' and 'data driven' processing. If the 1985 formulation is correct, it should be possible to construct tasks on which schizophrenics perform better than normals due to the latter forming expectancies which are inappropriate to the stimulus presented. However the magnitude of this effect must be great enough to counteract the generally lowered performance shown by schizophrenics as a result of such factors as poor motivation.

A disturbance of this kind is intriguingly reminiscent of earlier descriptions of the ways in which schizophrenics' perceptions and/or thinking are disturbed. As Cutting (1989) points out, Matussek (1952) and Conrad (1958) were among the first to argue that the early stage of schizophrenia could be explained in terms of a breakdown of Gestalt perception, and that such a disturbance could form the basis of delusional perception. Matussek describes a patient who was aware of

"a lack of continuity of his perceptions *both in space and over time* [c.f. failure to make use of spatial and temporal redundancy]. He saw the environment only in fragments. There was no appreciation of the whole. He saw only details against a meaningless background" (Matussek 1952, p. 92).

Arieti (1966) later used the term "perceptual and apperceptual frag- mentation" for such phenomena. Matussek also noted another patient's report that "I may look at a garden, but I don't see it as I normally do. I can only concentrate on details. For instance I can lose myself in looking at a bud on a branch, but then I don't see anything else" (p. 92). In similar vein, Shakow's experimental work had led him to the conclusion that a schizophrenic "can't see the wood for the trees ... and examines each tree with meticulous care" (Shakow 1950, p. 388).

In considering schizophrenics' disturbances of perception and cogni- tion, a number of theoretical models have been drawn upon, and these often differ radically in their assumptions concerning the nature of normal information processing. However several models of normal cognition sug- gest that awareness of redundant information is inhibited to reduce infor- mation processing demands on a limited capacity system. Thus Posner and his colleagues (e.g. Posner 1982) distinguish automatic processes and conscious attention, the former not giving rise to awareness, the latter involving awareness and closely associated with "a general inhibitory process" (p. 173). A related position, although derived from a very dif- ferent data base, is that of Schneider and Shiffrin (1977). They argue that the change from controlled to automatic processing on a task may be seen as including a gradual inhibition of awareness of redundant information.

Although it is clearly hazardous to attempt to interpret studies in a different framework from those in which they were designed, let us consider seven influential views (see Table 1) as to the nature of schizophrenics' cognitive impairment.

Two of the quotes in Table 1 (1 and 3) suggest that cognitive perfor- mance is disrupted by the intrusion of material normally below awareness. The others can be related to a weakening of spatial and temporal regulari- ties on perception. How might these views be brought together and linked to the abnormal experiences characteristic of schizophrenia? In a very general sense the models of Broadbent, Posner and his colleagues, and Shiffrin and Schneider, may be seen as illustrating the way in which the spatial and temporal regularities of past experience influence the pro- cessing, and more speculatively, awareness, of current sensory input. The present author has therefore argued (Hemsley 1987) that *it is a weakening of the influence of stored memories of regularities of previous input on current perception which is basic to the schizophrenic conditions*. Note, it is not claimed that the "memories of past regularities" are not stored, nor that they are inaccessible. They may indeed be accessed by consciously controlled processing. Rather the suggestion is that the rapid and automatic assess- ment of the significance, or lack of significance, of aspects of sensory input (and their implications for action) is impaired as a result of a weakening of the influence of stored past regularities. Such regularities would among other things, influence the awareness of redundant information. A distur- bance would result in the intrusion into awareness of aspects of the environment not normally perceived, as noted by Matussek (1952). Recent evidence in support of this proposal will now be considered, and will be followed by a more detailed exposition of the way in which it might result in the emergence of psychotic symptoms. However, it is of interest that a similar position has been put forward by Patterson (1987) who suggests that there is

"a failure in the automaticity with which prior experience may be re–created in parallel with current stimulus input in schizophrenia (with concomitant failures in future orientation or contextually generated expectancy)" (Patterson 1987, p. 555).

Table 1: Current views on the nature of schizophrenia's cognitive impairment (from Hemsley 1987).

1. "The basic cognitive defect ... it is an awareness of automatic processes which are normally carried out below the level of consciousness "(Frith 1979, p. 233).

2. "There is some suggestion that there is a failure of automatic processing in schizophrenia so that activity must at proceed the level of consciously controlled sequential processing" (Venables 1984, p. 75).

3. Schizophrenics "concentrate on detail, at the expense of theme" (Cutting 1985, p. 300).

4. Schizophrenics show "some deficiency in perceptual schema formation in automaticity, or in the holistic stage of processing" (Knight 1984, p. 120).

5. Schizophrenics show a "failure of attentional focussing to respond to stimulus redundancy" (Maher 1983, p. 19).

6. Schizophrenics are less able to make use of the redundancy and patterning of sensory input to reduce information processing demands" (Hemsley 1985).

7. "Schizophrenics do not maintain a strong conceptual organization or a serial processing strategy ... nor do they organize stimuli extensively relative to others" (Magaro 1984, p. 202).

3. Recent Research Relevant to the Basic Formulation

Although our research program continues to draw upon the literature on normal cognition, we have increasingly looked to animal learning theory in devising our experimental paradigms. The latter has become increasingly "cognitive", and the setting up of a viable animal model for schizophrenia no longer seems an impossibility. Clearly this would facilitate research into the biological bases of schizophrenics' cognitive dysfunction. We have focused on two behavioral phenomena, latent inhibition (LI; cf. Lubow et al. 1982) and Kamin's (1969) blocking effect, both of which can be regarded as instances of the "influence of stored memories of regularities of previous input on current perception" (Hemsley 1987, p. 182).

3.1 Latent Inhibition

Lubow et al. (1982) have argued that the LI paradigm is an effective way of manipulating attention in animals and that it may provide a link with the attentional disturbance prominent in schizophrenia. The paradigm is illustrated in Figure 1. In the first stage, a stimulus is repeatedly presented to the organism (PE), in the second stage, the pre–exposed stimulus is paired with reinforcement in any of the standard learning procedures, classical or instrumental. When the amount of learning is measured, relative to a group that did not receive the first stage of stimulus pre–exposure (NPE), it is found that the stimulus–pre–exposed group learn the new association much more slowly. This is interpreted as indicating a reduction in the deployment of attention to a predictable redundant stimulus. The 'regularity' operating is that the stimulus has no consequence.

Figure 1: Latent Inhibition Paradigm. In normals, pre–exposure to "A" reduces rate of learning A – X association. This is usually interpreted as reflecting a reduction in the deployment of attention to a redundant stimulus.

		Test
Pre–exposure (PE) group	A–A.................. A–A	A – X
Non–Pre–exposure (NPE) group	....	A – X

It has been shown in animals that this effect is disrupted if amphetamine is administered in both the pre–exposure and test phase (Solomon et al. 1981), and the effect can be reinstantiated with neuroleptics. Interestingly, it is also disrupted by damage to the hippocampal formation (Kaye and Pearce 1987), a point which will be returned to in the final section of the this paper. As Lubow et al. (1982) write,

"output is controlled, not like in the intact animal, by the integration of previous stored inputs and the prevailing situational conditions, but only by the latter" (Lubow et al. 1982, p. 103).

The distinction between *data–driven* and *conceptually–driven* processing was discussed above, optimal performance being dependent on an interaction between the stimulus presented and stored memories of regularities in previous inputs which result in expectancies or response biases. Lubow et al. (1982) suggest that animals under the influence of amphetamine may be viewed as unable to utilize acquired knowledge in a newly encountered situation. They write:

"Not having the capacity to 'use' old stimuli, all stimuli are novel. Therefore such an organism will find itself endlessly bombarded with novel stimulation, resulting perhaps in the perceptual inundation phenomena described in schizophrenia" (Lubow et al. 1982, p. 104).

Clearly this is similar to the suggestion that schizophrenics fail to make use of the redundancy and patterning of sensory input to reduce information processing demands, and the   prediction is therefore of disrupted LI in acute schizophrenia. This we have recently demonstrated (Baruch et al. 1988) and the results are presented in figure 2, where higher scores represent more rapid learning.

The acute schizophrenics tend to perform better in the pre–exposure (PE) condition, and it was argued that these results are consistent with their being in a hyperdopaminergic state. Chronic medicated patients performed more normally. In addition, LI for the acute group normalized following 6–7 weeks of antipsychotic medication, as can be seen from figure 3. All except the acute pre–exposure group showed a simple practice effect.

Figure 2: Comparison of three groups on LI task (from Baruch et al. 1988a).

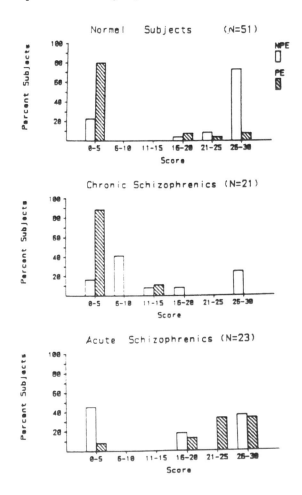

The performance of the acute group on the first occasion of testing was particularly interesting since in the pre–exposure condition they performed better than normal subjects, due to their continuing to attend to the redundant stimulus. It cannot therefore be attributed to a non–specific loss of efficient cognitive functioning.

It is important to note that LI does not simply represent a form of habituation. There is a major difference between the two: LI is disrupted by a change in context, whereas habituation is not. This may prove important for our understanding of schizophrenia, where a key disturbance may be the failure to relate specific associations to the context in which they occur. For LI, the association in question is one of stimulus—no consequence; a failure to link this association to its context should have the same consequences as a context shift, i.e. disruption of LI, and this may account for the performance of acute schizophrenics. Once again, Matussek's observations are relevant. He wrote:

"When the perceptual context is disturbed, individual objects acquire different properties from those which they have when the normal context prevails" (Matussek 1952, p. 94).

Figure 3: Changes in LI over time for schizophrenic groups (from Baruch et al. 1988a).

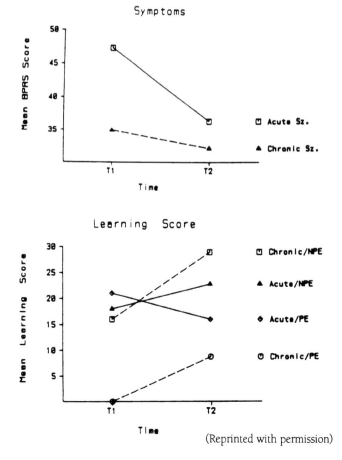

(Reprinted with permission)

Matussek suggested that the extent to which context is loosened crucially determines the severity of the disorder. Harrow and Silverstein (1991) also emphasize the failure to relate specific associations to the context, retrieved from long–term memory. They go on to discuss how such a weakening of long–term memory for contextual constraints might facilitate the schizophrenic's acceptance as 'real' of experiences which would be rejected by normal individuals.

3.2 Blocking Effect

A second paradigm, Kamin's (1969) blocking effect, possesses many of the same features as LI and is illustrated in Figure 4.

Figure 4: Blocking Paradigm. In normals, control group learns B – X faster than blocked group. Usually interpreted as reflecting reduction in attention to B in phase 2 for blocked group, because it is found to predict nothing additional to that predicted by A, i.e. it is redundant.

	Phase 1	Phase 2	Test
Blocking group	A – X	(A + B) – X	B – X
Control group	....	(A + B) – X	B – X

It again involves a pre–exposure phase in which the experimental group learns an association between two stimuli (A – X); control subjects learn either no association or a different one at this stage. Both groups are then presented with pairings between a compound stimulus (A + B) and X. Both groups are then tested for what they have learned about the B–X relationship. The pre–exposed group demonstrates less learning than controls; this is the blocking effect and it is generally agreed that it arises as a result of a process in which attention to B is reduced because it is found to predict nothing in addition to what is predicted by A (Pearce & Hall, 1980). It is viewed as *redundant* (c.f. Hemsley 1985). Like LI, the blocking effect in animals is abolished by amphetamine (Crider et al. 1982), and by damage to the hippocampus (Solomon 1977). It was predicted that the blocking effect would be reduced in acute schizophrenics. This was found to be the case (Jones et al. 1991a), and the results are summarized in Figure 5, which presents rank means on trials to criterion; here higher scores represent slower learning. Acute schizophrenics actually performed worse in the control condition, whereas normals showed the usual blocking effect. The scores of the chronic patients were somewhat difficult to interpret as they performed very poorly in both conditions. A second experiment therefore employed a simpler blocking task. On this, both normals and chronic schizophrenics exhibited a blocking effect; there was no effect however of pre–exposure in the acute schizophrenic group.

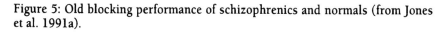

Figure 5: Old blocking performance of schizophrenics and normals (from Jones et al. 1991a).

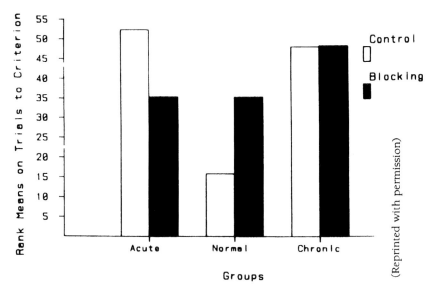

We have recently conducted one further study relevant to these issues, (Jones et al. 1991b). It is relevant both to the role of context in determining schizophrenic performance, but also to the question of whether it is correct to describe the cognitive abnormalities of acute schizophrenia as *attentional*. Hemsley's (1987) model deliberately avoided this terminology and instead emphasized the "weakening of the influence of past regularities", since there are tasks in which different predictions are generated by the two formulations. The experiment used a choice reaction time paradigm developed by Miller (1987) from one devised by Eriksen and Eriksen (1979). Subjects were required to make one of two responses to two visually presented letters (e.g. A or B). These targets were regularly accompanied by two flanking letters (e.g. X, Y, making displays of the form XAX or YBY). Occasionally the flanking letters were interchanged, (YAY or XBX) but the correct response was till cued by the target (A or B). Normal subjects show a reliable slowing of reaction time on such context shift trials; clearly their performance is being influenced by the 'past regularities' within the task. If acute schizophrenics were simply to demonstrate a broader span of attention, they should be more aware of the flankers, and hence show a greater than normal slowing of reaction time on context shift trials. However, if they are less influenced by past associations between focal stimuli and context, they should be less affected than normal subjects by context shift. The latter is the result found by Jones et al. (1991b) for acute but not chronic schizophrenics. Subsequent analyses by hand of response have unfortunately somewhat complicated the picture. Only with right hand responses did we observe the effect described above, which was interpreted as indicating, that acute schizophrenics fail to integrate context with target stimulus–response association. The result is however consistent with research indicating primarily left hemisphere dysfunction in schizophrenia. It is of interest that Kinsbourne suggests that

"it takes left hemisphere damage to impair the depth of conscious analysis ... By depth I mean relation of present to previous (and prospective) relevant experiences" (Kinsbourne 1988, p. 248).

We are currently exploring laterality effects within the latent inhibition paradigm.

4. The Cognitive Bases of Schizophrenic Symptoms

The present paper is concerned primarily with models of positive symptomatology, in particular recent research relevant to delusion formation. However, it is rare for schizophrenics to show only positive or negative symptoms. It remains unclear whether the distinction represents: (a) two underlying and distinct disorders; (b) differing severity of the same disorder; (c) individual differences in reaction to the same disorder; (d) different stages of the same disorder (acute vs. chronic), or a combination of (b), (c), and (d). Thus Pogue–Geile and Harrow conclude that

"the evidence is supportive of the view that negative symptoms may represent a severity threshold on a continuum of liability to schizophrenia" (Pogue–Geile and Harrow 1988, p. 437).

Within the present formulation, a more drastic weakening of the influence of stored regularities on current perception might result in a level of disorganization such as to render difficult any goal directed activities.

Relevant to (c) is Strauss' (1987) argument that certain aspects of schizophrenics' functioning may reflect the action of control mechanisms which

"involve conscious and unconscious psychological processes that focus on regulating the amount of demand faced to fit the adaptive capacity available" (Strauss' 1987, p. 85).

Such control processes were seen by Hemsley (1977) as crucial to negative symptomatology. Schizophrenics were viewed as being in a state of *information overload*; symptoms such as poverty of speech, social withdrawal and retardation, represented adaptive strategies, learnt over time so as to minimize the effects of the cognitive impairment. One may also speculate that the search for meaning in the altered experiences may diminish over time, as actions based on these prove ineffective or counterproductive. As Anscombe (1987, p. 254) puts it, "less and less the subject forms his own impressions, and more and more he is impinged upon by his environment".

The 1987 model is illustrated in figure 6. However the dotted line represents a modification which our recent experimental work suggests is necessary for our understanding of delusion formation. The earlier model followed Maher (e.g. 1974, 1988) in viewing delusions as essentially a product of normal reasoning, serving as explanations which the deluded individual uses to account for aberrant perceptual experiences. This emphasis on abnormal experiences as a basis for delusion formation is also prominent in the earlier writings of Matussek (1952). Following a loosening of the perceptual context, attention may be captured by inciden-tal details of the environment. Normally such an aspect of the situation would not reach awareness, but its registration prompts a search for reasons for its occurrence. Frith's (1979) model adopts a similar position. More recently Anscombe has extended this to suggest that certain of the patients thoughts may be imbued with a significance that is out of propor-tion to their real importance, simply because they happen to capture the attentional focus. He goes on to argue that both internally and externally generated perceptions "are not placed in a context of background knowledge" and that this "results in the coming to awareness of hasty and alarming appraisals by pre–attentive process". However, Spitzer (1990) has rightly cautioned that where patients are making statements about their own altered way of experiencing reality, these should not be labelled as delusions.

Figure 6: Model of cognitive abnormalities and symptoms of schizophrenia (modified from Hemsley 1987).

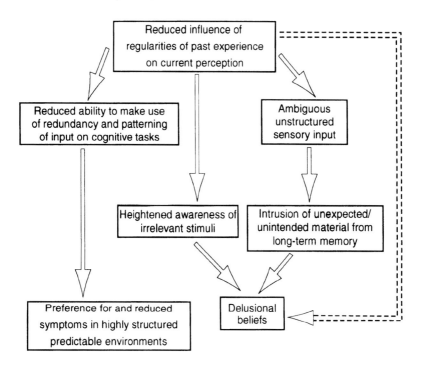

Maher's views cannot however be accepted uncritically. Chapman and Chapman (1988), in a study of the relationships of beliefs to experiences in a group of students, concluded that the processes by which subjects reach delusional or nondelusional interpretations of anomalous experiences are not equally reasonable. We have therefore carried out two studies exploring the reasoning of deluded individuals. A problem which is encountered is in setting a standard for correct or'normal reasoning. Fischoff and Beyth–Marom (1983) suggest that Bayesian inference provides a general framework for evaluating beliefs in the normal population, and that it may be used to describe a person's consistency with, or departure from, the model. Hemsley and Garety (1986) extended this approach to the inferences of deluded subjects. Bayesian procedures provide a model of different stages of the formation and evaluation of a hypothesis (belief): 1. The identification of data sources that are most useful for discriminating between competing hypotheses; 2. the assessment of the implications of an observed datum vis–a–vis the truth of competing hypotheses; 3. an aggregation of implications of different data with an overall appraisal of the relative likelihood of the truth of the hypothesis; 4. the selection, based on appraisal, of the appropriate course of action.

In our first study (Huq et al. 1988) a probabilistic inference task based on the paradigm outlined by Phillips and Edwards (1966) was employed. Pairs of jam jars containing colored beads constituted the stimulus material. In each pair there were in each jar two sets of colored beads in equal and opposite proportions. Thus Jar A would contain yellow (Y) and black (B) beads in the proportion, 85Y: 15B; Jar B would contain the beads in the ratio 85B: 15Y. Subjects were informed that evidence, in the form of single beads, would be drawn from one of the jars. They were required to indicate the probability of a particular jar having been chosen, and to say when they were sure of its identity. Deluded subjects requested less information before reaching a decision, and expressed higher certainty levels than either normals or non delusional psychiatric controls. There was however large variability within the deluded sample, half of whom responded in an extreme fashion. Abnormalities in reasoning may therefore be confined to a subgroup of deluded patients.

Our second study (Garety et al. 1991) employed a similar paradigm and replicated the earlier finding of a smaller number of draws to decision in both paranoid and schizophrenic groups. This is illustrated in figure 7.

However, this study included a further condition to examine belief maintenance or change. In this, the first ten beads supported one hypothesis, the final ten beads the alternative. The sequence was thus as follows

AAABAAAABA BBBABBBBAB

Among the variables examined was the effect of the first item of potentially disconfirmatory evidence (Item 4). Here the schizophrenic and paranoid subjects were more likely to respond by revising their probability estimates downwards, while the anxious and normal control groups tended either to make no change or continued to affirm their initial hypothesis by increasing their estimates slightly. After certainty was reached, deluded subjects were more likely to make a dramatic change in probability estimate following an item of disconfirmatory evidence.

Figure 7: Draws to Decision (from Garety et al. 1991).

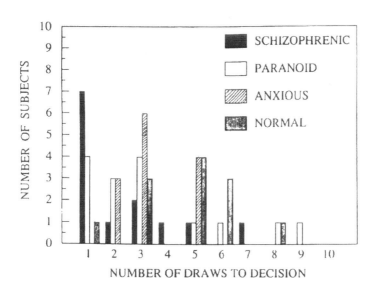

The findings of this second study therefore do not suggest that deluded subjects are characteristically incorrigible. Some members of the deluded groups are not clinging tenaciously to their hypotheses but rapidly changing them. This is consistent with those models of schizophrenia which emphasize the greater influence accorded to the immediate environmental stimuli compared with the effects of prior learning (Salzinger 1984, Hemsley 1987). Hence the need for modification of the present author's earlier view on delusion formation.

Among the most prominent features of delusional thinking is an abnormal view of the relationships between events. As Schneider (1930) put it,

"meaningful connections are created between temporarily coincident external impressions, external impression with the patient's present condition, or perceptions with thoughts which happen to be present, or events and recollections happening to occur in consciousness about the same time" (Schneider 1930).

Similarly Arieti (1966) observed "patients see nonfortuitous coincidences everywhere" (p. 231). Matussek (1952) quotes a patient as saying "out of these perceptions come the absolute awareness that my ability to see connections had been multiplied many times over" (p. 96). For example, objects showing certain qualities which had become prominent were seen as being linked in some significant way. Such feelings of relatedness, based on temporal or spatial contiguity between experiences, may proceed to an assumption of a causal relationship between them. Meehl, claims that schizophrenia prone individuals

"entertain the possibility that events which, according to the causal concepts of this culture, cannot have a causal relation with each other, might nevertheless do so" (Meehl 1964, quoted in Eckblad & Chapman 1983, p. 215).

A patient of the present author, recalling his psychotic experiences noted that the co–occurrence of two events often led immediately to an assumption of a causal relationship between them. It was as if previous non co–occurrences were completely ignored.

Table 2: A possible pathway to the perception of abnormal causal relationships (from Hemsley 1990).

1. A search for causal explanations takes place to *make sense* of the world. This frequently occurs when events violate expectations and achieve prominence.

2. Temporal order and contiguity tend to indicate causal relationships (e.g., x causes y) but in addition, normal subjects take into account the covariation between x and y. Thus for a particular conjunction of x and y, consideration is also given to the occurrence of x without y, and y without x on previous occasions (i.e. past regularities).

3. If schizophrenia is characterized by:

a) awareness of aspects of the environment not normally attended to, and
b) a reduction of the influence of past regularities on current perception,

then, abnormal causal relationships may be inferred on the basis of a single co–occurrence.
(Reprinted with permission)

How might such clinical observations relate to the present model? In reviewing the processes that underlie the judgement of causation, Einhorn and Hogarth (1986 p. 5) note that normal people engage in causal reasoning in order to make sense of the world, and that this is more likely to happen *when perceptions violate expectations and become prominent*. Spatial and temporal contiguity are clearly of great importance in concluding that there exists a causal relationship. However, in assessing the strength of such a relationship, account is also taken of instances of the occurrence of X in the absence of Y, and Y in the absence of X (i.e. past regularities). Consider now the case of the schizophrenic patient. Not only does the *weakened influence of past regularities of current perception* result in the intrusion of redundant material into awareness; it also influences the assessment of the covariation between X and Y. Hence abnormal causal relationship may be inferred on the basis of a single co–occurrence. This is illustrated more formally in Table 2 (from Hemsley 1990).

Most would accept that many delusional beliefs arise on the basis of hallucinatory experiences. I argued (Hemsley 1987) that the extensive literature on sensory/perceptual deprivation in normal subjects may be relevant to schizophrenic hallucinations. It is clear that unstructured input may result in abnormal perceptual experiences, which Leff (1968) suggested to "overlap considerably with those of mentally ill patients" (p. 1547). We have also been able to demonstrate the short term manipulation of auditory hallucinations in a group of schizophrenic patients by means of alterations in auditory input (Margo et al. 1981). The magnitude of the experiences reported was inversely related to the structure and attention commanding properties of the input. If, as proposed above, the schizophrenic condition is characterized by a reduction in the influence of the regularities of past experiences on current perception, the result would be ambiguous, unstructured sensory input. One might, therefore, argue that hallucinations are related to a cognitive abnormality which even under normal conditions results in ambiguous messages reaching awareness and hence fails to inhibit the emergence of material from long term memory (LTM) (c.f. figure 4). Given the constructive nature of normal recall, the intrusions would not necessarily be identical to previously presented material. In similar vein, George and Neufeld have referred to an inter-action between the

"spontaneous retrieval of information stored in LTM and sensory processing, the latter having an inhibitory effect on the former" (George & Neufeld 1985, p. 268).

Rund (1986) has also suggested that

"Schizophrenics, possibly because of a sensory overload, ... are more susceptible to such a direct flow between long term storage and the sensory storage level" (Rund 1986, p. 532).

5. Possible Links with Biological Models

It has frequently been suggested (e.g. Weinberger et. al. 1983, Huber 1986) that pathology of the limbic system is associated with schizophrenia. In particular, the hippocampus has been discussed as a possible region of the brain that might be affected. Although neuropathological studies have provided some support for this view (e.g. Falkai & Bogerts 1986), the findings are far from straightforward, and many other brain regions have been implicated. However, the possible functions if the hippocampus appear very relevant to the present model. Olton et al. have suggested that

"The hippocampus may be the brain structure that allows each of the various components of a place and an event to be linked together, and compared with other places and events" (Olton et al. 1986, p. 354).

In a related formulation Gray (1982) has argued for the role of the hippocampus in the comparison of actual and expected stimuli; if there is a mismatch, there is increasing attention to that input. A defect in this system could relate to a weakening of the effect of past regularities on current perception. This view has been elaborated by Schmajuk (1987) who argues for the utility of the hippocampally lesioned animal as a model for schizophrenia. It was noted previously that both *latent inhibition* and *blocking* are disrupted by damage to the hippocampal formation. Schmajuk argues that the dopamine theory of schizophrenia is reconcilable with his model since hippocampal dysfunction might result in an increase in dopamine receptors in related brain structures such as the nucleus accumbens.

Our most recent model (Gray et al. 1991a; 1991b) has attempted to link dopaminergic hyperactivity with temporal lobe pathology, and to relate both to the disturbances of information processing considered to underlie schizophrenic symptoms. Anatomically, the model emphasizes the projections from the septo–hippocampal system, via the subiculum, to the nucleus accumbens, and their interaction with the ascending dopaminergic projection to the accumbens. Psychologically the model emphasizes a disturbance, in acute schizophrenia, in the normal integration of stored memories of past regularities of perceptual input with ongoing motor programs and the control of current perception. Clearly psychological and biological models of psychotic symptomatology are converging in intriguing ways.

Summary

It is argued that schizophrenia is characterized by a weakening of the influence of regularities of previous input on current perception. The paper indicates how this formulation relates both to the experiences of schizophrenic patients and more general aspects of symptomatology, in particular delusion formation. Recent experimental work relevant to the model is summarized and is found to be broadly supportive. The use of paradigms derived from animal learning theory has facilitated links with biological models of the disorder.

References

Anscombe R: The disorder of consciousness in schizophrenia. Schiz. Bull. 11: 241–260, 1987
Arieti S: Schizophrenic cognitions. In: Hoch PH, Zubin J (eds): Psychopathology of Schizophrenia, pp. 37–48, New York, Grune & Stratton, 1966

Arieti S: Interpretation of schizophrenia, 2nd Edn. London, Crosby, Lockwood, Staples, 1974

Baruch J, Hemsley DR Gray JA (1988) Differential performance of acute and chronic schizophrenics in a latent inhibition task. J Nerv Ment Dis, 176: 598–606, 1988

Broadbent DE: Decision and Stress. London, Academic Press, 1971

Chapman LJ, Chapman JP: The genesis of delusions. In: Oltmanns TF, Maher BA (eds): Delusional Beliefs, pp. 167–183. New York, Wiley, 1988

Cohen R, Borst V: Psychological models of schizophrenic impairments. In: Häfner H, Gattaz WF Janzarik W (eds): Search for the Causes of Schizophrenia, pp. 189–202. Heidelberg, Springer, 1987

Crider A, Solomon PR, McMahon MA: Attention in the rat following chronic d-amphetamine administration: relationship to schizophrenic attention disorder. Biol Psychiat 17: 351–361, 1982

Cutting J: The Psychology of Schizophrenia. London, Churchill Livingstone, 1985

Cutting J: Gestalt theory and psychiatry. J Roy Soc Med 82: 429–431, 1989

Einhorn HJ, Hogarth RM: Judging probable cause. Psych Bull 99: 3–19, 1986

Eriksen BA, Eriksen CW: Effects of noise letters upon the identification of a target letter in a nonsearch task. Percept Psychophys 16: 143–149, 1974

Falkai P Bogerts B: Cell loss in the hippocampus of schizophrenics. Eur Arch Psychiat Neurol Sci 236: 154–161, 1986

Fischoff B Beyth–Marom R: Hypothesis evaluation from a Bayesian perspective. Psych Rev 90: 239–260, 1983

Frith CD: Consciousness, information processing and schizophrenia. Br J Psychiat 134: 225–235, 1979

Garety RA, Hemsley DR, Wessely S:Reasoning in deluded schizophrenic and paranoid patients. J Nerv Ment Dis 179: 194–201, 1991

George L, Neufeld, RWJ: Cognition and symptomatology in schizophrenia. Schiz Bull 11: 264-285, 1985

Gray JA: The neuropsychology of anxiety. Oxford, Oxford University Press, 1982

Gray JA, Feldon J, Rawlins JNP, Hemsley DR, Smith AD: The neuropsychology of schizophrenia. Beh Br Sci 14: 1–20, 1991a

Gray JA, Hemsley DR, Gray N, Feldon J, Rawlins JNP: Schizophrenia bits: Misses, mysteries and hits. Beh Br Sci 14: 56–84, 1991b

Harrow M, Silverstein M: The role of long term memory and monitoring in schizophrenia: multiple functions. (Commentary to Gray et al., 1991a). Beh Br Sci 14: 30–31, 1991

Hemsley DR: What have cognitive deficits to do with schizophrenic symptoms? Br J Psychiat 130: 167–173, 1977

Hemsley DR: Information processing and schizophrenia (paper presented at EABT conference, Munich). In: Straube E, Hahlweg K (eds): Schizophrenia, concepts, vulnerability and intervention, pp. 59–76. Heidelberg, Springer, 1990

Hemsley DR: An experimental psychological model for schizophrenia. In: Häfner H, Gattaz WF Janzarik W (eds): Search for the Causes of Schizophrenia, pp. 179–188. Heidelberg, Springer, 1987

Hemsley DR: What have cognitive deficits to do with schizophrenia? In: Huber G (ed): Idiopathische Psychosen, pp. 111–127, Stuttgart, Schattauer, 1990

Hemsley DR, Garety PA: The formation and maintenance of delusions: a Bayesian analysis. Br J Psychiat 149: 51–56, 1986

Huber G: Negative or basic symptoms in schizophrenia and affective illness. In: Shagass C et al. (eds): Biological Psychiatry, pp. 1136–1138. New York, Elsevier, 1986

Huq SF, Garety PA, Hemsley DR: Probabilistic judgements in deluded and non deluded subjects. Quart J Exp Psych 40A(4): 801–812, 1988

Jones S, Gray JA, Hemsley DR: Kamin blocking effect and incidental learning in acute and chronic schizophrenia. (paper submitted, 1991a)

Jones S, Hemsley DR, Gray JA (1991b) Contextual effects on choice reaction time and accuracy in acute and chronic schizophrenics: Impairment in selective attention or in the influence of prior regularities. British Journal of Psychiatry 159, 415–421, 1991b

Kamin LJ: Predictability, surprise, attention and conditioning. In: Campbell BA Church RM (eds): Punishment and Aversive Behaviour, pp. 279–296. New York, Appleton–Century–Crofts, 1969

Kaye H, Pearce JM: Hippocampal lesions attenuate latent inhibition and the decline of the orienting response in rats. Quart J Exp Psychol 39B: 107–125, 1987

Kinsbourne M: Integrated field theory of consciousness. In: Marcel AJ, Bisiach E (eds): Consciouness in contemporary science, pp. 239–256, Oxford, Clarendon Press, 1988

Knight RA: Converging models of cognitive deficit in schizophrenia. In: Spaulding WD, Cole, SF (eds.): Theories of Schizophrenia and psychosis, pp. 93–156, University of Nebraska Press, 1984

Leff JP: Perceptual phenomenon and personality in sensory deprivation. Br J Psychiat 114: 1499–1508, 1968

Lubow RE, Weiner I, Feldon J: An animal model of attention. In: Spiegelstein MY, Levy A (eds): Behavioural models and the analysis of drug action, pp. 89–107, Amsterdam, Elsevier, 1982

Maher BA: Delusional thinking and perceptual disorder. J Ind Psychol 30: 98–113, 1974

Maher BA: A tentative theory of schizophrenic utterance. In: Maher BA, Maher WB (eds): Progress in Experimental Personality Research, Vol. 12, pp. 1–52. New York, Academic Press, 1983

Maher BA: Anomalous experience and delusional thinking: the logic of explanation. In: Oltmanns TF, Maher BA (eds): Delusional Beliefs, pp. 15-33, New York, Wiley, 1988

Margo A, Hemsley DR, Slade PD: The effects of varying auditory input on schizophrenic hallucinations. Br J Psychiat 139: 122–127, 1981

Magaro PA: Psychosis and schizophrenia. In: Spaulding WD, Cole, SF (eds.): Theories of Schizophrenia and psychosis, pp. 157–230, University of Nebraska Press, 1984

Matussek P: Untersuchungen über die Wahnwahrnehmung. 2. Mitteilung. Archiv für Psychiatrieund Zeitschrift Neurologie 189: 279–318, 1952

McGhie A, Chapman J: Disorders of attention and perception in early schizophrenia. Br J Med Psychol 34: 103–115, 1961

Meehl PE: Manual for use with checklist of schizotypic signs. Unpublished manuscript, Univ.of Minnesota, 1964, quoted in Eckblad M, Chapman LJ: Magical ideation as an indicator of schizotypy. J Cons Clin Psychol 51: 215–225, 1983

Miller J: Priming is not necessary for selective attention failures: Semantic effects of unattended, unprimed letters. Percept Psychophys 41(5): 419–434, 1987

Norman DA, Bobrow DG: On the role of active memory processes in perception and cognition. In: Cofer CN (ed): The structure of human memory. San Francisco, Freeman, 1976

Olton DS, Wible CG, Shapiro MC: Mnemonic theories of hippocampal function. Beh Neurosci 100: 852–855, 1986

Patterson T: Studies towards the subcortical pathogenesis of schizophrenia. Schiz Bull 13: 555–576, 1987

Pearce JM, Hall G: A model for Pavlovian learning: variations in the effectiveness of conditioned but not of unconditioned stimuli. Psych Rev 87: 532–552, 1980

Phillips LD, Edwards W: Conservatism in a simple probabilistic inference task. J Exp Psychol 72: 346–354, 1966

Pogue–Geile MF, Harrow M: Negative symptoms in schizophrenia: their longitudinal course and prognostic importance. Schiz Bull 11: 427–439, 1988

Posner M: Cumulative development of attentional theory. Amer Psychol 37: 168–179, 1982

Rund BR: Verbal hallucinations and information processing. Beh Brain Sci 9(3): 530, 1986

Schneider C: Die Psychologie der Schizophrenen. Leipzig, Thieme, 1930

Schneider W, Shiffrin RM: Controlled and automatic human information processing – I. Detection, search and attention. Psych Rev 84: 1–66, 1977

Schmajuk NA: Animal models for schizophrenia: the hippocampally lesioned animal. Schiz Bull 13: 317–327, 1987

Shakow D: Some psychological features of schizophrenia. In: Reyment ML (ed): Feelings and Emotions, pp. 383–390, New York, McGraw Hill, 1950

Shallice T: Information processing models of consciousness: possibilities and problems. In: Marcel AJ, Bisiach E (eds): Consciousness in contemporary science, pp. 305–333, Oxford, Clarendon Press, 1988

Solomon PR: Role of the hippocampus in blocking and conditioned inhibition of rabbits nictating membrane response. J Comp Physiol Psychol 91: 407–417, 1977

Solomon PR, Crider A, Winkelman JW, Turi A, Kamer RM, Kaplan LJ: Disrupted latent inhibition in the rat with chronic amphetamine or haloperidol induced supersensitivity: Relationship to schizophrenic attention disorder. Biol. Psychiat., 16: 519–537, 1981

Spitzer M: On defining delusions. Comp Psychiat 31: 377–397, 1990

Strauss J: Processes of healing and chronicity in schizophrenia. In: Häfner H, Gattaz WF Janzarik W (eds): Search for the Causes of Schizophrenia, pp. 75–87, Heidelberg, Springer, 1987

Venables PH: Cerebral mechanisms, autonomic responsiveness and attention in schizophrenia. In: Spaulding WD, Cole, SF (eds.): Theories of Schizophrenia and psychosis, pp. 47–91, University of Nebraska Press, 1984

Weinberger DR, Wagner RL, Wyatt RJ: Neuropathological studies of schizophrenia: a selective review. Schiz Bull 9: 193–212, 1983

M. Spitzer, F.A. Uehlein
M.A. Schwartz, C. Mundt
(eds.): Phenomenology
Language & Schizophrenia.
Springer-Verlag, New York, 1992

Are Latent Thought Disorders the Core of Negative Schizophrenia?

Winfried Barnett & Christoph Mundt

1. Introduction: The Positive–Negative Dichotomy of Schizophrenia

Since its inception as a diagnostic entity, attempts have been made to divide schizophrenia into homogeneous subgroups. Kraepelin (1899) already distinguished more florid symptoms from those that were marked by losses or deficits; the latter were responsible for the term "dementia praecox". Bleuler (1911) is well known and influential in Anglo-American psychiatry and is often viewed as a forefather of the distinction between positive and negative schizophrenia. For example, Pfohl and Andreasen (1986), Crow (1982), and Sommers (1985) see present-day negative symptoms as a reduced version of Bleuler's fundamental or basic symptoms (disturbances of association and affect, ambivalence, and autism).

As Sass has pointed out, Gruhle (1922) already used arguments which anticipate some of the present day discussions:

"It seems undeniable to me that in many cases of dementia praecox there is a plus of impulses. Similar to the occurrence of sometimes a hypo-, sometimes a hyperphase in manic-depressive insanity... some courses or phases of schizophrenia are distinguished by a plus and others by a minus in mental activity" (Sass 1989, p. 29).

According to Gruhle (1929), both the increase and the decrease in mental activity are psychologically inexplicable symptoms caused by the schizophrenic process. Concerning the dichotomy positive versus negative, he judged negative symptoms to be similar to those belonging to the residual form of the illness, i.e. flattening of thought and affect, stereotypes, perseveration, apathy, and abulia. Gruhle (1929) qualified this theory by pointing out that numerous symptoms such as negativism and autism are not suitable for classification into negative and positive.

When researchers became increasingly concerned with improving the reliability of diagnosis and the concordance between American and European diagnostic practices (Kendell 1975), they began to place renewed emphasis on delusions and hallucinations, i.e. positive symptoms in the present terminology. The "first rank symptoms" of K. Schneider

(1939), which are given prominence in modern standard interviewing instruments such as the PSE (Wing 1970) and the SADS (Endicott & Spitzer 1978), stress the importance of these positive symptoms for the diagnosis of schizophrenia. In this context it seems worthwhile to state, as Andreasen and Flaum (1991) have recently emphasized, that Schneider used his first rank symptoms only as a diagnostic tool and never claimed that they were pathognomic for schizophrenia.

In the revisions of diagnostic criteria for schizophrenia that have been in process for several years, the need for an expanded view of this illness has become increasingly apparent. Based on factor analysis studies, Strauss et al. (1974) proposed that there were two separate symptom profiles in schizophrenia: positive symptoms, consisting of abnormal productions, and negative symptoms, consisting of deficits or loss of function. Following the renewal of interest in negative symptoms, there have been numerous speculations about their etiology as a fundamental aspect of schizophrenia.

Several investigators have claimed that negative symptoms derive from structural neurological changes in the brain, whereas positive symptoms reflect functional neurochemical changes (Crow 1980, Crow et al. 1982, Andreasen 1982). The hypothetical relationship between negative symptoms and more complex cognitive deficits is based primarily on an association between the negative features of schizophrenia and impaired cognitive functioning (Johnstone et al. 1978, Owens & Johnstone 1980, Andreasen et al. 1982, Cornblatt et al. 1985, Andreasen et al. 1990, Goetz & van Kammen 1986). Furthermore, deficits in certain cognitive tasks have been found to characterize schizophrenic patients in remission after a psychotic episode (Wohlberg & Kornetsky 1973, Asaranow & MacCrimmon 1978) as well as in a residual state (Asaranow & MacCrimmon 1981, 1982). In other studies, the severity of negative but not positive symptoms has been successfully predicted by deficits in laboratory tasks involving visual, nonverbal stimuli (Place & Gilmore 1980, Green & Walker 1984, Knight et al. 1985, Knight et al. 1986, Nuechterlein et al. 1986, Weiner et al. 1990) and by neuropsychological tests measuring motor and visual deficits (Green & Walker 1985). Silverstein and Arzt (1985) investigated the relationship in schizophrenia between neuropsychological dysfunction and associative thought disorder. Their findings suggest a correspondence between thought disorders and cognitive impairment, with the further implication that negative schizophrenic symptoms may be correlated with neuropsychological dysfunction. From these studies, all of which emphasize cognitive impairments, it can be hypothesized that attentional deficits and the absence of organizing cognitive aspects of language production may be the psychopathological "core" symptoms of negative schizophrenia. These disturbances, however, are too subtle to be noticed in conventional psychiatric examinations and are more likely to be detected by specific laboratory tasks of cognitive and language performance. Therefore, in order to characterize these psychopathological microsymptoms, we like to introduce the term "latent thought disorders".

On the other hand, social psychiatric research has shifted emphasis to the role of social factors in the genesis of negative symptoms. Wing and Brown (1970) demonstrated that these symptoms are common in an non-stimulating environment and furthermore are less severe after an "increase in the richness of social environment" (Wing 1978). Many negative symptoms such as anhedonia, loss of volition, psychomotor retardation and social withdrawal can be viewed primarily as the outcome of hospi-talization or of a non-responsive milieu. Goffmann (1961) coined the term "institutionalization" and Ciompi (1980) discussed chronic schizophrenia as an artifact caused by the psychosocial consequences of acute attacks. Moreover, negative symptoms have been seen as the product of psychogenic reactions to psychosis when acute, positive symptoms of illness have remitted ("postpsychotic regressive state" by Kayton et al. 1976). Especially when negative symptoms occur prominently during the successful drug treatment of positive symptoms, a pharmacogenic depres-sion can be assumed (Johnson 1969, Marjot 1969, Segal & Ropschitz 1969, Ayd 1975, Ananth & Chadirian 1980). Indirectly, drugs may generate Parkinsonian symptoms and produce the so-called "akinetic depression" (Rifkin et al. 1975, van Putten & May 1978). Postpsychotic depression, which can occur either as a reactive, secondary phenomenon or as a part of the schizophrenic disease process, is strikingly similar in its appearance to negative symptoms (Shanfield et al. 1970, Planansky & Johnston 1978, Johnson 1981, Möller & von Zerssen 1982, Strian et al. 1982, Siris et al. 1983, Hogarty & Munetz 1984). From this point of view, anhedonia and related depressive symptoms may be regarded as the underlying core psychopathology of negative schizophrenia.

Knights and Hirsch (1981) already noted that "it is difficult to dis-tinguish between depressive symptoms and negative symptoms of schizophrenia". Furthermore, some recent investigations have shown that negative symptoms occur quite frequently and in considerable severity in a variety of disorders, including all forms of depressive disorders, organic states with dementia, non-depressive neurosis, personality disorders and even in nonpsychiatric patients (Andreasen & Akiskal 1983, Pogue-Geile & Harrow 1984, Chaturvedi et al. 1985, Nestadt & McHugh 1985, Kulhara & Chadda 1987, Mundt et al. 1989, Kitamura & Suga 1991). Mundt and Kasper (1987) examined negative symptoms in four diagnostic groups (schizophrenia, endogenous depression, neuroses, and diabetes mellitus) and employed rating scales which successfully separated these diagnostic groups on the basis of subscores for language and certain thought disorders.

With respect to the very different points of view described above concerning negative symptoms, Carpenter et al. (1985) distinguished between primary (deficit) and secondary negative symptoms. They argued that certain negative symptoms such as emotional withdrawal and the reduction of initiative and interpersonal social involvement can be regarded as coping strategies and therefore may represent secondary aspects of schizophrenia. These negative symptoms occur in schizophrenics and also in patients with other diagnoses, and the perceived lack of motivation, withdrawal and resignation may be secondary pathological reactions to these disorders. On the other hand, a primary, more elementary and specific feature may only occur in schizophrenics, characterized by language disturbances and abnormalities of thinking and perception.

Regarding schizophrenic negative symptomatology, Hemsley (1990) recently hypothesized that "certain of the behavioral abnormalities shown by schizophrenics represent adaptive strategies to cope with the disorganization" (secondary negative symptoms) "resulting from the cognitive abnormalities" (primary negative symptoms). The primary negative symptoms are assumed to be caused by the absence of organizing cognitive factors and are specific for schizophrenia while the secondary negative symptoms result from non-specific coping strategies and occur ubiquitously.

2. Hypotheses on the Occurrence and Course of Negative Symptoms in Schizophrenics and Neurotic Controls

As reported above, negative symptoms occur in patients with various diagnoses.

A recent study demonstrated that negative symptoms in recently remitted acute schizophrenics and recently admitted acute neurotics were of similar severity and showed considerable overlap (Mundt et al. 1989). In fact, neurotics had even higher scores on self-reporting scales like the FBF, possibly due to their neurotic tendency to overreport language and thought disturbances. According to clinical experience and previous studies, negative symptoms of schizophrenics first become apparent in recently remitted acute schizophrenics.

The following hypotheses have been derived from the literature and from clinical experience (see figure 1): If it is true that the psychopathological core phenomena of schizophrenic negative symptoms are language and thought disturbances, while neurotic negative symptoms consist entirely of reactive attitudes and behaviors, the schizophrenic inpatient's performance in tests of cognition, perception, and language should be inferior to that of the neurotics. Assuming successful treatment, negative symptoms should decline in schizophrenics as well as in neurotic patients after a sufficient period of psychiatric care. If a primary, specific component of negative symptoms is linked to abnormalities of language, thinking or perception, this component should decline in parallel with improved performance on the corresponding tests. Therefore, is would be expected that negative symptoms would not diminish in those schizophrenics in whom cognitive impairment remains prominent. In schizophrenics in whom cognitive disturbances have largely remitted, negative symptoms should be much less marked at the time of retesting. For neurotic patients, however, a decrease in negative symptomatology should not be associated with improved performance on cognitive and language tasks.

Figure 1. Prevalence and course of negative symptoms and "latent thought disorder"—Hypothesis

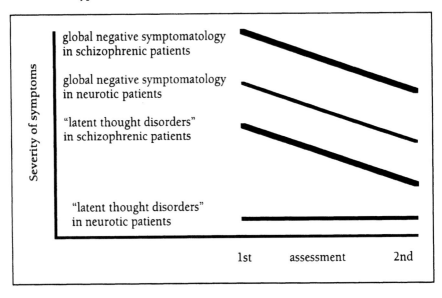

3. Subjects and Methods

3.1 Schizophrenic Patients

Following successful treatment of an acute episode of illness, twenty-five schizophrenic inpatients were recruited for this study a few days prior to their transfer to a rehabilitation ward. All patients were younger than age 30 years and had a psychiatric history of less than seven years duration. Patients with severe chronic courses and with negative symptoms that did not seem amenable to rehabilitation were excluded. The experimental procedure was described to all subjects. Consent was obtained for one assessment at the time of recruitment and for a second assessment eight weeks later. Diagnoses were determined by the ward psychiatrist using DSM–III–R criteria (American Psychiatric Association 1987). The sample consisted of eighteen patients having schizophrenia, paranoid type and seven patients with schizophrenia, disorganized type. Patients with a history of brain disease, prolonged drug or alcohol abuse, or other conditions likely to be related to brain dysfunction (e.g., mental retardation) were excluded. All of the schizophrenic patients were receiving conventional maintenance dosages of phenothiazine medications (mean chlorpromazine-equivalence dosage was 1.4 mg at the time of the first assessment and 0.3 mg at the time of the second assessment). The first evaluation took place on the acute ward and the second evaluation on the rehabilitation ward eight weeks later.

3.2 Neurotic Controls

Twenty-two neurotic inpatients were asked to participate in this study shortly after their admission to the hospital. According to DSM–III–R criteria, they suffered from dysthymia (four patients), major depression (ten patients), personality disorder (four patients), adjustment disorder (two patients), generalized anxiety disorder (one patient) and obsessive compulsive disorder (one patient). Typically, these patients received an negligible dosage of neuroleptics; a minority of them received tricyclic antidepressants. The first and second assessment took place on the hospital wards where these patients were admitted. As in the experimental group, neurotic patients with a history of brain disease, drug or alcohol abuse, or mental retardation were excluded from the study. There was no age limit for neurotic control cases.

3.3 Assessments

All tests and ratings were carried out by a psychiatrist with considerable diagnostic experience on inpatient psychiatric units. This psychiatrist was previously trained to use the test manuals and rating scales and, in a pre-test, successfully generated reliable symptom ratings. The rater was instructed to avoid making hypothetical inferences from case histories when rating symptomatology.

Investigators obtained a speech sample by requesting a monologue from subjects. Subjects were instructed to begin speaking about the reasons for his/her hospitalization, and to continue talking about any topic he/she wishes, such as his/her friends or hobbies, until told to stop. The monologue served both as a warm-up exercise and as a means of obtaining a tape-recorded monologue which could be examined through the use of a cloze procedure. Cloze methodology was developed by Taylor (1953) as a measure of readability. The cloze procedure represents the coherence of speech in terms of the conveyability of its meaning. It consists of having subjects guess words which have been systematically deleted from a given text. In the current investigation, the cloze procedure of Salzinger et al. (1964) was utilized. These investigators introduced cloze methodology as a research tool for the study of schizophrenic language. According to their cloze procedure, a typed script of the tape-recorded first 200 words of each monologue is prepared in which a blank of standard length is substituted for every fifth word. When independent raters are asked to guess the missing words, the speech samples of normal subjects have significantly higher correct guessing scores than those taken from schizophrenic patients. Salzinger et al. (1978) used cloze scores (the number of words correctly guessed) as a quantitative measurement of the degree of communicability and demonstrated that communicability was better for normal subjects than for schizophrenics. These investigators also showed that schizophrenics whose speech samples received higher cloze scores remained in the hospital for less time than those whose speech received lower cloze scores.

Following the monologue, all patients received a diagnostic interview which lasted for approximately forty-five minutes. This interview was evaluated on rating scales which are described below.

Next, patients were given the Konzentrations-Verlaufs-Test (K-V-T) (Abels 1961). In Germany, this is a well established card sorting test of concentration over time. The subject has to sort sixty cards into four heaps depending on whether the cards show one or the other of two different target numbers, both numbers, or none of them. The results measure concentration capacity and are judged by the speed of response, the number of errors and the carefulness of the subject (which is itself determined by a formula which takes speed as well as frequency of error into account).

Patients were then administered the Mehrfach-Wortschatz-Intelligenztest (MWT-B) (Lehrl 1977). This is a short paper-pencil intelligence test which provides reliable and valid information about Verbal IQ. The MWT-B was used as a screening instrument to determine the comparability of intelligence in subjects and controls.

Next, patients self-administered the Frankfurter Beschwerde-Fragebogen (FBF) (Süllwold & Huber 1986). This is a self-rating scale derived from the theoretical concept of "basic symptoms" of schizophrenia developed by Huber and his group (Gross et al. 1987). On the phenomenological level, there is extensive overlap between the so-called basic symptoms and most schizophrenic negative symptoms, although there are fundamental differences in their theoretical foundations. The Huber group assumes that positive symptoms develop from negative or basic symptoms which are regarded as being closely related to the "somatic substrate", i.e. the cerebral origin of schizophrenia. The FBF focuses on fluctuating cognitive microsymptoms such as mild derealization, cognitive gliding and loss of automatisms, all of which are considered essential for the theory of basic disturbances.

After the FBF, patients self-administered the German version of the Beck Depression Inventory (BDI) (Beck et al. 1981). The BDI is a well established instrument that detects depression in routine screening and in research.

Finally, subjects were administered a visual vigilance task, the Continuous Performance Test (CPT). We used the version of Wagner (1989), which was derived from the original work of Rosvold et al. (1956). In this version, the subject views 480 briefly presented numbers that appear in rapid succession at regular intervals over a continuous span of vigilance. The subject is asked to respond to a predesignated target (the number O) by pressing a button. The exposure time is 250 msec, the inter-stimulus interval 1 second, and the total vigilance period eight minutes. The target stimulus occurs in 25% of presented stimuli. Performance on the CPT is evaluated by examining errors of omission (missed targets), errors of commission (responses to non-targets), and reaction time.

Among many conceivable measures of sustained attention (e.g. shadowing tasks and crossmodal reaction time), the CPT was chosen because there is some evidence that CPT performance deficits co-vary with negative symptoms and are not correlated with delusions and hallucinations (Nuechterlein et al. 1986). Additionally, CPT performance deficits persist in relatively asymptomatic schizophrenics (Asarnow & MacCrimmon 1978, Wohlberg & Kornetsky 1973) and may therefore be a negative symptom-linked marker. Moreover, Nuechterlein et al. (1986) found an—albeit inconsistent—correlation between CPT performance and formal thought disorder. Accordingly, it is possible that impaired attention may be the fundamental or core cognitive deficit in negative schizophrenia from which the other symptoms are derived.

The entire evaluation procedure lasted one and a half to two hours. After the patient left the investigation room, the psychiatrist filled in several psychopathometric instruments. All patients were rated on the SANS (Andreasen 1982) as well as on the Positive and Negative Syndrome Scale (PANSS) (Kay et al. 1987), a scale with positive and negative subscales, the latter including blunted affect, emotional withdrawal, poor report, social withdrawal, difficulty in abstract thinking, lack of spontaneity and flow of conversation, and stereotyped thinking.

Patients were also rated on the Intentionalitätsskala (InSka; Mundt et al. 1985). The InSka qualitatively and quantitatively measures the patient's retreat from efforts towards goal attainment and the constitution of interpersonal reality. This scale contains subscores for psychomotor activity, language behavior, affective reactivity, delusion and autism, initiative and motivation, and social behavior.

Psychopathology was further documented by the AMDP-System (Arbeitsgemeinschaft für Methodik und Dokumentation in der Psychiatrie 1981), a comprehensive review of psychopathological manifestations using traditional descriptive psychopathology as its frame of reference. The AMDP-System contains thirteen major categories (intellectual deficit, disorders of consciousness, disturbances of orientation, disturbances of attention and memory, formal thought disorders, phobias and compulsions, delusions, disorders of perception, disorders of ego, disturbances of affect, disorders of drive and motor behavior, circadian disturbances, and other disturbances) and one hundred operationally defined items, each indicating a psychopathological symptom.

Finally, depressive symptoms were assessed on the Hamilton Depression Scale (Hamilton 1960).

3.4 Data Analysis

Subjects and controls were compared by independent t tests for each instance of assessment. To investigate the course of the symptoms, two-factorial repeated-measures analyses of variances (ANOVA) were conducted. Although the data analysis was informed by our directional hypotheses, the p-values, to be conservative, are two-tailed rather than one-tailed. For the statistical procedures, SAS (Helwig, w.y.) and BMDP (Dixon 1985) computer software programs were used.

4. Results

T test comparisons of psychiatric symptoms in schizophrenics and neurotic controls as assessed by rating scales at initial testing reveal the following findings:

On the basis of SANS scores, schizophrenics showed significantly more alogia ($p < .05$), attentional impairment ($p < .05$), and affective flattening ($p < .01$). No significant differences were detected in subscores for avolition-apathy and anhedonia-asociality. The PANSS differentiated schizophrenic from neurotic control groups on both positive and negative subscales ($p < .05$). On the InSka, subscales for psycho-motor activity and social behavior could separate schizophrenics from neurotic controls ($p < .05$), while subscores for language behavior, affective reactivity, delusion and autism, and initiative and motivation revealed no differences.

Other instruments, including the FBF, the AMDP, the BDI and the Hamilton Depression Scale failed to show significant differences between both groups.

Comparison of baseline psychopathology measures with those obtained on retest after eight weeks by analyses of variances (ANOVA) showed an interaction between diagnosis and time of assessment without statistically significant differences between the diagnostic groups at retest. This was the case for the SANS–subscales of alogia ($p < .05$), avolition-apathy ($p < .05$), anhedonia-asociality ($p < .05$), attentional impairment ($p < .05$), for the positive subscale of the PANSS ($p < .01$), for the InSka–subscores delusion/autism ($p < .05$) and social behavior ($p < .001$), and the AMDP–system category of drive and motor behavior ($p < .05$).

For some subscales, repeated-measures analysis of variances revealed statistically significant improvements of both neurotic and schizophrenic patients at the time of the second assessment without any significant difference between the diagnostic groups. This was the case with the InSka-subscores for language behavior ($p < .05$), affective reactivity ($p < .001$), and initiative and motivation ($p < .05$). In the AMDP-system, the major categories of disturbances of attention ($p < .01$), formal thought disorders ($p < .01$), and disturbances of affect ($p < .001$) showed significantly less symptomatology in both diagnostic groups when retested. In addition, depressive symptomatology as measured by both the BDI and the Hamilton Depression Scale was significantly less severe in neurotics and schizophrenics at the time of the second assessment (for both scales $p < .001$). Finally, the general psychopathological subscale of the PANSS showed an improvement in both groups ($p < .001$).

The results of tests for latent thought disorders are of interest. (To reiterate, latent thought disorders are conceived of as the core of schizophrenic negative symptoms. They are quantified by tests of language, attention, and concentration. Dysfunction of this type can be unobtrusive in every-day-communication with patients and can remain undetected and unrepresented in psychopathological scales.) Between–groups comparison using t tests revealed no significant differences on either the first or the second assessment for the following parameters: language as measured by the cloze procedure; concentration capacity and its course during the test period as measured by the K–V–T; and attention as measured by CPT performance using the subcategories errors of omission, errors of commission, and reaction time.

During the first assessment, there was merely a non-significant tendency for schizophrenics to show more errors of omission and longer reaction times. Although there were no differences between diagnostic groups at any assessment time, an analyses of variance revealed a significant improvement for schizophrenics in the number of errors on the K–V–T ($p < .05$) and in errors of omission on the CPT ($p < .001$) when first and second assessments were compared. In contrast, schizophrenics responded significantly poorer to non-targets in the CPT when they were retested, when compared with their responses during the first assessment ($p < .05$).

To summarize our results (see figure 2), the cross-sectional comparison of schizophrenic and neurotic patients revealed no difference in communicability as measured by the cloze procedure, concentration capacity as measured by the K-V-T, or sustained attention as measured by the CPT, neither at the time of the first assessment nor at the time of the second assessment eights weeks later. Negative symptomatology as measured by several rating scales, however, was significantly greater in schizophrenics on most subscales at the time of the initial assessment. Most subjects and controls had both negative and depressive symptoms, the latter measured by the Hamilton Depression Scale and the BDI. However, a between-group difference of depressive symptomatology could not be ascertained, neither at the time of baseline measures nor at retest.

The longitudinal within-group comparison showed no improvement of schizophrenics' monologues as evaluated by the cloze procedure and no improvement of reaction time in the K–V–T. However, the number of K–V–T errors improved significantly as did errors of omission as measured by the CPT. In contrast, schizophrenics made significantly more errors of commission on the CPT when retested.

In the neurotic group no differences occurred in communicability, concentration capacity, or sustained attention when first and second assessment scores were compared.

At retest, negative symptoms were significantly less marked on many rating scale subscores in both diagnostic groups, and the severity of negative symptomatology did not show any between–group differences at the time of retest, subscores of the SANS did correlate with diagnostic groups over time. Depressive symptomatology showed significant improvement in both groups.

In conclusion, our initial hypothesis of an association between schizophrenic negative symptomatology and abnormalities of language, attention, and perception could not be confirmed.

Figure 2: Prevalence and course of negative symptoms and "latent thought disorders"—Results

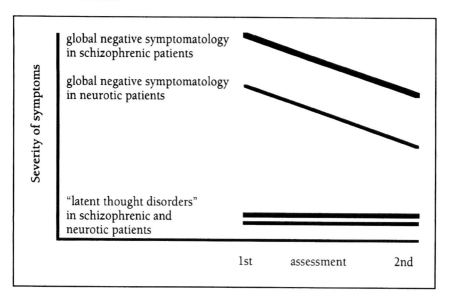

5. Discussion

Our inability to confirm our initial hypothesis raises various issues. In the first place, any comparison of our results with those of other investigators must include an analysis of differences in measurements and methods. Secondly, the impact of sampling artifacts must be considered. Thirdly, the problem of distinguishing primary from secondary negative symptoms arises, a problem which ultimately brings the whole concept of negative schizophrenia into question.

(1) Comparing our results with other reports in the literature, we must emphasize that different approaches can tap different subcomponents of information processing. Caution is warranted when generalizing from results obtained by particular measurement procedures. Many studies which demonstrate cognitive impairment in negative schizophrenia use measures of sustained attention, concentration capacity, and language behavior or communicability which differ from those which we have adopted. For example, in addition to the conventional version of the CPT which uses a simple and clearly focussed target, modified versions have been used which increase the difficulty of the task by adding distraction, a memory load, or stimulus degradation (Spring et al. 1990). As a result, many studies of schizophrenics and populations at risk for schizophrenia are now carried out with different versions of the CPT (Nuechterlein & Zaucha 1990). These studies have produced inconsistent results. Our version of the CPT was developed along the lines of the original version by Rosvold et al. (1956). Had we used a version of the CPT which more successfully challenges the cognitive deviance of schizophrenics, we might

have discovered the differences between schizophrenics and controls that we had initially anticipated. Our failure to detect differences of concentration and language between schizophrenics and controls can be interpreted in the same way. We also have to wonder if the cognitive and language tasks chosen by us sufficiently reflect the cognitive impairment and language disturbances found in schizophrenia. If the disturbances in schizophrenia are too subtle to show up on our tests, our investigations can never demonstrate differences between schizophrenics and controls.

On the other hand, while the tests in our battery have proven to be valid measures of cognitive and language impairment in many studies, other investigations have yielded results similar to ours. Allen (1982) found no evidence of attentional or cognitive impairment when comparing negative schizophrenia to other conditions. In the study of Green and Walker (1986), positive but not negative schizophrenics showed significant deficits on a digit–span task when compared to normal controls; schizophrenics with positive symptoms were the only group to show a significant decrease in digit-span performance when challenged with a distraction. A factorial study by Bilder et al. (1985) yielded no clear positive–negative differences in attentional and global cognitive impairment; instead, these differences co-varied with a factor that encompassed thought disorder, bizarre behavior and alogia. Recently, Harvey et al. (1988) and Harvey and Serper (1990) reported that cognitive deficits in schizophrenics correlate with the severity of positive but not negative thought disorders. Moreover, the latter study disclosed a strong association between verbal information processing deficits and positive thought disorder while no association could be detected between linguistic or communication measures and negative thought disorder. Finally, the relationship of verbal measures of associative dysfunction with positive rather than negative symptoms of schizophrenia has been reported by Silverstein and Arzt (1985).

Taking into account all these studies, we have to conclude that the empirical evidence is contradictory at present. Our results reflect the possibility that cognitive and language impairment in schizophrenia is not associated with the occurrence or severity of negative symptoms.

(2) Another important point is the comparability of sampling in different studies. Most studies revealing an association between negative symptoms and cognitive impairment begin with large samples from which subgroups with superior and inferior cognitive test performances or strongly and weakly manifested negative symptoms are selected and then compared. Most studies that fail to link negative schizophrenia with cognitive impairment use smaller samples which are not subdivided. Hence, we might regard cognitive impairment as a facultative rather than an obligatory part of negative symptomatology in schizophrenia.

Additionally, the seminal study of Andreasen and Olsen (1982) has been criticized because the negative schizophrenia group is significantly older than the positive one and has had much more electroconvulsive treatment (e.g. Kay 1991). Therefore, age or frequent electroconvulsive treatment might account for some of the cognitive and neurologic differences found in Andreasen and Olsen's study. In another attempt to explore the abnormalities of mental activity underlying schizophrenia, Liddle and Morris (1991) examined 43 patients with a mean duration of illness of 29 years. In this study, chronicity is a major determinant of neuropsychological impairment and duration of illness is also associated with cognitive deficits. Perhaps the low average age and short duration of illness of our schizophrenic sample is one reason why cognitive impairment was absent. Accordingly, we might speculate that negative symptomatology in our schizophrenics was mainly psychological (and therefore, by definition, of secondary nature), while cognitive impairment (and thereby, by definition, primary negative symptomatology) did not occur because we did not investigate long term patients with cerebral changes.

(3) This leads to the crucial question, whether primary and secondary negative symptoms can be differentiated. So far this distinction is based on theoretical assumptions rather than clinical observations. In the original paper of Crow (1980), based on the data of Johnstone et al. (1978), negative symptoms are assumed to withstand neuroleptic treatment. Crow (1980) argued that an illness characterized by predominantly negative symptoms must be irreversible because it is due to structural abnormalities of the brain. Since then, several studies have demonstrated the improvement of positive and negative symptoms with neuroleptic treatment (Breier et al. 1987, Tandon et al. 1990, Kane et al. 1988, Goldberg 1985). Defending Crow's concept, Carpenter and Conley (1991) have suggested that secondary negative symptoms should respond to present-day treatment while primary negative symptoms would hardly ever do so. However, this is a theoretically unclear concept since many pathogenetic processes can be influenced by treatment and by the spontaneous course of an illness. Moreover, it is not possible to distinguish between primary and secondary negative symptoms on the level of descriptive phenomenology.

A striking feature of our investigation is the presence of negative symptoms in both schizophrenics and neurotics (as reported in earlier studies) as well as the improvement of negative symptoms in both groups upon retesting. With effective treatment of the actual psychosis or neurosis, negative symptoms improve. Both groups do not differ on depression scores at the time of first assessment or when retested, and both groups show significant improvement in depression scores at the time of the second assessment. This seems to indicate that negative symptoms in both groups are related to a demoralized state and to depressive psychomotor retardation. Hence, although we failed to differentiate primary from secondary negative symptomatology, we can conclude that depressed affect functions as a retarding component within the overall framework of negative symptomatology. Our sample consists of patients who are younger and more short–term than patients in studies which find an association between negative symptoms and cognitive impairment. In these younger, more acutely ill patients, the affective component of illness and psychomotor retardation appear to represent the psychopathological core of the negative syndrome rather than cognitive dysfunction. This might not be the case in a population of older, chronic patients with cerebral alterations.

In conclusion, we assume that two different independent psychopathological processes can be responsible for the negative syndrome. This assumption conforms to clinical observations. In our rehabilitation ward we see patients whose main symptoms are blunted affect, retardation and lack of emotional rapport. When this syndrome arises following the remission of acute symptoms, it is possible for it to subside again soon. Utilizing Janzarik's structural–dynamic psychopathology, Kick (1991) recently called this clinical picture dynamic constriction. This syndrome may be basically different from the negative syndrome of chronic long term patients, although transitions can be visualized.[1]

Summary

The psychopathological nature of negative schizophrenia appears to be unclear since negative symptoms are not specific for schizophrenia and the distinction between primary and secondary negative symptoms is phenomenologically inconclusive. According to our previous results the initial hypothesis of this study was that a deficiency of cognitive organization is the core phenomenon of negative schizophrenia. 25 schizophrenic inpatients and 22 neurotic controls were investigated with psychopathological scales, language measures and cognitive tasks at the time of their recovery from acute symptoms and after eight weeks on the rehabilitation or psychotherapy wards. Although schizophrenic patients showed somewhat more marked negative symptoms on rating scales than neurotics at the time of their first assessment, the cognitive and language performance did not differ. Either group improved after eight weeks of treatment. Thus the initial hypothesis could not be confirmed. We conclude that affective retardation rather than cognitive deficiencies is the psychopathological core of the negative syndrome in our sample of young short term schizophrenic patients.

References

Abels D: Der Konzentrations-Verlaufs-Test K–V–T (the course–of–concentration–test, 2nd ed). Berlin, Springer, 1961
Allen HA: Dichotic monitoring and focussed versus divided attention in schizophrenia. British Journal of Clinical Psychology 21: 205-212, 1982

1 The authors wish to acknowledge the help of Dr. G. Witt, Psychosomatische Klinik des Zentralinstituts für Seelische Gesundheit Mannheim, for assistance in data collection and Dr. P. Richter, Psychiatrische Universitätsklinik Heidelberg, for statistical advice and computing assistance.

American Psychiatric Association: Diagnostic and Statistical Manual of Mental Disorders, third edition, revised (DSM–III–R). Washington, DC: American Psychiatric Association, 1987

Anath J, Chadirian A: Drug induced mood disorder. International Pharmacopsychiatry 15: 58-73, 1980

Andreasen NC: Negative symptoms in schizophrenia: definition and reliability. Archives of General Psychiatry 39: 784-788, 1982

Andreasen NC: Positive vs. negative schizophrenia: a critical evaluation. Schizophrenia Bulletin 11: 380-389, 1985

Andreasen NC Akiskal HS: The specificity of Bleulerian and Schneiderian symptoms: a critical re-evaluation. Psychiatric Clinics of North America 6: 41-54, 1983

Andreasen NC, Flaum M: Schizophrenia: the characteristic symptoms. Schizophrenia Bulletin 17: 27-49, 1991

Andreasen NC, Flaum M, Swayze VW, Tyrrell G, Arndt S: Positive and negative symptoms in schizophrenia. Archives of General Psychiatry 47: 615-621, 1990

Andreasen NC, Olsen SA: Negative vs. positive schizophrenia: definition and validation. Archives of General Psychiatry 39: 789-794, 1982

Andreasen NC, Olsen SA, Dennert JW, Smith JW: Ventricular enlargement in schizophrenia: Relationship to positive and negative symptoms. American Journal of Psychiatry 139: 297-302, 1982

Ayd FJ: The depot fluphenazines: a reappraisal after 10 years' clinical experience. American Journal of Psychiatry 132: 491-500, 1975

Arbeitsgemeinschaft für Methodik und Dokumentation in der Psychiatrie AMDP: Das AMDP-System: Manual zur Dokumentation psychiatrischer Befunde (The AMDP-System: Manual for the Assessment and Documentation of Psychopathology, 4th ed.). Berlin, Springer, 1981

Asaranow RF, MacCrimmon DJ: Residual performance deficit in clinically remitted schizophrenics: a marker of schizophrenia? Journal of Abnormal Psychology 87: 597-608, 1978

Asaranow RF, MacCrimmon DJ: Span of apprehension deficits during postpsychotic stages of schizophrenia. Archives of General Psychiatry 38: 1006-1011, 1981

Asaranow RF, MacCrimmon DJ: Attention/information processing, neuropsychological functioning, and thought disorder during the acute and partial recovery phases of schizophrenia: A longitudinal study. Psychiatry Research 7: 309-319, 1982

Beck AT: Depression Inventory. Philadelphia, Center for Cognitive Therapy, 1978

Beck AT, Rush AJ, Shaw BF, Emery G: Kognitive Therapie der Depression. München, Urban & Schwarzenberg, 1981

Bilder RM, Murkherjee S, Rieder, RO, Pandurangi, AK: Symptomatic and neuropsychological components of defect states. Schizophrenia Bulletin 11: 409-417, 1985

Bleuler E: Dementia praecox oder die Gruppe der Schizophrenien (Dementia Praecox or the Group of Schizophrenias). Leipzig, Deuticke, 1911

Breier A, Wolkowitz OM, Doran AR, Roy A, Boronow J, Hommer D, Pickar D: Neuroleptic responsivity of negative and positive symptoms in schizophrenia. American Journal of Psychiatry 144: 1549-1555, 1987

Carpenter WT, Conley RR: Treatment approaches to negative symptoms. In JF Greden, R Tandon (eds): Negative Schizophrenic Symptoms: Pathophysiology and Clinical Implications (pp. 205-214). Washington, DC: American Psychiatric Press, Inc., 1991

Carpenter WT, Heinrichs DW, Alphs LD: Treatment of negative symptoms. Schizophrenia Bulletin 11: 37-49, 1985

Chaturvedi SK, Prasad Rao G., Mathai JP: Negative symptoms in schizophrenia and depression. Indian Journal of Psychiatry 27: 237-241, 1985

Ciompi L: Ist die chronische Schizophrenie ein Artefakt? Argumente und Gegen-argumente (Is chronic schizophrenia an artefact? Arguments and counter-arguments). Fortschritte der Neurologie Psychiatrie 48: 237-248, 1980

Cornblatt BA, Lenzenweger MF, Dworkin, RH, Erlenmeyer-Kimling L: Positive and negative schizophrenic symptoms, attention, and information processing. Schizophrenia Bulletin 11: 397-407, 1985

Crow TJ: Molecular pathology of schizophrenia: more than one disease process? British Medical Journal 280: 1-9, 1980

Crow TJ: The biology of schizophrenia. Experientia 38: 1275-1282.

Crow TJ, Cross AJ, Johnstone ECD, Owen F: Two syndromes in schizophrenia and their pathogenesis. In: Henn FA, Nasrallah HA (eds.): Schizophrenia as a Brain Disease, pp. 196-234. New York, Oxford University Press, 1982

Dixon WJ: BMDP Statistical Software. Berkley, University of California Press, 1985

Endicott J, Spitzer RL: A diagnostic interview: the Schedule for Affective Disorders and Schizophrenia. Archives of General Psychiatry 35: 837-844, 1978

Goffmann E: Asylums. New York, Anchor Books, 1961

Goetz KL, van Kammen DP: Computerized axial tomography scans and subtypes of schizophrenia: a review of the literature. Journal of Nervous and Mental Disease 174: 208-213

Goldberg SC: Negative and deficit symptoms in schizophrenia do respond to neuroleptics. Schizophrenia Bulletin 11: 453-456, 1985

Green M, Walker E: Attentional performance in positive and negative schizophrenia. Journal of Nervous and Mental Disease 174: 208-213, 1986

Green M, Walker E: Neuropsychological performance and positive and negative symptoms in schizophrenia. Journal of Abnormal Psychology 94: 368-377, 1985

Green M, Walker E: Susceptibility to backward masking in schizophrenics with positive and negative symptoms. American Journal of Psychiatry 141: 1273-1275, 1984

Gross G, Huber G, Klosterkötter J, Linz M: Bonner Skala für die Beurteilung von Basissymptomen BSABS (The Bonn Scale for the Assessment of Basic Symptoms). Berlin, Springer, 1987

Gruhle HW: Die Psychologie der Dementia praecox (The psychology of dementia praecox). Zentralblatt für Neurologie 78: 454-471, 1922

Gruhle HW: Psychologie der Schizophrenie (Psychology of Schizophrenia). In: Berze J, Gruhle HW (eds): Psychologie der Schizophrenie (Psychology of Schizophrenia), pp. 73-168. Berlin, Springer, 1929

Hamilton M: A rating scale for depression. Journal of Neurology, Neurosurgery, and Psychiatry 23: 56-62, 1960

Harvey PD, Earle-Boyer EA, Levinson JC: Cognitive deficits and thought disorder: a retest study. Schizophrenia Bulletin 14: 57-65, 1988

Harvey PC, Serper MR: Linguistic and cognitive failures in schizophrenia. Journal of Nervous and Mental Disease 178: 487-493, 1990

Helwig J: Einführung in das SAS. transl. by G. Frenzel. Cary, North Carolina: SAS Institute Inc.

Hemsley DR: Information processing and schizophrenia. In: Straube ER, Hahlweg K (eds): Schizophrenia. Concepts, Vulnerability, and Intervention, pp. 59-76. Springer, Berlin, 1990

Hogarty GE, Muntzer MR: Pharmacogenic depression among schizophrenic out-patients: a failure to substantiate. Journal of Clinical Psychopharmacology 4: 17-24, 1984

Huber G, Gross G, Schüttler R: Schizophrenie. Eine verlaufs- und sozialpsychiatrische Langzeitstudie (Schizophrenia. A long-term study of course and social psychiatric effects). Berlin, Springer, 1979

Janzarik W: Dynamische Grundkonstellationen in endogenen Psychosen (Dynamic basic constellations of endogenous psychoses). Berlin, Springer, 1959

Janzarik W: Schizophrene Verläufe. Eine strukturdynamische Interpretation (Schizophrenic courses. A structural-dynamic interpretation). Berlin, Springer, 1968

Johnson DAW (1981). Studies of depressive symptoms in schizophrenia: I. The prevalence of depression and its possible causes. British Journal of Psychiatry 139: 89-93, 1981

Johnson J: Depressive changes after fluphenazine treatment. British Medical Journal 3: 718, 1969

Johnstone EC, Crow TJ, Frith CD, Carney MWP, Price JS: Mechanisms of the anti-psychotic effect in the treatment of acute schizophrenia. Lancet I: 848-851, 1978

Kane J, Honigfeld G, Singer J, Meltzer H, & the Clozapin Collaborative Study Group (1988). Clozapine for the treatment-resistant schizophrenic. Archives of General Psychiatry 45: 789-796, 1988

Kay SR: Longitudinal course of negative symptoms in schizophrenia. In: Greden JF, Tandon R (eds): Negative Schizophrenic Symptoms: Pathophysiology and Clinical Implications, pp. 21-40. Washington DC, American Psychiatric Press, 1991

Kay SR, Fiszbein A, Opler LA: The Positive and Negative Syndrome Scale (PANSS) for Schizophrenia. Schizophrenia Bulletin 13: 152-160, 1987

Kayton L, Beck J, Koh S: Postpsychotic state, convalescent environment, and thera-peutic relationship in schizophrenic outcome. American Journal of Psychiatry 133: 1269-1274, 1976

Kendell RE: The Role of Diagnosis in Psychiatry. Osney Mead, Oxford, Blackwell Scientific Publications, 1975

Kick AH: Psychopathologie und Verlauf der postakuten Schizophrenie (Psycho-pathology and Course of Postacute Schizophrenia). Berlin, Springer, 1991

Kitamura T, Suga R: Depressive and negative symptoms in major psychiatric disorders. Comprehensive Psychiatry 32: 88-94, 1991

Klosterkötter J: Basissymptome und Endphänomene der Schizophrenie (Basic symptoms and final phenomena of schizophrenia). Berlin, Springer, 1988

Knight RA, Elliot D, Freedman, E: Short term visual memory in schizophrenics. Journal of Abnormal Psychology 94: 427-443, 1985

Knight RA, Elliot D, Roff DJ, Watson CG: Concurrent and predictive validity of components of disordered thinking. Schizophrenia Bulletin 12: 427-446, 1986

Knights A, Hirsch SR: "Revealed" depression and drug treatment for schizophrenia. Archives of General Psychiatry 38: 806-811, 1981

Kraepelin E: Psychiatrie, 6th ed., Leipzig, Barth, 1899

Kulhara P, Chadda R: A study of negative symptoms in schizophrenia and depression. Comprehensive Psychiatry 28: 229-235, 1987

Lewine RJJ, Fogg L, Meltzer HY: Assessment of negative and positive symptoms in schizophrenia. Schizophrenia Bulletin 9: 368-376, 1983

Liddle PF, Morris DL: Schizophrenic syndromes and frontal lobe performance. British Journal of Psychiatry 158: 340-345, 1991

Marjot DH: Depression following fluphenazine treatment. British Medical Journal 3: 780, 1969

Möller HJ, von Zerssen D: Depressive states occurring during the neuroleptic treat-ment of schizophrenia. Schizophrenia Bulletin 8: 109-117, 1982

Mundt Ch, Fiedler P, Pracht B, Rettich R: (1985). InSka (Intentionalitätsskala)—ein neues psychometrisches Instrument zur quantitativen Erfassung der schizo-phrenen Residualsymptomatik (InSka—a new questionnaire for the quantitative registration of schizophrenic residual symptomatology). Nervenarzt 56: 146-149, 1985

Mundt Ch, Kasper S: Zur Schizophreniespezifität von negativen und Basissymptomen (specifity of negative and basic symptoms in schizophrenia). Nervenarzt 58: 489-495, 1987

256   W. Barnett, Ch. Mundt

Mundt Ch, Kasper S, Huerkamp M: The diagnostic specificity of negative symptoms and their psychopathological context. British Journal of Psychiatry 155 (Suppl 7): 32-36, 1989

Nestadt G, Mchugh PR: The frequency of and specifity of some "negative" symptoms. In: Huber G (ed): Basisstadien endogener Psychosen und das Borderline-Problem, pp. 183-193. Stuttgart, Schattauer, 1985

Nuechterlein KH, Edell WS, Norris M, Dawson ME: Attentional vulnerability indicators, thought disorder, and negative symptoms. Schizophrenia Bulletin 12: 408-426, 1986

Nuechterlein KH, Zaucha KM:Processing abnormalities in patients and high-risk children. In: Straube ER, Hahlweg K (eds): Schizophrenia. Concepts, Vulnerability, and Intervention, pp. 77-96. Springer, Berlin, 1990

Owens DGC, Johnstone EC: The disabilities of chronic schizophrenia—their nature and the factors contributing to their development. British Journal of Psychiatry 136: 384-395, 1980

Pfohl B, Andreasen N: Schizophrenia: diagnosis and classification. In: Hales FA (ed): Psychiatry update, vol. 5, pp. 38-51. Washington DC, American Psychiatric Press, 1986

Pfohl B, Winokur G: The micropsychopathology of hebephrenic/catatonic schizophrenia. Journal of Nervous and Mental Disease 171: 296-300, 1983

Pfohl B, Winokur G: The evaluation of symptoms in institutionalized hebephrenic/catatonic schizophrenics. British Journal of Psychiatry 141: 567-572, 1982

Place J, Gilmore GC: Perceptual organization in schizophrenia. Journal of Abnormal Psychology 89: 409-418, 1980

Plananski K, Johnston R: Depressive syndrome in schizophrenia. Acta Psychiatrica Scandinavica 57: 207-218, 1978

Pogue-Geile MF, Harrow M: Negative and positive symptoms in schizophrenia and depression: a follow up. Schizophrenia Bulletin 10: 371-387, 1984

van Putten T, May PRA: "Akinetic depression" in schizophrenia. Archives of General Psychiatry 35: 1101-1107, 1978

Rifkin A, Quitkin F, Klein SF: Akinesia, a poorly recognized drug-induced extrapyramidal behaviour disorder. Archives of General Psychiatry 32: 672-674, 1975

Rosen WG, Mohs RC, Johns CA, Small NS, Kendler KS, Horvath TB, Davis KL: Positive and negative symptoms in schizophrenia. Psychiatry Research 13: 277-284, 1984

Rosvold HE, Mirsky A, Sarason I, Bransome ED, Beck LH: A continuous performance test of brain damage. Journal of Consulting Psychology 20: 343-350, 1956

Salzinger K, Portnoy S, Feldmann RS: Communicability deficit in schizophrenics resulting from a more general deficit. In: Schwartz S (ed): Language and Cognition in Schizophrenia, pp. 35-53. Hillsdale, Erlbaum, 1978

Salzinger K, Portnoy S, Feldmann RS: Verbal behavior of schizophrenics and normal subjects. Annals of the New York Academy of Sciences 105: 845-860, 1964

Sass H: The historical evolution of the concept of negative symptoms in schizophrenia. British Journal of Psychiatry 155 (Suppl 7): 26-31, 1989

Schneider K: Psychischer Befund und psychiatrische Diagnose (Mental state and psychiatric diagnosis). Leipzig, Thieme, 1939

Segal M, Ropschitz DH: Depressive changes after fluphenazine treatment. British Medical Journal 4: 169, 1969

Shanfield S, Tucker GJ, Harrow M, Detre T: The schizophrenic patient and depressive symptomatology. Journal of Nervous and Mental Disease 151: 203-210, 1970

Silverstein ML, Arzt, AT: Neuropsychological dysfunction in schizophrenia. Journal of Nervous and Mental Disease 173: 341-346, 1985

Siris SG, Rifkin A, Reardon GT, Endicott J, Pereira DH, Hayes R, Casey E: Course-related depressive syndromes in schizophrenia. American Journal of Psychiatry 141: 1254-1257, 1983

Sommers E: "Negative symptoms": conceptual and methodological problems. Schizophrenia Bulletin 11: 364-378, 1985

Spring B, Lemon M, Fergeson P: Vulnerabilities to schizophrenia: information-processing markers. In: Straube ER, Hahlweg K (eds): Schizophrenia. Concepts, Vulnerability, and Intervention, pp. 97-114. Berlin, Springer, 1990

Strauss JS, Carpenter WT, Bartko JJ: The diagnosis and understanding of schizo-phrenia, II: speculations upon the process that underlie schizophrenic symptoms and signs. Schizophrenia Bulletin 11: 61-76, 1974

Strian F, Heger R, Klicpera C: The time structure of depressive mood in schizophrenic patients. Acta Psychiatrica Scandinavica 65: 66-73, 1982

Süllwold L, Huber G: Schizophrene Basisstörungen (Basic disturbances in schizophrenia). Berlin, Springer, 1986

Tandon R, Goldman RS, Goodson J, Greden JF: Mutability and relationship between positive and negative symptoms during neuroleptic treatment in schizophrenia. Biological Psychiatry 27: 1323-1326, 1990

Tandon R, Greden JF: Conclusion: is integration possible? In: Greden JF, Tandon R (eds): Negative Schizophrenic Symptoms: Pathophysiology and Clinical Implications, pp. 233-239. Washington DC, American Psychiatric Press, 1991

Taylor WL: Cloze procedure: a new tool for measuring readability. Journalism Quarterly 30: 415-433, 1953

Wagner M: Experimentelle Verfahren zur Aufmerksamkeitsprüfung (EVA): CPT und SAT (Experimental measures of attention: CPT and SAT). München, Psychiatrische Universitätsklinik, 1989

Weiner RU, Opler LA, Kay SR, Merriam AE, Papouchis M: Visual information processing in positive, mixed, and negative schizophrenic syndromes. Journal of Nervous and Mental Disease 178: 616-626, 1990

Wing JK: A standard form of psychiatric Present-State Examination and a method for standardizing the classification of symptoms. In: Hare EH, Wing JK (eds): Psychiatric Epidemiology: An International Symposium, pp. 93-108. London, Oxford University Press, 1970

Wing JK: Schizophrenia: Towards a New Synthesis. London, Academic Press, 1978

Wing JK, Brown GW: Institutionalization and Schizophrenia. Cambridge, Cambridge University Press, 1970

Wohlberg GW, Kornetsky C: Sustained attention in remitted schizophrenics. Archives of General Psychiatry 28: 533-537, 1973

M. Spitzer, F.A. Uehlein
M.A. Schwartz, C. Mundt
(eds.): Phenomenology
Language & Schizophrenia.
Springer-Verlag, New York, 1992

Clinical and Experimental Analysis of Motor Phenomena in Schizophrenia

Theo C. Manschreck

1. Introduction

Disturbed motor behavior in schizophrenia has been a hallmark of the disorder since it was first conceptualized in the nineteenth century. Well before the clinical introduction of neuroleptic medication in the 1950s, psychiatrists and others had documented numerous movement anomalies, voluntary and involuntary, which affected the limbs, the whole body, posture, coordination, and purposeful behavior (Kraepelin 1919). Despite the array of descriptions, we have remarkably limited knowledge of the pathogenesis of these movements or their relationship to other features of schizophrenia (Manschreck 1986).

Table 1: Catatonic Features

Excitement		Stupor
Violence	Stereotypies	Catalepsy (postural persistence)
Exhaustion	Mannerisms	Rigidity
	Echopraxia/Echolalia	Negativistic Motor Behavior
	Psychomotor	Last Minute Responses
	Retardation	Mutism

While the dramatic, extreme manifestations of catatonic behavior in schizophrenia (Table 1) are known to most; other forms of movement disorder, often of a more subtle character, have been reported widely (Table 2). Such movements have been classified in terms of the degree of activity (increased or reduced), patterns, bodily distribution, and association with voluntary or involuntary initiation of movement. The richness of descriptive commentaries, however, has not inspired much clinical or experimental investigation. Indeed one may conclude that until recently the puzzles of motor disturbance have been largely neglected.

Several factors have contributed to the neglect. The first was Bleuler's proposal (1911/1950) of a psychological explanation for the psychopathology of schizophrenia. Bleuler focused on "inner, psychic" disturbances affecting the verbal or symbolic sphere of intellect, and specifically proposed loosening of associations as the pathogenetic mechanism. This was an understandable choice in that disturbances of verbal or symbolic behavior are accessible and somehow more familiar, certainly more so than the often inconspicuous patterns of motor response. Emphasis on what became known as *formal thought disorder* was associated with reduced clinical interest in motor anomaly in schizophrenia. Motor disturbances were viewed as secondary consequences to a primary disturbance of thinking. Therefore, active characterization and investigation of motor features stagnated, ignored in the effort to explain the nature of disturbed thought.

Table 2: Abnormalities of Spontaneous Motor Behavior in Schizophrenia

Decreased Motor	Increased Motor	Postural
Activity	Activity	Disturbance
General	*General*	
Retardation	Restlessness	Rigidity
Poverty of Movement	Excitement	Catalepsy
Stupor		Stereotypic/
		Manneristic Postures
		Clumsiness
Patterned	*Patterned*	
Motor Blocking	Tremor	
Cooperation	Stereotypies/Mannerisms	
Opposition	Spasms	
Automatic Obedience	Choreiform Movements	
Negativism	Athetoid Movements	
Ambitendency	Parkinesia	
Echopraxia	Perseverative Movements	
Last Minute Responses	Impulsive Movements	
	Carphologic Movements	
	Agitation	
	Tics	
	Mannerisms	

A second factor was the introduction of neuroleptic treatment. This innovation made the evaluation of motor disturbance more complicated, because neuroleptic-induced side effects are frequent, easily detected, yet difficult at times to distinguish from intrinsic motor anomalies. On the other hand, drug-induced Parkinsonian features and acute dystonias rekindled interest in the motor phenomena of schizophrenia, albeit an interest centered largely in the neuropharmacology of extrapyramidal side effects. The detection and characterization of tardive dyskinesia, also associated with neuroleptic drug treatment, have stimulated neuropharmacology and clinical studies, but again the focus has been the effect of treatment.

A third factor has been the reduced occurrence of dramatic catatonic features and of the catatonic subtype of schizophrenia. This apparent drop in incidence has added challenge to the investigation of motor anomalies and has raised a question about the value of such work.

The fourth factor is the remarkable complexity of motor behavior itself, even the most superficially simple forms of movement response. Experimental studies (Wulfeck 1941, King 1954) indicate that motor action is governed by multiple, often independent, influences and that its experimental analysis is dauntingly complex.

Despite neglect, the need to understand motor disturbances remains clear. First, motor disturbances more subtle than catatonic posturing are common in schizophrenia and require explanation. Secondly, one of the major methodological problems in studying schizophrenia is that the most characteristic features of psychopathology, such as forms of delusion, hallucination, and thought disorder, require the patient's verbal report to establish their presence, a formidable methodological confound. The evaluation of non-language forms of abnormality, therefore, has special significance. Third, systematic clinical research with objective techniques has been sparse. Despite this, motor disturbance represents a major frontier for several disciplines. For instance, the domains and interests of neurology, psychology, and psychiatry clearly encompass the psychopathology of motor abnormalities. One need only think of Huntington's disease, depression, and Parkinson's disease wherein motor, cognitive, and mood features arise in association. Interdisciplinary collaboration to address the nature of these intriguing phenomenological associations is consistent with trends toward greater convergence and integration of scientific endeavor in neuroscience, cognition, and biological psychiatry.

The purpose of this essay is threefold: 1) to specify the tasks research should address concerning motor disturbances in schizophrenia; 2) to summarize recent developments on these tasks; and 3) to indicate future directions for investigative effort.

A broader theme is that the methodological challenges that confront the science of psychopathology are especially evident in the study of motor behavior. A need to emphasize experimental techniques is an important priority. As the field moves from the bedside to the laboratory, the means of measurement will need to shift, especially toward greater reliance on measures or techniques that are not dependent on human judgment, such as rating scales; rather, quantitative measures, open to experimental analysis and variation, represent a sounder approach. Ultimately, the correlation of quantitative, peripheral measures with measures of central physiologic or anatomic brain features will offer the prospect of resolving fundamental questions.

2. Research Tasks

One can frame the fundamental research tasks in schizophrenic motor disturbance by pointing to three challenges. The first is *to determine the kinds and frequencies of motor anomalies* in these conditions. This task has to do with clinical assessment and requires progress in description and definition, as well as reliability and discrimination, in the assessment of motor behaviors. A second and related task is *to distinguish forms of abnormal motor behavior* associated with drug treatment from those that are intrinsic to schizophrenia and *to understand their pathogenesis.* This task has been highlighted by Rogers (1985) who describes much of the opinion in this area as a "conflict of paradigms", meaning that strong theoretical perspectives influence what we see and what we fail to see in motor psychopathology. Stated in the extreme, there are those who see all motor disturbance as related to treatment or other factors, but not to schizophrenia itself. And there are those who see motor disturbance as a reaction to the illness. Still others see it as part of schizophrenia. The third task and ultimately the most significant one is *to understand what motor anomalies have to do with schizophrenia* and how knowledge of them can help us understand this enigmatic disorder. Progress has been made on each of these tasks.

Our efforts and those of others who work in this interdisciplinary area are based on the principle that a scientific account of schizophrenia requires an adequate explanation of the variety and frequency of motor disturbances observed in this illness.

2.1 Study One: Kinds and Frequencies

Our efforts to assess the kinds and frequencies of motor disturbances in schizophrenia began with an empirical investigation of clinically ill patients (Manschreck et al. 1982). There had been a few such studies previously, but they had been unsystematic and focused on different issues. This study hypothesized that formal thought disorder and disturbances in voluntary motor behavior would be positively associated. This hypothesis was derived from three propositions that:

1. the attentional deficit hypothesis has explanatory value in the understanding of speech, reaction time, and other behaviors;
2. attention has a critical role in motor activity; hence disturbed attention has impact on motor activity; and
3. a parsimonious account of schizophrenia would propose one pathology rather than several.

Using a rating technique inspired by the clinical literature, we identified classically described categories of spontaneous motor anomaly and assessed their severity in schizophrenic and depressed patients. We tested patients for evidence of difficulty in simple and complex motor actions, such as the ability to perform a sequence of actions and to switch from one movement to another. We adopted procedures suggested by Freeman (1969), Luria (1966), and standard neurologic techniques (DeJong 1967). Instruments for examining psychopathology and drug effects (Table 3) were also employed.

Table 3: Methods: Clinical Studies

Assessment	Procedure/Test*
Diagnosis:	DSM-III & Research Diagnostic Criteria
Motor assessments:	1-hour spontaneous motor activity examination
	10-minute examination of elicited movements—simple (general motility) and complex motor tasks (switching): observations of disorganization, delayed response, lengthy completion, postural persistence.
Drug-induced effects:	AIMS[1], TAKE[2]
Formal thought disorder:	ratings from SADS[3] interview
Delusions:	ratings from SADS interview
Affective blunting:	Abrams & Taylor scale (1978)
Neurologic sensory signs:	standard assessment of graphesthesia, stereognosis
Cognitive functions:	Mini-mental state examination

* Reliabilities assessed for all procedures

The findings were briefly:
1. In a heterogeneous sample of 37 schizophrenic patients, 36 had evidence of abnormal voluntary movements; patients with the paranoid subtype (n = 13) displayed less severe disturbance; among mood disorder patients (n = 16), movement abnormality was considerably less frequent;

---

1 Abnormal Involuntary Movement Scale
2 Targeting Abnormal Kinetic Effects
3 Schedule for Affective Disorders and Schizophrenia

2. Motor disturbance in schizophrenic subjects was associated with a number of other features, specifically formal thought disorder, emotional blunting, and non-localizing neurologic signs;
3. The motor impairments observed were not dramatic, rather they were often subtle or inconspicuous features of movement that might be easily missed or ignored in routine clinical evaluation. Three general forms of disturbance in voluntary motor behavior emerged: persistent disruption in the smoothness and coordination of spontaneous movements; the frequent occurrence of spontaneous, intermittent, highly repetitive movements; and disturbances in motor action sequences elicited on examination.
4. Although drug-induced motor effects were evident, a number of analyses demonstrated they had distinct characteristics compared to intrinsic disorders. In fact, neuroleptic medication appeared to produce marginal improvements in intrinsic motor disturbances.

We concluded that disturbed motor activity of the forms classically associated with schizophrenia occur frequently in contemporary patients with schizophrenia, and that they are associated with a number of psychopathological features, especially formal thought disorder. These observations suggest that schizophrenic motor abnormalities share a common pathogenesis with other features of the illness.

2.2 Study Two: Motor Anomaly and Clinical Cognitive Deficit

A further investigation of motor abnormality (Manschreck and Ames 1984) corroborated the earlier study, yielding data that approximately 88% of a schizophrenic sample displayed abnormal voluntary movements. This study also explored the connection of movement disturbance to other disease features, especially cognitive abnormalities. The main findings were:

1. Formal thought disorder, especially poverty of information, is associated with abnormal movements in schizophrenia;
2. Cognitive functioning is disturbed in relation to abnormal motor movements. This was shown with respect to overall mental status performance and to poor recall performance in particular, which is associated with abnormal movements, independent of the presence of movements associated with tardive dyskinesia.

This study, therefore, extended the observations of the first study by showing that motor abnormalities are associated with specific cognitive difficulties.

Other studies have attempted to apply laboratory techniques for more objective assessment of motor and cognitive disturbances; specifically, techniques were sought with greater reliability, the reduction or elimination of the influence of human judgment, and quantifiability.

2.3 Study Three: Motor Anomaly and Speech Disorganization

In this study (Manschreck et al. 1981) we utilized a measure of language disorganization, the type token ratio (TTR), as a quantitative index of formal thought disorder to examine its relationship to clinical motor disturbance as identified by the previously described approaches. This ratio is a simple, reliable measure of different words uttered in a speech sample and reflects the flexibility or variability in lexicon usage. It is generally lower in schizophrenic subjects than in normal controls. The main findings were:

1. The type token ratio was negatively related to motor disturbance (r = -.58, p < .01), meaning that the less variable the vocabulary used, the more disturbance was evident in motor behavior. This index of speech deviance replicated our prior findings of an association between clinically rated formal thought disorder and motor deviance;

2. The correlation between motor abnormality and poverty of information was itself especially high (r = .78, p < .001). We concluded that disruption in language behavior in schizophrenia is associated with clinical evidence of disruption in motor behavior.

At this point, to improve on the clinical assessment of motor features, we sought to develop a laboratory technique to quantify motor anomalies in schizophrenia. To do so required that we first select and defend the best out of many possible laboratory measurement techniques of motor anomaly; second, that we establish the validity and reliability of that measure. A useful technique would permit us to test further the hypothesis that motor anomalies are related to features of psychopathology.

To select an appropriate measurement, we relied on the concept of redundancy in schizophrenia as a guidepost (Cromwell 1968). This concept had already proved useful in the study of speech in schizophrenia. As it is in speech, redundancy is a key feature of skilled motor performance. In information theory, any event can be regarded as redundant to the extent that its occurrence and characteristics are predictable from observation of immediately preceding events. Simple rhythmic movements such as hammering a nail are examples of high-redundancy activities. Adequate responses to redundant stimuli may be made with relatively little demand upon attention. Thus, the detection and use of redundancies that determine responses are adaptive and efficient mechanisms of the mind.

Substantial evidence exists that schizophrenic patients are unable to make effective use of the redundancies inherent in many tasks, while normal and non-schizophrenic controls materially improve their performance when tasks include redundant features (e.g. King 1962).

We, therefore, chose to test schizophrenic patients using motor responses involved in synchronization with a rhythmic auditory stimulus, predicting that schizophrenic subjects would be less able than controls to synchronize motor movements with rhythmic stimuli, which of course are characterized by considerable redundancy (Table 4).

Table 4: Additional Methods: Laboratory Studies

Material: Verbal sample, description of Brueghel's "The Wedding Feast"	
Assessment	Procedure/Test
Quantitative index of language disorganization:	—type-token ratio (TTR)
Motor assessment:	—tapping synchronously to acoustic stimuli. —Mean interval accuracy—subject compared to programmed stimuli. —Synchronization accuracy—uniformity of intervals between beats.

2.4 Studies Four/Five: Deficient Motor Synchrony

We have published two studies (Manschreck, Maher, Rucklos et al. 1981, Manschreck et al. 1985) employing the laboratory measure of motor synchrony as an index of motor disorganization in schizophrenia. The results of these two studies, the first using a mechanical device for measuring motor synchrony and the second, a computerized measure, are congruent. The findings were:

1. At certain rates of rhythmic stimuli, schizophrenic subjects, when compared to normal and other controls, failed to achieve equivalent inter-beat intervals, that is, to rhythmize their tapping to the stimulus beat. This suggests that schizophrenic subjects fail to adapt their attentional responses to the redundancies of this motor task. Rather, they tend to exhibit relatively inefficient and non-uniform performance.

2. Deficient motor synchrony correlated with clinical assessment of motor and thought disturbance and with such rating scale items as "messy in eating habits", "muttering to self", and "emotional withdrawal".

These data indicate that deficient motor synchrony is associated with other key aspects of psychopathology in schizophrenia. Specifically, abnormal voluntary movements are associated with those clinical features that characterize the so-called defect state of schizophrenia and with those neurologic and cognitive features that suggest impairment in brain functioning and information processing.

2.5 Study Six: Redundancy Associated Deficits in Motor and Memory Response

Indeed, we have recently completed a study (Manschreck et al. 1991 unpublished) relevant to this suggestion. In this study we tested the proposition that certain subtle memory anomalies found frequently in schizophrenia are not a separate pathology but are related to other psychopathological features, specifically motor and thought disturbances. The experimental results indicate that schizophrenic subjects matched for memory ability with normal controls demonstrate a common, reduced ability to take advantage of the predictable or redundant features in two different tasks, one involving simple word recall and another the performance of motor synchrony. These same subjects demonstrate increased levels of formal thought disorder.

When capacity to utilize the predictable or redundant features of a stimulus pattern is deficient or compromised, diverse forms of adaptive behavior are affected. In this example, these encompass disturbances in form of speech, motor performance, and memory for words.

Concurrent difficulties of schizophrenic subjects in motor, memory, and speech tasks are notable on two counts. First, they are not likely to be the result of a generalized deficit; and second, there is no a priori reason to expect associated deviances in these functions as they reflect different forms of cognitive activity. Indeed, evidence from the motor task avoids the possible confound of using language as the source of performance measures, because schizophrenic subjects frequently produce disturbed utterances.

The capacity to identify characteristics of schizophrenia associated with motor anomalies provides a basis then on which to build a richer picture of the nature and complexity of them. Increased specification and precise measurement of these features, in the clinic and laboratory, promise to provide insights concerning why these connections are present; that is, why motor, memory, and speech (thought) disturbances overlap in this disorder. From such observations and elaboration of our understanding of these phenomena, a more precise localization of the anatomic correlates of these disturbances will be possible.

3. Preliminary Summary

The studies discussed above focused on abnormal voluntary movements (AVMS) that occur in schizophrenia. From these and other studies, several conclusions can be made about such movements. First, high risk studies indicate they may be present prior to onset of psychosis in individuals who receive this diagnosis (Fish 1987, Watt et al. 1984). Second, although not pathognomonic for this disorder, they occur frequently among patients with schizophrenia (Manschreck et al. 1982, Manschreck & Ames 1984). Third, they can be reliably distinguished from abnormal involuntary movements. Fourth, they are associated with formal thought disorder, affective blunting, and disturbed cognition. And finally, they appear to improve marginally with drug treatment.

4. Abnormal Involuntary Movements: Toward Convergent Explanations

There has been a parallel interest in abnormal involuntary movements (AIMS) in schizophrenia. The study of these movements has been especially complicated due to the effects of neuroleptic drugs. Most psychiatrists have, until recently, considered abnormal involuntary movements to be synonymous with drug side effects. However, this view is inconsistent with a number of observations. Long before neuroleptic treatment, Kraepelin (1919) described involuntary movements indistinguishable from those now reported as tardive dyskinesia (Crow et al. 1983). And, a number of recent studies have found abnormal involuntary movements in psychotic patients never treated with neuroleptics (e.g. Owens et al. 1982, Rogers 1985).

Like AVMS, AIMS may be a part of the psychopathology of schizophrenia (Crow et al. 1983, Iager et al. 1986). Evidence of more intellectual impairment and ventricular enlargement among schizophrenic patients with AIMS than in patients without such movements has been documented (Waddington & Youseff 1986).

These parallel developments raise the possibility of a relationship between abnormal voluntary movements and abnormal involuntary movements. Two general hypotheses could be put forward concerning this relationship. The first is that the two kinds of motor anomaly are independent, resulting from at least two different processes or sets of processes. The second, that they are related, assumes a common underlying process or set of processes. Currently, there is no guide to help us select from these alternatives. Nevertheless, Manschreck (1989b) has proposed that the two are related for several reasons. Patients with abnormal involuntary movements (AIMS), and those with abnormal voluntary movements (AVMS) show problems in intellectual functions and thought production (Table 5). And, the principle of parsimony favors a single process explanation particularly when we know so little about the underlying pathophysiology of these anomalies. Several predictions could be made on the basis of these proposals.

First, the presence of AVMS may be a predictor for the onset of abnormal involuntary movements with chronic neuroleptic treatment. Secondly, the occurrence of AIMS may predict a severe course of schizophrenic illness. A corollary prediction would be that the presence of AIMS would be associated with cognitive deficits of a similar kind to those occurring in patients with AVMS but distinguished by greater severity. And third, the increased cognitive abnormality in schizophrenic patients with

AIMS may be characterized by qualitative, i.e. different kinds, as well as quantitative, (i.e. worse) differences compared with patients with AVMS.

Table 5: Features of Abnormal Voluntary Movements (AVMS) and Abnormal Involuntary Movements (AIMS) in Schizophrenia

Feature	AVMS	AIMS
Prevalence	Virtually all	10-15%*
Onset	Early in course	Late in course
Sex	? Males increased risk	? Females increased risk
Relation to schizophrenia	Intrinsic	Unclear; association to antipsychotic [medication??]
Presence prior to antipsychotic treatment	Present	Small percentage with "spontaneous dyskinesias" Present
Effect of anti– psychotic treatment	Reduce	Sometimes eliminate ("mask")
Prognosis	Variable	Often poor, more severe deficit features (negative symptoms)
Associated cognitive changes	Yes	Yes

* Corrected for the 5-10% prevalence of spontaneous dyskinesias.

4.1 Study Seven: The Relationship of AIMS and AVMS in Schizophrenia

We recently studied (Manschreck et al. 1990) the clinical psychopathology, cognitive features and neurologic characteristics of a group of chronic schizophrenic patients. We evaluated dyskinesia using the Abnormal Involuntary Movement Scale (AIMS) and abnormalities of voluntary motor response according to the techniques described above. All patients were on neuroleptic medication for at least one year prior to this study. The main findings (see Table 6) are:

1. Patients with involuntary dyskinesias had significantly greater evidence of abnormal voluntary movements than those without.
2. Moreover, this group had more negative symptoms, lower premorbid intelligence, and poorer recall on mental status examination.

3. The non-dyskinetic group showed similar abnormalities in psychopathological features; their disturbances were less severe.
4. The dyskinesias detected did not reach a threshold of severity required to meet criteria for tardive dyskinesia according to current definitions (Schooler & Kane 1982).
5. Estimates of drug treatment exposure did not differ in the two groups.

These observations are consistent with the hypothesis that abnormal involuntary and voluntary movements are related, and that the presence of the former is associated with greater severity in both voluntary motor disturbances and a number of non-motor clinical features (Manschreck 1989b).

In the report of this study (Manschreck et al. 1990) we proposed that the association between abnormal involuntary and involuntary movements may indicate a common pathogenesis. Similar proposals have been put forward elsewhere (Crow et al. 1983, McKenna et al. 1991). Crow's argument is that AIMS are part of schizophrenia, especially the Type II subsyndrome. Our data are consistent with this proposal. Other associations are, however, worth noting. For example, schizophrenic patients with AIMS may have an earlier onset of clinical illness (reflected in lower premorbid intellectual ability) and a more profound deterioration in personality functioning and cognition (reflected in negative symptoms and memory changes).

These results do not address specifically the impact of neuroleptics on the pathogenesis of AIMS; however, they suggest that a causal model implicating neuroleptics as the single source is inadequate. The possibility that some pathology, common to drug effects and schizophrenia itself, may be at work is intriguing and consistent with such findings.

In agreement with Rogers's (1985) "conflict of paradigms" hypothesis, we may conclude that while motor abnormalities in schizophrenia are indisputably present, they are not pathognomonic for the condition; and their source (i.e. drug-induced or intrinsic to the disorder) is far from clear. The ultimate discovery of the origin of these movements, however, appears to go well beyond the capacities of current rating techniques alone. A reasonable hypothesis is that these movements arise from a common origin, possibly closely connected anatomical sites of pathology (e.g. basal ganglia and other subcortical areas; Albin et al. 1989). Such a proposal has been put forward for other disorders wherein cognitive, mood, and movement disturbances coincide (McHugh 1989). In this view, diseases of the basal ganglia, such as Huntington's and Parkinson's, are syndromically related because similar functional symptoms are present yet differ because each reflects the distinct disruption of local pathology in complex, interacting and integrated systems subserving motor control, cognition, and affective state.

In a similar manner, McKenna and colleagues (1991) propose that the phenomenological overlap of extrapyramidal movements and those associated with schizophrenia itself (Lund et al. 1991) may be the result of common or closely connected anatomic sources. They suggest specifically the ventral-striatal-pallidal complex citing work by Heimer et al. (1982), and Nauta (1979). The nuclei of this complex are located in close proximity to the nuclei of the basal ganglia; like them, they receive innervation from ascending dopaminergic pathways. In functional terms there is evidence from animal studies that hyperkinesia and stereotypy are associated with lesions in this area, thus giving some credibility to this proposal.

Table 6: Differences and Similarities in Schizophrenic Subjects With and Without Abnormal Involuntary Movements

Features Differing for Subjects with Involuntary Movements	Features Similar for both Groups
Psychopathology Greater negative symptomatology More severe formal thought disorder	General psychiatric symptomatology
Neurological Features More voluntary motor abnormalities	Sensory function Motor synchrony Perceptual organization
Cognition Lower premorbid intellectual activity Lower current intellectual functioning Possible poorer recall on mental status	Language, attention, orientation Effect of contextual constraint on immediate recall Recognition memory Visuospatial memory

5. Future Directions

Brain imaging techniques may help identify the relevant and distinct pathophysiology of extrapyramidal movements and movements intrinsic to the disorder. The experimental analysis of motor behavior abnormality may also be useful in resolving these complicated questions. Unique or characteristic motor responses may well reflect the specific effects of homogeneous pathologies. Thus comparative studies of patients with different basal ganglia disorders might be a useful step in discovering disease-specific motor patterns (Albin et al. 1989, Manschreck 1983). In terms of clinical research, the study of syndromes such as Crow's Type I and Type II, the positive and negative syndromes, and Peter Liddle's three neuropsychologically defined syndromes (Liddle & Morris, 1991) offer additional tools to map the clinical inter-relationships of motor and other features. High risk samples might be another source of advances, and for similar reasons, early onset (prior to age 20) cases. Such samples offer the prospect of examining the earliest "pure" manifestations and unfolding natural history of movement anomaly.

It is evident that there has been change in the fortunes of motor abnormalities in schizophrenia. Long neglected, they now increasingly demand explanation. Nevertheless, investigation needs to be directed towards understanding their varied and frequent occurrence in schizophrenic disorders. Clarifying the relationship of cognitive and other disturbances to disordered movements, may help unravel the puzzle of pathogenesis and illuminate important aspects of the clinical phenomenology and natural history of these conditions. In such a setting a more comprehensive view of schizophrenia may emerge.

The steps in this process will of necessity be numerous. We need to enlarge our knowledge of the descriptive characteristics, natural history, and organization of abnormal motor action sequences for both abnormal voluntary and involuntary movements. Longitudinal studies of motor features in relation to other components of the psychopathology of schizophrenia are in order. The laboratory is a critical arena for this investigative focus. It will provide the measures to examine anatomic, pathophysiologic, and cognitive mechanisms. Disciplines such as robotics and artificial intelligence should inspire increasingly sophisticated models of motor behavior. The use of computer based technology can enhance the assessment and reliability of investigation. Indeed integration of information and approaches from various kinds of research offers the best prospects for advancing knowledge.

Summary

Motor abnormalities, long neglected, are now an important target for interdisciplinary investigation in schizophrenia. Despite formidable methodological challenges, research has demonstrated their frequent occurrence and association with a variety of psychopathological features. Recent studies have also provided a framework for proposals about anatomic and physiologic underpinnings that should guide further empirical effort. The evidence indicates that motor anomalies constitute a core, if not unique, disturbance in schizophrenia. For a satisfactory understanding of schizophrenic development, deviances of movement must be accounted for.[4]

4 Acknowledgement: The author wishes to thank Elaine M. Sword for her assistance in the preparation of this paper. In rendering this report, studies from the Laboratory for Clinical and Experimental Psychopathology (formerly located at Massachusetts General Hospital and Harvard Medical School) at New Hampshire Hospital and Dartmouth Medical School as well as from other investigators was used to illustrate progress on each task. Work in this laboratory has been conducted with the collaborative involvement of many individuals, most notably Brendan Maher. Among a number of others, Donna Ames, Nancy Keuthen, Craig Latham, Mary Rucklos, and Don Vereen deserve special mention.

References

Abrams R, Taylor MS: A rating scale for emotional blunting. American Journal of Psychiatry 135: 226-229, 1978

Albin RL, Young AB, Penney JB; The functional anatomy of basal ganglia disorders. Trends in Neurosciences 12: 366-375, 1989

Bleuler E: Dementia Praecox or the Group of Schizophrenias, New York, International University Press, 1950 (originally published in 1911)

Cromwell R: Stimulus redundancy in schizophrenia. Journal of Nervous Mental Disease 146: 360-375, 1968

Crow TJ, Owens DGC, Johnstone EC, Cross AJ, Owen F: Does tardive dyskinesia exist? Modern Problems in Pharmacopsychiatry 21: 206-219, 1983

DeJong R: The Neurological Examination, New York, Harper & Row, 1967

Fish B: Infants predictors of the longitudinal course of schizophrenic development. Schizophrenia Bulletin, 13: 395-409, 1987

Freeman T: Psychopathology of the Psychoses, New York, International Universities Press, 1969

Heimer L, Switzer RD, van Hoesen GW: Ventral striatum and ventral pallidum: components of the motor system? Trends in Neurosciences 5: 83-87, 1982

Iager AC, Kirch DG, Jeste DV, Wyatt RJ: Defect symptoms and abnormal involuntary movements in schizophrenia, Biological Psychiatry 21: 751-755, 1986

King HE: Anticipatory behavior: temporal matching by normal and psychotic subjects. Journal of Psychology 53: 425-440, 1962

King HE: Psychomotor Aspects of Mental Disease: an Experimental Study. Cambridge, MA, Harvard U. Press, 1954

Kraepelin E: Dementia Praecox and Paraphrenia (translated by E Barclay & W Barclay), Edinburgh, Livingston, 1919

Liddle PF, Morris DL: Schizophrenic syndromes and frontal lobe performance. British Journal of Psychiatry 158: 340-345, 1991

Lund CE, Mortimer AM, Rogers D, McKenna PJ: Motor, volitional, and behavioral disorders in schizophrenia, 1:Assessment, using the modified Rogers scale, British Journal of Psychiatry 158: 323-327, 1991

Luria AR: Highen Cortical Function in Man, New York, Basic Books, 1966

Manschreck T: Motor abnormalities in schizophrenia. In: Nasrallah H, and, Weinberger D (eds), Handbook of Schizophrenia, Vol 1, The Neurology of Schizophrenia, pp. 65-96, New York, Elsevier, 65-96, 1986

Manschreck TC: Psychopathology of motor behavior in schizophrenia. Progress in Experimental Personality Research 12: 53-99, 1983

Manschreck TC, Ames D; Neurologic features and psychopathology in schizophrenic disorders. Biological Psychiatry 19(5): 703-719, 1984

Manschreck TC, Keuthen NJ, Schneyer ML, Celada MT, Laughery J, Collins P: Abnormal involuntary movements and chronic schizophrenic disorders. Biological Psychiatry 27: 150-158, 1990

Manschreck TC, Maher BA, Ader DN: Formal thought disorder, the type-token ratio, and disturbed voluntary motor movements in schizophrenia. British Journal of Psychiatry 139: 7-15, 1981

Manschreck TC, Maher BA, Miller-Ventor C, Rosenthal JE, Berner J: Memory and motor disturbances in schizophrenia: evidence for a redundancy associated deficit, unpublished, submitted, 1991

Manschreck TC, Maher BA, Rucklos ME, Vereen DR, Ader DN: Deficient motor synchrony in schizophrenia. Journal of Abnormal Psychology 90(4): 321-328, 1981

Manschreck TC, Maher BA, Rucklos ME, Vereen DR: Disturbed voluntary motor activity in schizophrenic disorders. Psychological Medicine 12: 73-84, 1982

Manschreck TC, Maher BA, Waller NG, Ames D, Latham CA: Deficient motor synchrony in schizophrenic disorders: clinical correlates. Biological Psychiatry 70: 990-1002, 1985

Manschreck TC; Motor abnormalities and the psychopathology of schizophrenia, In Kirkaldy B (ed): Normalities and Abnormalities in Human Movement, pp. 100-127, Basel, Karger, 1989a

Manschreck TC; Motor and cognitive disturbances in schizophrenic disorders, In C Tamminga C, Schulz SC (eds) Schizophrenia: Scientific Progress, pp. 372-380, New York. Oxford, 1989b

McHugh PR: The neuropsychiatry of basal ganglia disorders, Neuropsychiatry, Neuropsychology, and Behavioral Neurology 2: 239-247, 1989

McKenna PJ, Lund CE, Mortimer AM, Biggins CA: Motor, volitional, and behavioral disorders in schizophrenia 2: the "conflict of paradigms" hypothesis. British Journal of Psychiatry 158: 328-336, 1991

Nauta WJH: A proposed conceptual organization of the basal ganglia and telencephalon, Neuroscience 4: 1875-1881, 1979

Owens DGC, Johnstone EC, Frith CD: Spontaneous involuntary disorders of movement. Archives of General Psychiatry 39: 452-481, 1982

Rogers D: The motor disorders of severe psychiatric illness: a comflict of paradigms. British Journal of Psychiatry 147: 221-232, 1985

Schooler N, Kane JM: Research diagnoses for tardive dyskinesia. Archives of General Psychiatry 39: 486-487, 1982

Waddington JL, Youseff HA: Late onset involuntary movements in chronic schizophrenia: relationship of "tardive" dyskinesia to intellectual impairment and negative symptoms. British Journal of Psychiatry 149: 616-620, 1986

Watt NF, Anthony EJ, Wynne LC, Rolf J (eds): Children at Risk for Schizophrenia, New York, Cambridge University Press, 1984

Wulfeck WH: Motor function in the mentally disordered 1 A comparative investigation of motor function in psychiatrics, psychoneurotics, and normals. Psychological Record 4: 271-323, 1941

M. Spitzer, F.A. Uehlein
M.A. Schwartz, C. Mundt
(eds.): Phenomenology
Language & Schizophrenia.
Springer-Verlag, New York, 1992

Lateralized Information Processing and Emotional Stimulation in Schizophrenia and Depression

Matthias Fünfgeld, Rose A. Fehrenbach, Rainer Wilkening, Ute Wichmann-Francke, Helga Maes, Godehard Oepen

1. Introduction

Diverging neuropsychological models of hemispheric dysfunction in schizophrenia and depression as well as the moderating role of emotion on the onset and course of these disorders are the subject of investigation of this study. Deficits in patients with acute schizophrenic psychosis have usually been interpreted as indicating primarily left hemispheric dysfunction (Flor-Henry 1969, Gur 1978, Magaro & Chamrad 1983, DeLisi et al. 1989). This view has been challenged by some authors who have suggested a primary deficit in the right hemisphere (Schweitzer 1982, Venables 1984, Oepen et al. 1987, Cutting 1990), or dysfunction involving both hemispheres (Kolb & Whishaw 1983, Gruzelier 1984, Taylor 1984). Quite apart from any brain pathology, family studies of schizophrenia have demonstrated that patients who live in families with high levels of expressed emotionality have a greater risk of relapse than patients living in other families (Brown et al. 1972; Leff & Vaughn 1976). This finding emphasizes the importance of psychosocial factors on the course of schizophrenic illness.

Most neuropsychological models of depression stress dysfunction in the right cerebral hemisphere (Moskovitch et al. 1981, Johnson & Crockett 1982), while studies of patients with focal cortical lesions provide strong evidence for a left hemispheric contribution to depression (Gainotti 1972, Robinson et al. 1984, Robertson 1986). Coffey (1987), in a review of the literature on hemispheric dysfunction in depression, concludes that bilateral deficits are involved in depression with more emphasis on the right hemisphere.

Performance asymmetries in neuropsychological tasks with hemispheric specificity have been used to make inferences about the underlying pathology in psychiatric disorders. This view of "hemisphere superiority" is influenced by Moscovitch (1976, 1986), who, while acknowledging that many higher cortical functions are located in both hemispheres, nonetheless emphasizes that the cognitive process itself is carried out by the hemisphere that can more efficiently perform the task while the contralateral hemisphere is inhibited. The rudimentary language functions of the right hemisphere in split brain patients are consistent with this model as well as observations that small lesions of the left hemisphere often lead to more severe language disturbances than larger lesions (Kinsbourne 1974). This can additionally be understood as a release of inhibition of right hemispheric language capabilities from left hemispheric control.

In a previous study of schizophrenic and depressed patients (Oepen et al. 1990), using a divided visual field paradigm, we found unstable but not differently lateralized performances in a word/nonsense syllable decision task with left hemispheric superiority and in a face/scrambled face decision task with right hemispheric superiority. However, following an emotionally ambivalent stimulation, distinct patterns of asymmetrical changes were found in both disorders: In schizophrenic patients, stimulation led to an increase in right visual field (RVF) performance, while in depressed patients, stimulation led to increase in left visual field (LVF) performance. The different effect of emotional stimulation in both disorders, which indicates that lateral processing asymmetries can be altered by emotional material, was interpreted as specific for underlying schizophrenic or depressive pathology.

In this study, improved versions of the same two hemispheric tasks are used in order to replicate the previous findings of basically unaltered hemispheric asymmetrical functioning in schizophrenia and depression. Additionally, the investigators assess the impact of neutral and emotionally negative stimulation on asymmetries and performance in these two tasks in order to draw conclusions about the underlying pathology of schizophrenia and depression.

2. Method

2.1 Tasks and Procedures

Tasks: 1. Word/non-word decision task, with a previously demonstrated RVF advantage (Regard et al. 1985), utilizing German words (prepositions, conjunctions and indefinite pronouns) and pronounceable nonsense syllables. 2. Face/non-face decision task, with a previously demonstrated LVF advantage (Regard & Landis, 1986), using photographs of faces together with photographs of the same faces with intermingled features. Both studies were run in a divided visual field paradigm.

In order to study the effects of additional emotional stimulation, both tasks were modified to include stimuli which had been rated to be either emotionally "neutral" (i.e., merely provoking an arousal reaction as a result of surprise) or emotionally "negative" (i.e., provoking not only surprise, but also fear or anxiety). The emotional valence of this additional visual stimulus material had been rated tachistoscopically by two independent samples of normal control subjects. For these ratings, the stimulation material was presented centrally for 100 ms. Only pictures that had been identified by all subjects, and that had been rated consistently as negative or neutral, and not positive, were included as emotional stimuli. As emotionally negative stimuli the authors chose a realistic drawing of a spider, a photo of a human skull, and a drawing of a house on fire. Neutral stimuli chosen for the experiment were a drawing of a bucket, a photograph of a small bottle, and a drawing of a pair of glasses. These stimuli were paired in the contralateral hemifield with a word or face stimulus to make up a trial resembling the rest of the word– or face–trials.

These additional trials were included at fixed places in the trial sequences of the word– and the face–tasks. The reactions in trials with additional emotional stimulation were not counted when calculating the performance in these runs. Thus, in runs with and without additional emotional stimulation, responses to the same trials were measured. The first trial with emotional stimulation was placed before the first original item, preceded by 3 items, the reaction to which was not recorded either.

Stimuli were presented in a double simultaneous manner. The stimuli were presented in such a way that the visual angle between the outer parts of the stimuli and the central fixation point was between 1 to 3 degrees. Subjects were instructed to respond manually with their index-fingers ipsilateral to the side of a target stimulus word or face, respectively. When bilateral non–target stimuli were shown, no response was required (Go/Nogo paradigm). The stimuli were presented for 120 ms in the word/nonword task and for 60 ms in the face/nonface task. Immediately after the stimulus a visual masking stimulus was presented for 6 seconds, during which the response could be made. One test consisted of 36 such trials with 12 targets left, 12 targets right, and 12 bilateral non-targets. Manual reactions were registered for 3 seconds only, beginning with onset of the word– or face–stimulus.

A testing session began with two identical runs of the same task, i.e., involving either words or faces, followed by a third run in which the additional trials with emotional significance were introduced. Later, the subject had to carry out the other task (word– or face–decision), again with two identical runs followed by a run with additional trials containing emotionally negative or neutral stimuli. For each subject group the task sequence was balanced with respect to type of task (word or face) and type of stimulation (negative or neutral). Additionally, the task sequence was arranged so that the same tasks (word vs. face) and emotional additional stimulations in the third trial (neutral vs. negative) did not follow directly after each other. To prevent carry–over effects between the task triplets, breaks of 1 to 2 hours were introduced between them.

2.2 Subjects

In all subject groups both gender and years of formal education were evenly distributed. All subjects were right-handed as demonstrated by a measure of hand-preference (Edinburgh Handedness Inventory, EHI; Oldfield 1976); and a paper and pencil tracking test of hand function (Hand-Dominanz-Test; Steingrüber 1971). The normal control subjects were screened for a personal or family history of neurological and/or psychiatric disorder. Persons with uncorrected impaired vision (Visus < .9) were excluded. Patients were diagnosed according to the German version of the DSM-III-R (Wittchen et al. 1989). Among the group "schizophrenia" only patients with acute paranoid schizophrenia were selected. Subjects selected for the group "depression" all fulfilled the criteria for a present major depressive episode. Patients were included in the study only if the diagnosis could be verified by external raters through the Structured Clinical Interview for DSM-III-R (SCID) in the German version (Wittchen et al. 1990). In addition to this, only patients with severe symptoms according to the Inpatient Multidimensional Psychiatric Scale (IMPS, German version; Hiller et al. 1986) were tested (cut-off: severity higher than the 40th percentile of the corresponding diagnostic group of acute inpatients). The majority of patients tested were taking standard doses of neuroleptic or antidepressant medication.

Tachistoscopic data consist of the frequencies and reaction times of correct responses in both visual fields. Since false positive responses were equally more frequent in the left visual field in both patients and controls, relative frequencies of correct responses, which are commonly used, overestimate the performance in the left visual field in both tasks. To correct for this, an individual chance correction procedure was developed in which the expected frequencies were substracted from the observed frequencies of correct responses, divided by the number of stimuli of the category. This ratio which is presented as the data in the experiments stands for the relative frequency of correct responses above chance level in the visual field (see figures 1a, 2a, 3a). Statistical evaluation of data was calculated using a multivariate analysis of variance for repeated measurements (MANOVA) with the Group-Factor (schizophrenia, depression, control) as independent variable, and performance in the hemifields as dependent variables. As the evaluation of left–right performance asymmetries, retest-reliabilities, and stimulation effects involve multiple testings of the same subjects, these effects had to be included as within–subjects-factors in the repeated mesurements design. To avoid the reporting of chance findings as significant, the authors refrain from comparing all groups with each other and limit themselves to statisitically independent comparisons using orthogonal contrasts for the inter-group comparisons: Contrast PC compares patients with controls, Contrast SD compares schizophrenia with depression.

3. Results

Table 1 shows the age, gender, and handedness distribution in the three experimental groups. In table 2, the IMPS ratings of the two patient groups are summarized. The results of tachistoscopic tasks in schizophrenic and depressed patients, and in controls are shown in figures 1 through 3. Figures (a) present chance corrected relative frequencies, and figures (b) present means of reaction time medians.

Table 1: Age, gender, and handedness in the experimental groups

Group	N	Female	Male
Schizophrenia	24	12	12
Age		29.7 ± 7.8	28.8 ± 7.8
EHI		95.7 ± 10.0	89.3 ± 14.4
Depression	19	10	9
Age		44.8 ± 12.3	36.7 ± 10.1
EHI		95.7 ± 10.5	98.0 ± 12.3
Controls	18	9	9
Age		24.5 ± 2.1	28.2 ± 5.9
EHI		100.0 ± 0.0	97.8 ± 6.6

Reliability: The experimental design permits two approaches to the issue of the reliablity of the tasks used: 1. To control for sequence effects, the order of the presentation of triplets of word and face tasks was balanced. Consequently, no systematic effects should be expected comparing the performance and asymmetries in two identical tests immediately following each other. 2. As effects of two different types of stimulation are to be compared at a later stage of data analysis, it is crucial that there are no systematic differences between identical pairs of tasks preceded by neutral or negative stimulation. No significant performance or asymmetry differences were found using these methods, neither in repeated identical runs nor in identical pairs of the word or face runs. Therefore, there are no indicators that the reliability of the tasks used in the balanced design is questionable. Hence, it is justified to evaluate the effects of neutral vs. negative stimulations on performance in the two tasks.

Sex differences: There were no significant sex differences in any of the groups studied, nor were there correlations of visual field performances with gender. Hence, no evidence was found for different lateralization in women compared to men.

Table 2: IMPS ratings of the patients

IMPS	Schizophrenia Mean ± Sdev		Depression Mean ± Sdev	
Excitement	3.4	3.8	5.0	5.9
Hostility	4.0	3.1	2.5	4.6
Paranoid Projection	11.7	3.1	1.2	1.5
Grandiosity	1.2	1.7	.0	.0
Perceptual Distort.	4.3	3.2	.2	.7
Anxious Depression	6.5	3.7	10.3	3.9
Retardation/Apathy	2.6	3.3	3.8	3.9
Disorientation	.0	.0	.0	.0
Motor Disturbances	1.1	1.6	.1	.4
Conceptual Disorg.	1.2	1.9	.0	.0
Impaired Functioning	8.3	3.7	12.9	3.8
Obsessive-Phobic	1.5	1.5	1.8	1.6

Performance asymmetries and stimulation effects: In order to assess stimulation effects on general performance and visual field asymmetries the authors compared second runs without additional emotional stimulation with corresponding runs with additional negative and neutral emotional stimulation (see tables 3 and 4).

Word Task: The relative frequencies of correct responses above chance level are summarized in Table 3: Not surprisingly, the word tasks demonstrate significant differences in general performance between patients and controls (PC). The absolute performance of patients with schizophrenia in the word tasks is substantially lower than that of patients with depression (SD). In fact, performance levels in schizophrenia range around levels predicted by chance. On the other hand, depressives perform at high levels not significantly different from the levels of normal controls. There is, however, a significant general effect of emotional stimulation (STIM) on the overall performance level: Emotional stimulation—regardless whether neutral or negative (NE)—lead to overall performance gains in all groups. The interaction 'schizophrenia vs. depression x effect of general stimulation' (SD x STIM) indicates that depressive patients do show larger gains under stimulation than schizophrenic patients.

Figure 1a: Normal Controls: Relative frequencies of correct responses above chance level in word/nonword and face/nonface decision tasks.

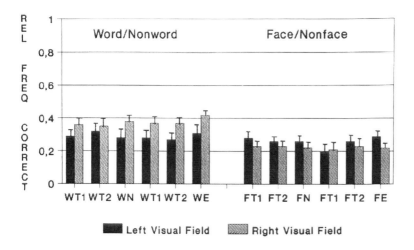

Figure 1b: Normal Controls: Reaction times of correct responses in word/nonword and face/nonface decision tasks.

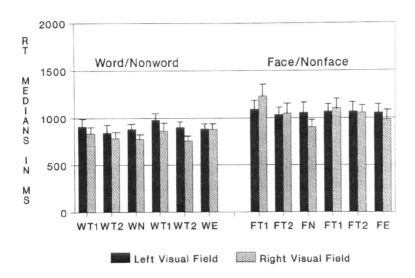

Reaction time (RT) data are summarized in Table 4. There is a highly significant RT difference between schizophrenic and depressed patients (SD), i.e., schizophrenic patients are slower producing correct manual responses. None of the other main effects reached statistical significance. As can be seen in figure 2b, schizophrenic patients do show faster RTs in the runs with neutral stimulation (WN & FN) as compared to the runs immediately preceding than in the runs with negative stimulation (WE & FE) as compared to the runs immediately preceding. In figure 3b, the opposite RT–pattern is seen, though less prominently, in patients with depression: There is a tendency for the runs with neutral stimulation (WN & FN) to become slower as compared to the runs immediately preceding, and for the negative stimulation runs (FE & WE) to become faster as compared to the runs immediately

280   M. Fünfgeld et al.

preceding. It is noteable that this effect can only be seen in reaction time data. In chance corrected accuracy data the differential effect of neutral vs. negative stimulation can no longer be observed, because part of it has been removed through the chance correction procedure. A significant three–way interaction SD x STIM x NE was observed, i.e., RTs in patients with schizophrenia are faster with any kind of stimulation than without; at the same time patients with schizophrenia are faster under neutral stimulation than under negative stimulation, while the reverse was found in depressed patients.

Figure 2a: Acute, paranoid Schizophrenia: Chance corrected relative frequencies of correct responses in word/nonword and face/nonface decision tasks.

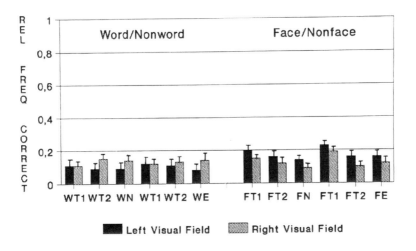

Figure 2b: Acute, paranoid Schizophrenia: Reaction times of correct responses in word/nonword and face/nonface decision tasks.

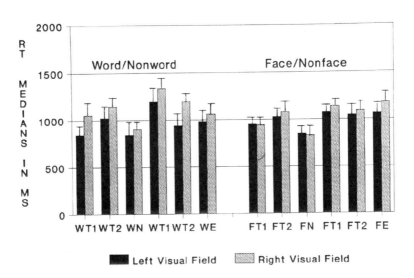

Figure 3a: Major Depression: Chance corrected relative frequencies of correct responses in word/nonword and face/nonface decision tasks.

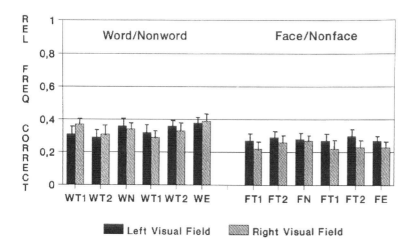

Figure 3b: Major Depression: Reaction times of correct responses in word/nonword and face/nonface decision tasks.

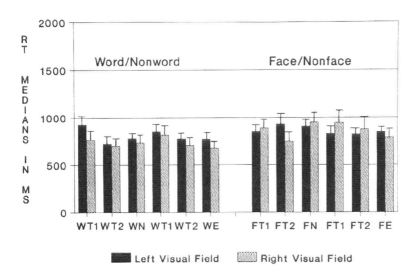

The data on the effects of the visual field (VF) in all groups taken together show only a trend towards a right visual field advantage in relative frequencies of correct responses, and not even a trend in RTs. This points to diverging visual field asymmetry measures in the three groups: In controls accuracy and reaction time data run synchronously, i.e., visual field advantages in both measures indicate left hemispheric superiority. Descriptively, without subjecting the data to any post hoc statistical analysis, schizophrenic patients' accuracy data point to the expected RVF advantage whereas RTs are consistently faster in the LVF, thus pointing in the opposite direction! In depressed patients there seem to be no clear visual field advantages in accuracy data with nothing more than a slight tendency for a RVF advantage in RT data.

Table 3: Performance and Asymmetry Effects in Relative Frequencies Above Chance Level in Word and Face Decision Tasks. Comparisons between the second run of each task with the runs with additional neutral or emotionally negative stimulation in two repeated measurements MANOVAs. Interactions are only listed when significance levels (p) reached less than .10.

	Word Decision		Face Decision	
Effect	F(1,58)	p	F(1,58)	p
PC	9.36	.003	2.78	.101
SD	34.56	.000	18.98	.000
VF	3.24	.077	8.57	.005
STIM	5.20	.026	.03	.871
NE	1.52	.222	.00	.964
SD x STIM	5.70	.020	.00	.965

legend:
PC   (schizophrenia and depression) vs. controls
SD   schizophrenia vs. depressive patients
NE   neutral vs. emotionally negative stimulation
STIM general stimulation effect
VF   left vs. right visual field

Table 4: Performance and Asymmetry Effects for Reation Times of Correct Responses in Word and Face Decision. Comparisons between the runs 2 with the runs with additional neutral or emotionally negative stimulation in two repeated measurements MANOVAs. Interactions are only listed when significance levels (p) reached less than .10

	Word Decision		Face Decision	
Effect	F(1,58)	p	F(1,58)	p
PC	.18	.673	.81	.371
SD	10.10	.002	2.33	.132
VF	.00	.963	8.51	.005
STIM	.79	.378	.02	.878
NE	1.10	.298	1.30	.260
SD x NE	.81	.372	4.82	.032
SD x NE x STIM	5.18	.026	5.52	.022

legend: (as in table 3)

Face Task: In relative frequencies of correct responses above chance level we find generally high performance levels for normal controls and depressed patients, whereas schizophrenic patients show an impairment in the detection of faces (SD). This impairment, however, is less marked than the impairment in the word decision task. Word decision tasks are easier than face decision tasks for normal controls, whereas schizophrenic patients perform better in face tasks than in word tasks (data on RTs and accuracy).

In contrast to the word task there are no RT differences between normal controls and patients (PC) and between schizophrenia and depression (SD). Depressed patients are even faster than normal controls. In the runs with additional emotional stimulation, schizophrenic patients show a marked improvement in reaction times under neutral stimulation and slower reaction times under negative stimulation. In depression the opposite was found, i.e., longer RTs under neutral and faster RTs under negative stimulation. The different effects of emotional stimulations in schizophrenic and depressed patients are also shown in the three-way interaction of SD x NE x STIM.

In all groups, a highly significant LVF advantage, both in accuracy and RT data, was detected. This is in contrast to the differential visual field effects (VF) in accuracy and RT data in the word decision task.

4. Discussion

4.1 Schizophrenia

Performance levels of schizophrenic patients show an impairment in both word and face decision tasks. Compared to the performance of controls, who show superior performance in word decisions, schizophrenic patients perform better in face decisions. The severe impairment of schizophrenic patients in the word task cannot be explained in terms of low educational level, as these patients even had marginally higher formal education than the patients with depression, who performed on a very high level in that task.

In the word task, the small RVF advantage in accuracy data is contrasted by a LVF advantage in the reaction time data. This reversed asymmetry pattern in RTs in schizophrenic patients might have contributed to the fact that the main effect of the visual field on RTs remained far from reaching statistical significance. It is possible that the low accuracy performance of the schizophrenic patients has reduced the expected RVF advantage in word decision (bottom effect). However, this fact in itself would not lead to a LVF advantage in reaction times. Hence, in our view, a more plausible interpretation of the data takes the difficulty of the task into account: The word task is very hard for patients with schizophrenia, as can be seen from their low performance (around chance level). This might lead to a different processing strategy in these patients relying more on RH faculties, such as guessing and holistic processing, which, however, are less effective for word stimuli. In general, it is possible that asymmetries in accuracy and reaction time cover different aspects of hemisphere function, and hence, can dissociate under certain circumstances.

In the face task, patients with schizophrenia show only a minor impairment. There are highly significant LVF advantages in all groups, and no dissociation of accuracy and reaction time asymmetries could be observed. The relatively minor impairment in accuracy in face decision and the lack of any reaction time impairment in the schizophrenic patients when compard to controls represent surprising findings. The lack of any reaction time deficit in the face task seems to disagree with most of the literature on cognitive tasks performed by schizophrenic patients, because larger reaction times are one of the best reproduced findings in research on schizophrenic patients. It should be mentioned here that the patients were acutely paranoid and that most of them received rather high doses of neuroleptics. Despite the slower reaction times in the word task, we did not find a reaction time deficit in the face task. This points towards a task-specific reaction time impairment of the schizophrenic patients in the word task.

Taken together, we interpret the data on schizophrenic patients along the lines of Gur's (1978) hypothesis of bilateral hemispheric dysfunction which is more prominent in the left hemisphere. This view is supported by our findings of severely reduced performance in the detection of function words. The data on face decisions, with only a slight impairment of right hemisphere performance as compared to controls, can be interpreted as a relative preservarion of right hemisphere function, especially in the context of lowered general performance levels in schizophrenia. The question remains, however, which of the interpretations—severe left hemispheric impairment, or relative right hemispheric preservarion—is more closely related to the observed pathology.

4.2 Depression

Although the prominent feature of depression is a disturbance of mood, problems with memory or concentration are common in depression and have been included as a diagnostic cirterion for Major Depression in the DSM-III-R. Reversable deficits in short-term memory, transfer of information from short-term memory to long-term memory, difficulties of stimulus encoding, as well as a conservative response bias have been proposed to account for poor performance on cognitive tasks in depression. Some authors have used cognitive tasks with "effortful vs. automatic" processing demands and found that depressive patients were impaired in the effort-demanding tasks only (Weingartner et al. 1981; Roy-Byrne et al. 1986; Tancer et al. 1990). Golinkoff and Sweeney (1989), however, were unable to replicate these findings. Watts et al. (1987) showed memory deficits in a sample—with 75% of the patients having a diagnosis of endogenous depression—which could not be explained in terms of different age, educational level, verbal intelligence, or response bias.

As most of the studies testing cognitive function in depression used memory tasks, these deficits are hardly comparable to our tasks in which the stress on memory is minimal. Nevertheless, given the severe psychopathological impairment of these patients, most of whom were on antidepressant drugs (which are known to have sedative effects), the high performance of the depressive patients in word and face decisions (RT and accuracy data) is remarkable. Although all of our patients were inpatients and dysfunctional in handling their everyday affairs, they were capable of achieving performance levels similar to, or even better than, normal controls.

In line with Weingartner et al. (1981), we tend to attribute the lack of a performance deficit in our sample of depressed patients to the highly structured tasks used in our experiment. Such structure was provided by the limited complexity of the task, the reduced number of manual reaction choices, and by the instruction, which encouraged subjects to guess when they were uncertain whether they had perceived the critical stimulus in one hemi-field.

In addition to the above reasons for the unexpectedly high performance of the depressed patients, it may be argued that depressed patients often feel highly tense and agitated. Moreover, there is evidence that depression is biologically paralleled by hypercortisolism (Holsboer 1989), which corresponds to a stress reaction. Heightened responsiveness to experimental situations which could be interpreted as vaguely threatening might be the result. It is striking that depressed patients do not show the expected RVF advantages in word tasks, whereas they show stable and expected LVF advantages in face decisions. In word decisions we find generally instable lateralization and prevailing LVF superiority. This finding might point to right hemispheric overactivity, which many authors consider associated with negative affect in depression (Flor-Henry 1979, Yozawitz et al. 1979, Coffey 1987). This is also in accordance with the findings of an earlier study (Oepen et al. 1990), in which a tendency was found in depressed patients for the right hemisphere to become more readily activated.

4.3 Effects of Additional Emotional Stimulation

For the discussion of general effects of additional emotional stimulation, we would like to refer to our findings utilizing accuracy data without individual chance correction, which were not reported above. (As already mentioned, chance corrections were considered desirable because the rates of manual reactions in the left and right hemifield, and therefore also the rates of false positive reactions in both hemifields, were disproportionate, with a predominance of more false positive reactions in the LVF.) In accuracy data without chance correction there is a highly significant effect of stimulation on the word task (STIM: p = .006), with a trend towards a more pronounced impact of emotionally negative stimulation on test performance (NE: p = .057). In chance corrected data, however, the general stimulation effect is reduced but still significant (see table 3: STIM:

p = .026), while the differential effect of negative vs. neutral stimulation is no longer statistically significant (p = .222). This means, that in all subject groups, additional emotional stimulation leads to an increase in false positive reactions. After chance correction, the performance gains under additional emotional stimulation are diminished but remain present in controls and depressives, while in schizophrenic patients these gains are no longer present. In our opinion, the performance gains observed under additional emotionally negative stimulation in uncorrected data can be attributed to two factors, both of which are related to attention: In the first place there is an attentional factor, which allocates more and adequate processing resources to the resolution of the task. Secondly, a nonspecific increase of arousal mediated by the right hemisphere occurs with a raised readiness for motor responses on the left side of the body.

Our finding of differential reaction time benefits upon additional emotional stimulation in schizophrenic patients (who benefit from neutral stimulation only) and in depressed patients (who benefit from negative stimulation only) is new (significant interactions SD x NE x STIM, present in reaction time data only). As a tentative explanation for this finding, we suggest, that neutral stimulation is mild enough to raise attentional capacities resulting in shorter RTs, while negative emotional stimulation does not have this effect. Such additional stimulation may even promote fearful and negative associations, but, in any event, does not mobilize attentional resources for stimulus processing. From a clinical point of view this might explain why in acute schizophrenic patients emotional stress can lead to dysfunctional behavior, and does not mobilize efficient coping abilities.

Contrary to our hypothesis we did not find a qualitatively different general effect of neutral vs. negative emotional stimulation. However, depressive patients seem to improve more under emotionally negative stimulation, while schizophrenic patients have greater performance gains under neutral stimulation. This can be seen in relation to findings that depressives have a negative recall bias when exposed to the same number of positive and negative self–referral adjectives (Bower 1981). Schizophrenic patients do not profit from negative stimulation; they show little or no changes compared to the neutral stimulation condition.

4.4 General Considerations

A divided visual field paradigm involving the detection of words and faces was used to draw conclusions about hemispheric functioning in schizophrenia and depression. The results are largely in line with authors who found a bilateral deficit in schizophrenia (Kolb & Winshaw 1983, Gruzelier 1984, Taylor 1984) and a major right hemispheric involvement in depression (Moskovitc et al. 1981, Johnson & Crockett 1982). The contribution of subcortical, and especially limbic and paralimbic structures to pathology in schizophrenia (Bogerts et al. 1987) are also consistent with our findings of impaired attention and increased nonspecific arousal under stimulation.

In contrast to earlier findings of unstable but not differently lateralized performance in both tachistoscopic tasks in schizophrenia and depression (Oepen et al. 1990) we found evidence for a dissociation of functional lateralization measures, namely accuracy and reaction time, in the word/nonword task in schizophrenic patients. The dissociations of general performance levels and visual field advantages, in schizophrenia as well as in depression, reveal a drawback in the neuropsychological assessment of laterality: As mentioned above, accuracy level, accuracy asymmetry, and reaction time asymmetry cannot be cited interchangeably, because they can become dissociated in psychiatric patients. Rather than neglecting such findings as inconsistencies, we should inquire about the conditions under which such dissociations occur and try to learn more about the underlying processes. For the future, combining neuropsychological methods with electrophysiological methods (such as event–related potentials) seems to be a promising line of research.

Summary

The role of lateralized information processing in patients with acute paranoid schizophrenia and major depression as well as in normal controls is investigated. In a divided visual field paradigm hemispheric function is studied in a word/nonword and a face/nonface decision task, with previously demonstrated right and left visual field advantages. Both tasks are presented twice and are followed by a final task with additional emotionally negative or neutral stimulation. Data evaluation includes reaction times and relative frequencies of correct responses above chance–level. In the word recognition task schizophrenic patients show the expected right visual field advantages with respect to the accuracy of their performance. However, comparisons to the depressed patients and the normal control subjects reveal, that general performance in this task is severely impaired. Moreover, reaction time asymmetries are reversed, i.e., show a left visual field advantage. In depressed patients, the expected asymmetry patterns is found in respect to reaction times. In the face decision task, general performance of both patient groups is less prominently impaired. Depressed patients show the expected left visual field advantages. They perform both tasks unexpectedly well compared to controls. Additional emotional stimulation produces a general accuracy benefit in all subject groups in the word tasks. Depressed patients improve more under emotionally negative stimulation whereas schizophrenic patients show more performance gains under neutral stimulation. The results are largely in line with previous findings of a bilateral hemispheric deficit in schizophrenia and reports of a major right hemispheric involvement in depression. Our findings of dissociated general performance levels, accuracy asymmetry, and reaction time asymmetry in schizophrenia and depression reveal a drawback in neuropsychological assessment of laterality and demonstrate that performance level, accuracy asymmetry and reaction time asymmetry data cannot be cited interchangeably.[1]

References

Bogerts B, Wurthmann C, Piroth HD: Hirnsubstanzdefizit mit paralimbischem und limbischem Schwerpunkt im CT Schizophrener. Nervenarzt 58: 97-106, 1987
Bower GH: Mood and Memory. American Psychologist 36: 129-148, 1981
Brown GW, Birley JLT, Wing JK: Influence of family life on the course of schizophrenic disorders: A replication. British Journal of Psychiatry 121: 241-258, 1972
Coffey CE: Cerebral laterality and emotion. The neurology of depression. Comprehensive Psychiatry 28: 197-219, 1987
Cutting J: The Right cerebral hemisphere and psychiatric disorders. Oxford, Oxford University Press, 1990
DeLisi LE, Buchsbaum MS, Holcomb HH, Langston KC, King C, KesslerR, Pickar D, Carpenter WT, Morihisa JM, Margolin R, Weinberger DR: Increased temporal lobe glucose use in chronic schizophrenic patients. Biological Psychiatry 25: 835-851, 1989
Flor-Henry P: Psychosis and temporal lobe epilepsy. A controlled investigation. Epilepsia 10: 363-395, 1969
Flor-Henry P: On certain aspects of the localization of the cerebral systems regulating and determining emotion. Biological Psychiatry 14: 677-698, 1979
Gainotti G: Emotional behaviour and hemisphere side of lesion. Cortex 8: 41-55, 1972
Golinkoff M, Sweeney JA: Cognitive impairment in depression. Journal of Affective Disorders 17: 105-112, 1989
Gur RE: Left hemisphere dysfunction and right hemisphere overactivation in schizophrenia. Journal of Abnormal Psychology 87: 226-238, 1978
Hiller W, Zerssen D von, Mombour W, Wittchen HU: Inpatient Multidimensional Psychiatric Scale (IMPS). Eine multidimensionale Skala zur systematischen Erfassung des psychopathologischen Befunds. Weinheim, Beltz, 1986
Holsboer F: Psychiatric implications of altered limbic-hypothalamic-pituitary-adreno-cortical activity. European Archives of Psychiatry and Neurological Sciences 238: 302-322, 1989
Johnson O, Crockett D: Changes in perceptual asymmetries with clinical improvement of depression and schizophrenia. Journal of Abnormal Psychology 91: 399-413, 1982
Kinsbourne M: Mechanisms of hemispheric interaction in man. In: Kinsbourne M & Smith WL (eds): Hemispheric disconnection and verbal function, pp 260-285. Springfield, Illinois, 1974
Kolb B, Whishaw I: Performance of schizophrenic patients on tests sensitive to left or right frontal temporal or parietal function in neurological patients. Journal of Nervous and Mental Disease 171: 435-443, 1983
Leff J, Vaughn C: Expressed emotion in families: Its significance for mental illness. Guilford Press, New York, 1985
Lorr M, Klett CJ: Major psychotic disorders: A cross-cultural study. Archives of General Psychiatry 19: 652-658, 1968
Magaro PA, Chamrad DL: Information Processing and lateralization in schizophrenia. Biological Psychiatry 18: 29-44, 1983

1 This study has been supported by a grant (OE 112/1-3) from the Deutsche Forschungsgemeinschaft, DFG.

Moscovitch M, Strauss E, Olds J: Handedness and dichotic listening performance in patients with unipolar endogenous depression who received ECT. American Journal of Psychiatry138: 988-990, 1981

Oepen G, Fünfgeld M, Höll T, Zimmermann P, Landis T, Regard M: Schizophrenia—an emotional hypersensitivity of the right cerebral hemisphere. International Journal of Psychophysiology 5, 261-264, 1987

Oepen G, Harrington A, Fünfgeld M, Schulte M: Emotion and Hemisphere Dynamics in Schizophrenia and Depression. In: Stefanis CN et al. (eds): Psychiatry: A World Perspective, Vol 2, pp. 225-230, New York, Amsterdam, Elsevier, 1990

Oldfield RC: The assessment and analysis of handedness: The Edinburgh Inventory. Neuropsychologia 9: 97-113, 1971

Regard M, Landis T, Graves R: Dissociated hemispheric superiorities for reading stenography vs. print. Neuropschologia 23: 431-435, 1985

Regard M, Landis T: Affective and cognitive decisions in normals. In: Ellis HD, Jeeves MA, Newcombe F & Young A (eds): Aspects of face processing. Dordrecht, Nijhoff Publ., pp. 363-369, 1986

Robinson RG, Kubos KL, Starr LB, Reo K, Price TR: Mood disorders in stroke patients. Brain 107: 81-93, 1984

Robertson MM: Ictal and interictal depression in patients with epilepsy. In: Trimble MR & Bolwig TG (eds): Aspects of epilepsy and psychiatry, pp. 213-234. Chichester, Wiley, 1986

Roy-Byrne PP, Weingartner H, Bierer LM, Tompson K, Post RM: Effortful and automatic cognitive processes in depression. Archives of General Psychiatry 43: 265-267, 1986

Schweitzer L: Evidence of right cerebral hemisphere dysfunction in schizophrenic patients with left hemisphere overactivation. Biological Psychiatry 17: 655-673, 1982

Steingrüber HJ: Hand-Dominanz-Test. Göttingen, Hogrefe, 1971

Taylor AM, Abrams R: Cognitive impairment in schizophrenia. American Journal of Psychiatry 141: 196-201, 1984

Tancer ME, Brown TM, Evans DL, Ekstrom D, Haggerty JJ, Pederson C, Golden RM: Impaired effortful cognition in depression. Psychiatry Research 31: 161-168, 1990

Venables PH: Cerebral Mechanisms, autonomic responsiveness, and attention in schizophrenia. In: Spaulding WD & Cole JK (eds): Nebraska Symposium on Motivation: Theories of Schizophrenia and Psychosis, pp. 47-89, 1984

Watts FN, Morris L, MacLeod AK: Recognition memory in depression. Journal of Abnormal Psychology 96: 273-275, 1987

Weingartner H, Cohen RM, Murphy DL, Martello J, Gerdt C: Cognitive processes in depression. Archives of General Psychiatry 38: 42-47, 1981

Wittchen HU, Zaudig M, Schramm E, Spengler P, Mombour W, Kluge J, Horn R: SKID—Strukturiertes Klinisches Interview für DSM-III-R. The Structured Clinical Interview for DSM-III-R, Weinheim, Beltz, 1990

Yozawitz A, Bruder G, Sutton S, Sharpe L, Gurland B, Fleiss J, Costa L: Dichotic perception: Evidence for right hemisphere dysfunction in affective psychosis. British Journal of Psychiatry 135: 224-237, 1979

M. Spitzer, F.A. Uehlein
M.A. Schwartz, C. Mundt
(eds.): Phenomenology
Language & Schizophrenia.
Springer-Verlag, New York, 1992

Preattentive Perception? Limited Capacity Channel System? What is Different in Schizophrenic Information Processing?

Rainer Hess, Ulrich Schu, Peter Müller, Reinhold Schüttler

1. Introduction

Attentional deficits have long been regarded as central in schizophrenic patients' cognitive functioning. Kraepelin already regarded an attentional deficit as a common finding in schizophrenic patients (Kraepelin 1919). Of course this is not surprising, because attention is a function central to any cognitive operation, be it perception, the recall of information, or the planning of motor acts. Theories of schizophrenic cognition that have seemingly nothing to do with attention, such as Bleuler's formulation of the "loss of associative threads", or Shakov's "loss of major set", to name but two, can also be interpreted from the view point of an attentional deficit.

What do we mean by the term attention? Originally, it was practically synonymous with *selective attention*, meaning that while we attend to one aspect of a stimulus display (in one or more modalities), we at the same time disattend to others (Wundt 1912, Broadbent 1958, Treisman 1964, Posner 1982). Therefore, to attend means to chose, to select, and to filter one aspect from others for more detailed or precise perception. In order to perceive a complex display completely, one must attend to various features or aspects one after the other, which means that the task is time consuming. The more complex the display is, or the more detailed the analysis, the more time is needed to scan it with scrutiny in order to perceive it completely (c.f. Broadbent 1982, Julesz 1984).

One important step towards understanding the process of attention is Broadbent's model of perception (1958), with the crucial feature being a *limited capacity channel*. Only information that has been processed through such a channel of limited capacity reaches the level of consciousness, or is ready to be stored in long term memory, or elicits suitable motor reactions. The incoming information is first filtered and then categorized. Finally, a bias is applied to certain categories—a process called *pigeon-holing* by Broadbent (1982), which means that certain categories "will be triggered off by less evidence than they would normally need" (Broadbent 1982, p. 260). It seems important to point out that previous experience retrieved from memory and the emotional coloring of past or present experience are also part of this attentive selection process. Hence, a disturbance of attention can affect all aspects of cognition.

Aside from selective attention, the term attention is used to describe the state of continuous vigilance or readiness to respond, i.e., *general attention* (see Nuechterlein & Dawson 1984). In this sense, attention is a prerequisite for perception and cognition. With increasing fatigue or clouding of consciousness, it diminishes. When this occurs during the course of an experiment on selective attention, it is quite likely that performance will be reduced. This may be misinterpreted as a deficit of selective attention unless general attention is properly controlled for.

Neisser (1966, p. 89) has already pointed out that focal attention cannot operate by itself, but must be preceded by a process he called *preattentive*. The preattentive process works "holistically" and immediately, and it operates as a guideline for the focal attentive process for detailed analysis of the perceptive field. Over the past 10-15 years this preattentive process has gained much interest, and outstanding experimental work in visual psychophysics has been reported by Anne Treisman and Bela Julesz (Treisman & Gelade 1980, Treisman 1988, Bergen & Julesz 1983, Julesz 1984, see also Hurlburt & Poggio 1985).

According to the hypotheses of Treisman and Julesz, only certain features described as "local conspicuous features" are perceived immediately and simultaneously within the entire visual field, irrespective of the size or information content of the image. They "catch the eye", which does not mean that they initiate eye movements. Rather, there is a neuronal process which operates very fast (50 ms), and has been compared to a spotlight that illuminates the conspicuous elements of a visual field. (Julesz 1984, Hurlburt & Poggio 1985). Julesz called these elements *textons*, and has stated that there should be no more than a total of about 20 of such elements (personal communication). Examples of textons are differences in color, orientation of lines, ends of lines (terminators), and crossings. In contrast to the focal attentive process, which seems to require serial neuronal processing, and is therefore time consuming, the preattentive process operates in parallel and rapidly.

Preattentive perception has not yet been studied in schizophrenic patients. We shall report on some preliminary results of experiments on preattentive vision in schizophrenic patients as compared to normal controls.

Although there are numerous reports on the deficits of schizophrenics in tasks that require selective attention, there are certain drawbacks in the experimental design of some of these studies: In the first place, general attention has not always been controlled for, so that the results are difficult to interpret. Secondly, it is a common finding that schizophrenics perform more slowly than normals on most tasks (see e.g. Marshall 1973, Frith 1981), but it remains unclear whether this is just a general or a specific deficit. It would be instructive to compare schizophrenic patients and normal control subjects matched not only for demographic variables, such as age, gender, and education, but also for general performance (for the problem of adequate matching see Chapman & Chapman 1973). In such a design, one may expect to find more specific perceptual deficits than merely slower performance.

Treisman and Schmidt (1982) published a test which was designed to prove the separate neuronal processing of information on the shape and color of objects. Subjects have to report both, (1) two numbers to the left and right of the stimulus display, and (2) letters and their colors, while the processing capacity is overloaded in a previoulsly defined particular way (see below). This test appears to have several advantages: General attention is continuously controlled for (naming of numbers); attention is spread across the entire display; the information processing capacity is overloaded in an individually defined way. Therefore one would expect that if a deficit is observed it should be specific to the perceptual process under study, and not nonspecific due to secondary influences on attention and thereby on perception.

2. Methods

2.1 Preattentive Visual Perception

10 schizophrenic inpatients (DSM-III-R) and 10 normal controls matched for age, sex, and years of education were investigated. The test consisted of 108 slides which were presented tachistoscopically with an inter-stimulus-interval of about 2 seconds. In 36 slides, the target was the letter "L" randomly placed among 35 letters "T" (non texton difference), in 36 additional slides the target L was among 35 plus signs "+" (texton difference, see figure 1). The rest of the slides contained only T (without target). The sequence of presentation was random (Bergen & Julesz 1983, Hess & Ahrens 1991).

Subjects were asked to fixate upon a point placed in the middle of the projection screen. Slides were projected for 40 msec. followed by a second slide (called mask) containing 36 elements like ╒╤ (a combination of the relevant features of ┌, ┬, and +). The stimulus onset asynchrony (SOA) between the two slides was varied between 200 and 800 milliseconds (ms). (see figure 1). The mask served the purpose of extinguishing the retinal afterimage and thus limiting the stimulus-time accurately. Subjects were asked to report whether they saw a target and, if so, where the target was located.

2.2 Visual Perception at a Defined Overload of Visual Processing Capacity

This test, adapted from Treisman and Schmidt (1982) was constructed as follows: Slides contained 2 one digit numbers (1 to 9) and 3 letters out of the five S, T, O, N, and X. The numbers were written in black ink, while the letters were written in different colors (yellow, green, blue, brown, and red). The slides were presented tachistoscopically and were immediately followed by a black and white noise mask in order to limit the retinal afterimage. Subjects were asked to report immediately after each stimulus whether they saw a target, and, if so, where the target was located. It turned out that when subjects recognized a target correctly, they could always indicate its location.

Fig. 1: Stimulus arrangement for the test on preattentive perception. (A) Texton target (L in +s). (B) Non texton target (L in Ts). (C) Time sequence of stimuli. Preparatory interval means that the subject is asked to concentrate on the fixation point on the projection screen. The stimulus then follows within approximately 1 second. The mask was composed of FF elements.

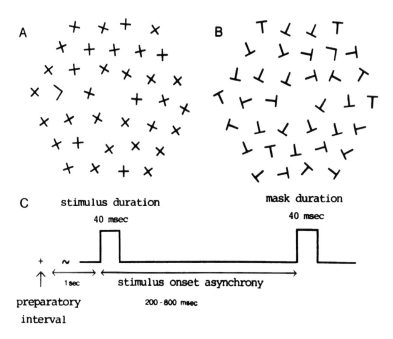

In order to enable each subject to perform at a similar level, the exposure duration necessary for correctly reporting the numbers and two additional items (either two letters or two colors or a letter and a color) with 10% errors was determined individually for each subject in pretests.

294   R. Hess et al.

Initially, 10 slides were presented with an exposure duration of 200 ms. If more than 2 correct items were reported, the exposure duration was shortened by steps of 20 ms; if the criterion was not met, the exposure duration was prolonged. The resulting individual exposure duration for fulfilling the criterion was then used to present all 64 slides. The items, positions of items, and the conjunctions of letters and colors, reported by subjects after each slide, were noted as the result.

23 outpatients fulfilling research diagnostic criteria (RDC) for schizophrenia participated in this experiment (18 paranoid, 1 hebephrenic, 2 latent schizophrenic and 2 schizoaffective). 15 of these patients were in complete remission at the time of the trial, the rest had mild paranoid hallucinatory symptoms or presented with a residual syndrome.

Subjects in the control group were paired for age, sex, and years of education. On average, subjects were 35 years old and had spent 13 years in school (for a more detailed description of the method see Schu et. al. 1991 and Schu, in preparation).

There was no significant difference in exposure duration, the type of errors, or in the error rates between medicated schizophrenic patients and patients without neuroleptics for at least one week (Schu et al. 1991), so data was pooled for the present analysis.

3. Results

3.1 Preattentive Visual Perception

Schizophrenic patients reported fewer correct (texton) targets with all SOAs from 200 to 800 ms (figure 2).

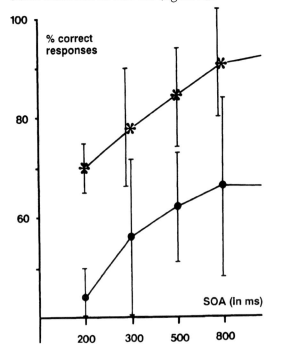

Figure 2: Mean and standard deviation of correct responses of patients (•) and matched controls (∗) at different stimulus onset asynchronies (SOAs). The differences were significant at all SOAs (t-test, p < 0.01).

While controls generally improved the number of correct responses with increasing SOA, this trend was not generally seen in the patient cohort: Some patients also improved their performance with increasing SOA, but others actually reported fewer correct targets at longer SOAs. This was never seen with controls. At the brief stimulus durations (40 ms) and SOAs (< 800 ms) used, the non-texton targets were identified correctly only by chance by both patients and controls.

3.2 Perception with Overloaded Channel Capacity

The individual exposure duration in the schizophrenic outpatients was on average longer than that of the controls (table 1). However, many of the patients' exposure durations were well within the range of the controls (figure 3). This is in contrast to results obtained with schizophrenic inpatients, where there was a complete separation between patients and controls (Hess et al. 1989, Seidlitz, in preparation).

Table 1: **Mean performance of schizophrenic patients and normal control subjects in the Treisman test (see text).**
features: letters or colors (average number reported per slide).
locations: location of the features.
conjunctions: report of a letter and its color.
wrong location: correct letter or color reported in wrong location.
illusory conjunction: wrong combination of correct letter and color.

$n1 = n2 = 23$	Schizo-phrenics	control subjects	$p_{Wilcoxon}$
exposure duration (ms)	425.2	226.1	0.0007
total errors (%)	11.9	13.2	0.2
features	3.4	3.4	0.8
locations	2.5	2.8	0.2
conjunctions	1.2	1.2	0.8
wrong location (%)	16.6	28.1	0.002
illusory conjunction (%)	15.5	24.9	0.004

During the main test, 98% of the numbers were reported correctly, which confirms that the entire stimulus display was perceived, and at the same time, that a constant level of general attention was sustained throughout the experiment. Similarly, the adequacy of the individual exposure duration was confirmed during the main experiment because controls and patients reported equally many items with the same percentage of errors. In this way, both groups were matched for performance (table 1). There was a slight (but not significant compared to the control group) tendency of schizophrenic patients to leave out an item (omission error: report less than 2 items) rather than to report a wrong one. Beyond reporting the same number of letters and colors with 10% errors, for which both groups were matched, the *position* of letters and colors and *conjunctions* between letters and colors were also reported equally frequently by both groups. The schizophrenic group, however, made fewer errors (i.e., position errors and/or conjunction errors), as indicated in table 1. This part of the task was completed more accurately by schizophrenic patients who, nonetheless, *needed more time*.

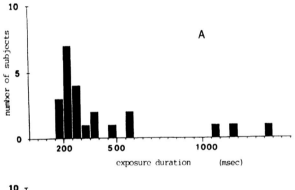

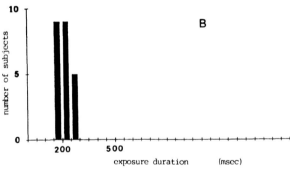

Fig. 3: Frequency distributions of individual exposure duration necessary to report two numbers and 2 further items from the stimulus display (Treisman test, pretest condition, for further explanation see text). (A) Patients, (B) matched controls. Mean exposure duration and level of significance, see table 1.

Within the patient group, the required exposure duration correlated with the severity of the disease as measured by the Brief Psychiatric Rating Scale (BPRS) anxiety/depression, thought disorder, and hostility/suspiciousness subscores, and by the Clinical Global Impression (CGI; see table 2). The type of errors (omission or incorrect report of items) seemed to be related to premorbid adjustment as evaluated by the Phillips Scale: The worse the adjustment, the more frequently omissions occurred and the more infrequently items were reported erroneously (table 2).

Table 2: Correlation coefficients between clinical parameters and the results in the Treisman test. Only significant correlations are reported (p < 0.05). omissions: If subjects reported less than 2 correct items during the main part of the experiment, this was regarded as an omission error.

n = 23	exposure duration	omissions	feature errors
premorbid adjustment (Phillips)		0.47	-0.58
Clinical Global Impresssions 1	0.55		
BPRS anxiety/depression	0.43		
anergia			
thought disorder	0.52		
activation		0.43	
hostility/suspiciousness	0.54		

rank-correlation (Spearman)

4. Discussion

4.1 Preattentive Perception

What is wrong with attention in schizophrenic patients? In preattentive visual perception, certain local conspicuous features—the textons—are perceived rapidly and independently. They appear to be processed in parallel and perception seems to occur automatically, or at least does not require the focusing of attention. In experimental tasks where information processing occurs largely automatically, schizophrenic patients are known to show very little impairment (Nuechterlein & Dawson 1984). Therefore one would expect preattentive vision to function normally in schizophrenics. In contrast to this expectation, our schizophrenic patients performed poorly on the test of preattentive vision.

It is premature, however, to conclude that preattentive processing malfunctions in schizophrenic patients. One has to consider that in order to limit the exposure duration accurately, a mask was used to limit the retinal afterimage. With two stimuli presented tachistoscopically within brief periods of time, it has been found in normal subjects that at intervals of up to about 300 ms between the two stimuli, only the second stimulus can be seen, even though the first one was seen when presented alone. This phenomenon has been referred to as *backward masking*. With the method of backward masking, Braff and Saccuzzo (1985) found in schizophrenic patients that the masking effect of the second stimulus (mask) is present at intervals up to about 500 ms. At longer intervals, there were no group differences, i.e., the masking effect was not found in both groups.

In our experiments on preattentive vision, the mask was used to accurately limit the retinal after image. Because the SOAs between stimulus and mask used were similar to the ones where backward masking occurs, one has to consider that this effect also played a role in our experiments. It may explain the differences between schizophrenic patients and controls at SOAs between 300 and 500 ms. At the longer interval of 800 ms, however, we still found differences between schizophrenic patients and controls. We observed that some patients' performances declined at 800 ms SOA. This was not seen in our control group, and it has not been reported in the literature for normal subjects. These two aspects may point to a genuine deficit of preattentive vision in schizophrenic patients, but the finding needs to be verified in a larger sample of both patients and controls. The number of normal subjects so far reported in the literature is small, and it is not known for example, whether age might influence the results.

It remains unclear how backward masking is related to the preattentive process. The locus within the neuronal pathway where such masking occurs has hypothetically been located at the transcription from iconic storage to short term memory (Braff & Saccuzzo 1985) or very early in short term memory, but the actual neuronal mechanisms are not known (Saccuzzo & Braff 1986).

In conclusion, one may say that the experiments on preattentive vision revealed a similar prolongation of the interference between mask and stimulus in schizophrenic patients as is known from the backward masking paradigm. How these two techniques relate to each other and whether a genuine difference remains in preattentive vision awaits further study.

4.2 Visual Perception of Schizophrenic Patients at a Defined Overload of Processing Capacity

The method described by Treisman and Schmidt (1982), which was chosen for these experiments, resembles the *span of apprehension technique* in which an array of letters is presented tachistoscopically and subjects have to report what they have seen. Using the span of apprehension test, various authors have reported deficits in schizophrenic patients (for reviews, see Cromwell & Spalding 1978, Nuechterlein & Dawson 1984). For the experiments reported here, the method of Treisman and Schmidt (1982) was chosen because it offers several advantages with respect to controlling two aspects of attention. Firstly, general attention is controlled for throughout the experiment because in each single stimulus a part of the elements, namely the numbers, have to be reported. Secondly, by determining the time needed by each subject to report two further items in addition to the numbers, patients and controls are also matched for performance on this task. This matching for performance on a task has been outlined by Chapman and Chapman (1973, pp. 99-101) as an important prerequisite for finding actual deficits in schizophrenics' thought and information processing that cannot be a consequence of their general reduction in performance.

In our experiment, we expected the schizophrenic patients to make more errors in naming conjunctions between color and shape, e.g. naming a red N where the N is actually yellow and some other letter in the display is red. The naming of conjunctions of color and shape is the most difficult task in the test because the information on color and shape are initially separated and processed independently in the visual pathway, as Treisman and Schmidt (1982) have shown. At a later stage of neuronal integration the information on both is brought together again. It can be assumed that during the time period when color and shape are processed separately, there is a greater risk of interference from other simultaneously ongoing activity in the brain. Therefore, more errors in reporting conjunctions occur. From a clinical point of view, interference, i.e., the disruption of a coherent line of thought by some other mental content, was found to be one of the characteristics of schizophrenic thought disorder (Buss & Lang 1965, for reviews see Callaway 1970, Chapman & Chapman 1973).

Regarding its control functions, the test fulfilled its purpose. Patients named the same number of items as normal subjects, also equally as many conjunctions of items, and they made a comparable number of errors. With regard to the type of errors, there was only a tendency for schizophrenic patients to leave out an answer rather than name an item incorrectly, but this was not significantly different in comparison to controls.

Schizophrenics also reported equally as many positions of items and conjunctions of color and shape, but in contrast to expectations, they did not make errors in this more difficult task. Like the controls, they named few conjunctions, but they did so even more correctly.

With respect to possible deficits in the processing of visual information in schizophrenic patients, our results appear to be disappointing, because there was little difference compared to controls when general attention was properly controlled for and subjects were matched for performance on the task. The only clear difference was that schizophrenics needed more time to respond at an equal level of accuracy. In previous experiments with schizophrenic inpatients who still suffered from delusions or hallucinations, the exposure durations necessary to fulfill the required criterion did not even overlap with those of the normal controls (Hess et al. 1989).

Similar results were obtained with the color-word test (Stroop 1935). In the color-word test either the word has to be read avoiding distraction from its incongruent color, or the color has to be named without being distracted by the meaning of the word. Using regular consecutive stimulus presentation where there is limited time to respond, schizophrenic patients also needed more time to respond to fulfill the required criterion of less than 10% errors (Hess et al. 1988). Both studies indicated that there was no basic difference in handling information, but that the *amount of information* that can be handled per time unit was limited in schizophrenic patients. Only when this upper margin of performance was exceeded did errors appear in fulfilling the required task.

Let us further illustrate these matters with the analogy of the functioning of a photocamera. A camera's shutter normally has exposure times from infinity down to about 1/300th of a second. Rapidly moving objects have to be exposed briefly, otherwise their image is blurred. Stationary objects such as landscapes will appear as sharp pictures even with long exposure time like 1/15th of a second. If we imagine a camera with an exposure time limited to no faster than 1/15th of a second, then the speed of moving objects will determine whether the pictures taken with this camera will be sharp or blurred.

If this model is valid, then it may be wrong to assume that schizophrenic patients should have a conspicuous information processing deficit. Because prominent symptoms of schizophrenia, such as hallucinations and delusions, deviate so much from normal experience, equally prominent differences in information processing have been suggested as a basic feature of schizophrenia. However, this is not necessarily true. It is conceivable that, if patients need slightly more time to process a certain amount of information, a mismatch between information load and processing capacity per time will lead to disturbances of perception. Delusions and hallucinations may then arise from this partially disturbed image of the outer world as a desperate attempt to achieve a consistent inner representation by adding illusory perceptual components or imaginary explanations.

4.3 Conclusions

In conclusion, it appears from our experiments that neither preattentive vision nor the reduction of information for further processing through the limited capacity channel system consistently malfunctions in schizophrenic patients. Disturbed perception may rather result from a mismatch between information load and processing capacity per unit of time. The possibility that schizophrenics mostly need more time to deal with sensory information (or less information per unit of time) can give us hints about the treatment of schizophrenia or about the prevention of relapse. If we can determine schizophrenics' individual information processing capacity per unit of time, and then connect this to the requirements of their everyday life, we may find a way to enable them to relate more normally to their environment.

Summary

Preliminary data are presented on preattentive visual perception in schizophrenic patients and in a normal control group. In a search paradigm, a target letter (L) had to be searched in either 35 + (texton difference) or in 35 T (non-texton difference). Stimuli were presented for 40 ms followed by a mask at various stimulus onset asynchronies (SOA) between 200 and 800 ms. At all SOAs, patients reported fewer correct responses than controls.

In a second paradigm on selective attention, subjects had to report two numbers and, in addition, two more items from a display containing three letters written in different colors and two numbers to the right and left of the letters. Subjects in both groups were matched on performance operationalized as the number of correct responses. Simultaneously, a defined information overload was introduced. Constant general attention (readiness to respond) and spread of attention across the entire display were controlled for by the particular design used. Errors in reporting letters, colors, positions of letters and colors, and conjunctions of letters and colors were noted as results.

With this particular design, nonspecific attentional influences were excluded. Because of the defined information overload, it was expected that subtle differences in attentional capacity could be detected. The results on preattentive perception indicate a poorer performance of schizophrenics at all SOAs. This finding can be interpreted in terms of the backward masking effect. However, while no differences have been found between schizophrenic patients and normal controls in backward masking at intervals of 500 ms and more, we did find a significant difference at 800 ms SOA. Whether this indicates an additional deficit not related to backward masking remains an open question which should be further investigated.

In the experiment on selective attention, schizophrenic patients needed on average longer presentation times to fulfill the criterion. Once matched for performance, there remained surprisingly little difference in the number and type of errors reported by patients and controls. Hence, it is possible that the only attentional deficit in schizophrenic patients consists of the need for slightly more time to process information. A mismatch between information load and individual processing capacity may result in distorted perception which may then form the starting point for a delusional interpretation of the world.

References

Bergen JR, Julesz B: Parellel versus serial processing in rapid pattern discrimination. Nature 303: 696-698, 1983

Braff DL, Saccuzzo DP: The Time Course of Information-Processing Deficits in Schizophrenia. Am J Psychiatry 142: 170-174, 1985

Broadbent DE: Perception and Communication. London: Pergamon Press, 1958

302   R. Hess et al.

Broadbent DE: Task Combination and Selective Intake of Information. Acta Psychologica 50: 253-290, 1982
Buss AH, Lang PJ: Psychological Deficit in Schizophrenia. J of Abnormal Psychology 70: 2-24, 1965
Callaway E: Schizophrenia and Interference. Arch Gen Psychiat 22: 193-208, 1970
Chapman LJ and Chapman JP: Disordered Thought in Schizophrenia. Englewood Cliffs, New Jersey, Prentice-Hall, 1973
Cromwell RL, Spaulding W: How Schizophrenics Handle Information. In: Fann WE, Karacan I, Pokorny AD, et al (eds): Phenomenology and Treatment of Schizophrenia. New York, Spectrum Publications, 1978
Frith CD: Schizophrenia: An abnormality of consciousness? In: Underwood G, Stevens R (eds): Aspects of Consciousness. Vol II, pp. 149-168, London, Academic Press, 1981
Hess R, Ahrens O: Ist bereits die praeattentive Wahrnehmung Schizophrener gestört? Biologische Psychiatrie. Laux G, Gaebel W (eds), Berlin, Springer, in press
Hess R, Reinhold B, Seidlitz M: Leistungsverhalten von Schizophrenen im Farb-Wort-Test (Stroop) im Vergleich zu einer normalen Kontrollgruppe. In: Oepen G (ed): Psychiatrie des rechten und linken Gehirns. Köln, Deutscher Ärzte Verlag,, 1988
Hess R, Seidlitz M, Reinhold B, Schu U, Müller P: Psychophysiologische Untersuchungen zur Informationsverarbeitung Schizophrener. In: Saletu B (ed): Biologische Psychiatrie, Vol. 2, Stuttgart, Thieme, 1989
Hurlbert A, Poggio T: Spotlight on Attention. Trends Neurosci 8: 309-311, 1985
Julesz B: A brief outline of the texton theory of human vision. Trends Neurosci 7: 41-47, 1984
Kraepelin E: Dementia Praecox and Paraphrenia (1913), translated by Barclay RM, Livingston E, Livingston S, Edinburgh, Livingston, 1919
Neisser U: Cognitive Psychology. New York, Appleton-Century-Croft, 1967
Marshall WL: Cognitive Functioning in Schizophrenia. Brit J Psychol 123: 413-433, 1973
Nuechterlein KH, Dawson E: Information processing and attentional functioning in the developmental course of schizophrenic disorder. Schizophrenia Bulletin 10: 160-203, 1984
Posner MI: Cumulative Development of Attentional Theory. American Psychologist 37: 168-179, 1982
Saccuzzo DP, Braff DL: Information-Processing Abnormalities: Trait- and State-Dependent Components. Schizophrenia Bulletin 3: 447-458, 1986
Seidlitz M: Dissertation, in prep.
Schu U: Dissertation, in prep.
Schu U, Hess R, and Müller P: Visuelle Wahrnehmung Schizophrener an der Grenze der Kanalkapazität. In: Laux G, Gaebel W (eds): Biologische Psychiatrie. Berlin, Springer, in press
Stroop RJ: Studies of interference in serial verbal reactions. Journal of Experimental Psychology 18: 643-662, 1935
Treisman A: Features and Objects: The Fourteenth Bartlett Memorial Lecture. The Quarterly Journal of Experimental Psychology 40A: 201-237, 1988
Treisman A: Selective Attention in Man. Brit. Med. Bull. 20:12-16, 1964
Treisman A, Gelade G: A Feature-Integration Theory of Attention. Cognitive Psychology 12: 97-136, 1980
Treisman A, Schmidt H: Illusory Conjunctions in the Perception of Objects. Cognitive Psychology 14: 107-141, 1982
Wundt W: Introduction to psychology. London, George Allen, 1912

Delusions

M. Spitzer, F.A. Uehlein
M.A. Schwartz, C. Mundt
(eds.): Phenomenology
Language & Schizophrenia.
Springer-Verlag, New York, 1992

The Phenomenology of Schizophrenic Delusions

Michael Alan Schwartz & Osborne P. Wiggins

1. Introduction: Doubt about the Certainty of Delusions

Writers on delusions, such as Karl Jaspers and Kräupl Taylor, have rather consistently seen certainty and incorrigibility of belief as two of their defining characteristics (Jaspers 1963, Kräupl-Taylor 1966, 1983, American Psychiatric Association 1987). In this paper we shall challenge this by now customary view. More specifically, we shall challenge this view *as its applies to a particular sub-class of delusions: the delusions of patients suffering from schizophrenia.* We shall, on the other hand, concede that certainty and incorribility of belief do indeed characterize another species of delusions, the delusions of delirious patients. Moreover, we shall admit that schizophrenic patients regularly claim that they are certain about their delusions or that they "know" some things to be the case that normal people would regard as delusional. We shall interpret these pervasive claims, however, as expressions on the part of schizophrenics that are motivated by *a determination to believe* something *indubitably* precisely because they both believe it and doubt it while they seek to eradicate their doubt. More simply put, their assertions of absolute conviction do not depict their actual experience but rather a *desired* one, an experience they seek to make real precisely by insisting that it is now real.

Karl Jaspers has noted a crucial component of the schizophrenic's experience that, when fully appreciated, will allow us to describe how both belief and disbelief plague the patient. Jaspers has called this feature the schizophrenic's "double orientation to reality" (Jaspers 1963, p. 150, 172, 296). Taking note of Jaspers' insight, we shall briefly review our own account of the initial stages of schizophrenia. We shall then briefly chart the transition from the "primary delusions" of the patient to the "secondary delusional elaboration." Tracing this course of the illness, however, will permit us to explicate the schizophrenic's "double orientation to reality" while demonstrating the roles that certain and incorrigible beliefs play in this troublesome orientation. We shall seek to substantiate our claims by showing how they help to explain two typical examples of schizophrenic behavior. We shall then contrast this intertwining of belief and doubt involved in schizophrenia with the uncomplicated certainty of belief characteristic of the delusions of delirious patients. The features of schizophrenia that we point out will allow us to delineate a path toward the effective use of psychotherapy for treatment of the illness.

Throughout the discussion the reader should remain aware of some crucial qualifications to our claims. These qualifications render our present findings provisional and preliminary. (1) This paper is an exercise in what we would like to characterize as "clinical phenomenology." Our aim is to describe some clinical features of deluded patients. Here we do not, for example, try to quantify our concepts and subject them to empirical confirmation. Furthermore, all cases have not been systematically collected, and we do not employ formal diagnostic criteria. (2) All the patients considered are receiving conventional treatment. (3) We do not claim that the "double orientation to reality" is present in all cases of schizophrenia. This phenomenon is frequently absent in individuals whose schizophrenic illness has a strong affective coloring. Furthermore, chronic patients often lack any double orientation.[1]

In the face of these manifold qualifications, we must concede that we are here engaged simply in generating and refining clinical concepts. In clinical research in psychiatry, however, beginnings as tentative as ours are often unavoidable, at least as a first step. Of course, in order to be justified this first provisional step must subsequently be subjected to empirical testing.

2. The "Double Orientation to Reality" in Schizophrenia

We shall develop our views regarding the mixture of belief and doubt in schizophrenic delusions by drawing on Jaspers' thesis concerning "the double orientation to reality" in schizophrenic patients. Jaspers has described this "double orientation" in the following manner:

> "Either the experiences (of the schizophrenic) are *unified*: there is only one reality for the patient, the psychotic one. Or there occur experiences—particularly the fantastic ones—in which the patient lives in two worlds simultaneously, the real one which he can correctly see and judge and his psychotic one. In his *double orientation* he may move in reality more or less correctly inspite of his cosmic experiences. The psychotic reality, however, is the actual reality for him. The real world has become an illusion (*Schein*) for him which he can correctly survey to the extent that he knows: these are doctors, and I am in the insane asylum, I am deluded by an illusory religious world, etc. It often happens that the patient in an acute psychosis is completely

---

1 Prior to the modern era of psychopharmacology, Jaspers observed: "The schizophrenic world of acute psychosis with its double orientation is something quite different from the world of the chronic state. This can grow into a system of ideas which for the patient carries memories of unforgettable occurrences in the acute state, and take deep effect. However in the end the double orientation vanishes" (Jaspers 1963, p. 296). Today, undoubtedly due to the efficacy of conventional treatment, the situation portrayed by Jaspers has changed somewhat. We observe the double orientation to reality in many chronic schizophrenics as well as in patients who are acutely ill. Other chronic patients continue to behave in conformity with Jaspers description.

filled for a time with his psychotic experiences and forgets who he was, where he is, etc. But he is apt to be ripped out (of this illusionary world) by harsh events or profound impressions (admission to an institution, visits by relatives). An emphatic word (*Anruf*) may lead the patient back to actual reality for a moment. Then immediately the double orientation reasserts itself: everything he does is doubly motivated, he himself is double and manifold" (Jaspers 1963, p. 150, translation modified).

We can see that, according to Jaspers, the schizophrenic is oriented toward *both* his psychotic world and the real world.[2] At times the patient may be consumed in his delusional world and sustain no awareness of the other world, the consensually validated world. This can occur when the patient is caught up in powerful emotions. At other times, however, the schizophrenic lives in both spheres simultaneously. Notice that Jaspers contends that, even when the consensually validated world is experienced as an illusion by the patient, he can still correctly survey its features. Although the world is an illusion for him, he still maintains an accurate understanding of its workings and properties. He even knows that from the perspective of the consensually validated world his religious experiences—the experiences he deems the most real—are considered delusions. This doubleness of reality entails that the patient's own motives are two-sided: a single action by the schizophrenic may aim at achieving both a goal in his delusional world and a goal in the shared world. The schizophrenic's self is also double: a single feature of his personality may have one meaning in the delusional world and a different—perhaps even contrary—significance in the shared world.

We shall now try to confirm and extend Jaspers' description of this double orientation to reality in schizophrenia by sketching some features of the course of the illness, beginning with its earliest stage.

3. From Primary Delusions to Secondary Delusional Elaboration

In the primary delusions the schizophrenic is directly presented with states of affairs that conflict with one another and with previous experiences (Jaspers 1963, pp. 98-99, Slater & Roth 1969, pp. 273-273, Wiggins et al. 1990). This conflict is pervaded with doubt and uncertainty, not only about a few mundane objects and states of affairs, but also about *reality in its entirety,* including one's own personal identity and one's whole past life (Wiggins et al. 1990). Along with this doubt and uncertainty arises anxiety, panic, and even terror. The senseless chaos that the schizophrenic now experiences is deeply unsettling. Even those aspects of things that have remained relatively familiar shadow forth an ominous sense that they too are at root different, alien, and unreal. The disorder and unreality that

---

2 Throughout this article we have followed Jaspers in speaking of two "worlds" or "realities" for the schizophrenic. The reader should not understand our use of these terms "world" and "reality" in any technical or precise sense. They have seemed to us only convenient colloquial ways to express features of the schizophrenic's experience that we have not paused to analyze here.

pervade everything can be called "ontological" because they affect even the most fundamental structures of events and things, such as space, time, causality, and substantiality (Wiggins et al. 1990). This foreboding chaos is experienced as only provisional, however, because the schizophrenic's mental life is already pervaded by an *expectancy* that some as yet unimaginable and unforeseeable order is emerging from the future.

This emerging order, however, remains opaque and indecipherable. But despite its opacity it captivates and preoccupies the schizophrenic's attention. He or she cannot turn away from it because it *demands* that he or she come to terms with it. The schizophrenic must actively and completely devote his or her attention to discerning the profound but inscrutable relationships among events and things. What normally occurs automatically in a person's mental life, below the level of active attention, namely, the constitution of an ordered world and a personal identity, must now be actively and explicitly brought about with great intellectual and emotional effort. The schizophrenic strenuously devotes him- or herself to discerning and interpreting an overall structure to things. This is the beginning of secondary "delusional elaboration" (Hamilton 1984, p. 52, Slater and Roth 1969, pp. 272-273). Such delusional elaboration generates order, consistency, and harmony: it must successfully constitute a new world and a new self that are both unified and coherent. Only such a world and self can be experienced free of intense uneasiness and discomposure.

This secondary delusional elaboraton requires too great a human effort, however. The insuperable difficulty lies in the fact that it must encompass in a coherent and unified pattern *both* the primary delusions *and* the consensually validated world. The subject must take "facts" that are *given* from both sources and construct an overall framework that connects them with one another in an intelligible and consistent arrangement. This framework must be actively constructed; it will not be automatically given by direct experience. But the framework must arise within constraints imposed by what is directly given.

Normal people have it considerably easier. Our overall interpretation of the world is largely inherited ready-made from our social environment. We can as we grow up simply internalize the socially accepted and consensually validated view of reality. The work of constructing a world view has already been accomplished by others through an ancient and far-reaching division of interpretive labor. We need merely imbibe it.

The most difficult problem for the schizophrenic is this: the two worlds that the schizophrenic is trying to systematically combine are inconsistent with one another. The other people who inhabit the consensually validated world will repeatedly disconfirm the schizophrenic's delusional world, and events will occur in the shared world that conflict with the schizophrenic's delusions. Consequently, the schizophrenic will repeatedly experience items that contradict one another. This repetitous conflict motivates further dedicated attempts to rearrange or extend the encompassing delusional system.

Because events directly occur in the schizophrenic's delusional world that contradict the shared world, he or she will disbelieve in the reality of the shared world. But because the schizophrenic also directly experiences the shared world, he or she will believe in its reality. And because events directly occur in the shared world that contradict the schizophrenic's delusional world, he or she will doubt the reality of the delusional world. But because the subject also directly experiences and is consumed by the delusional world, he or she will believe in its reality. *The schizophrenic thus both believes and disbelieves in the reality of the consensually validated world, and he or she both believes and disbelieves in the reality of the delusional world.* Not only is the schizophrenic "oriented" toward two worlds at once, but each orientation in itself mixes conviction with doubt.

This co-experience of doubt and belief in the same thing produces a heightened anxiety. This anxiety can be alleviated only if one of the worlds gives way entirely to the other. Only if a single self-consistent world emerges can the patient experience certainty and thereby escape doubt and its concomitant anxiety. There are then two alternatives: either (A) the subject closes off the shared world and dwells solely in the delusional world, or (B) the schizophrenic relinquishes the delusional world and abides exclusively in the shared world.

Alternative (A) can be temporarily realized. The schizophrenic can for a period of time ignore the shared world and devote him- or herself wholeheartedly to the delusional world. But the shared world inevitably reasserts its actual existence, and the schizophrenic experiences its incompatibility with the reality of the delusions.

Alternative (B) is unrealizable for two reasons.

First, the primary delusions continue to be unavoidably encountered and to consume the patient's attention. The schizophrenic's delusions preoccupy him or her. They *demand* that the subject focus on them and respond to them. The schizophrenic's own will has grown too weak to resist this demand, and they remain too insistent: one *must* devote one's effort and thought to them.

Second, the delusional system that the schizophrenic devises acquires a great personal value. Frequently, the system allows the patient to ascribe a positive value to actions and facts that would otherwise exhibit a negative value. For example, a person who is weak willed and fearful may develop patterns of behavior in which he or she constantly submits to the wishes and preferences of others. This self-sacrificial submission to the pettiness and whims of others can be interpreted as Christ-like. The subject is Christ. Being weak willed and fearful is bad. Being Christ is good. Consequently, enormous positive value lies in the delusional system that allows the person to interpret his or her self-abnegation as that of a greater Spirit who, out of superior power and love, can freely take on the sins of the whole world. The negative value of the alternative self-interpretation is unacceptable. To relinquish the delusional self-understanding is to confess that one's life has consisted in a cowardly submission to the demands of others. Therefore, as protection from the realization that he or she is weak willed and fearful, the schizophrenic *must* believe in his or her divine being with firm and incorrgible conviction.

We can now explain why schizophrenics often assert the absolute certainty of their belief in their delusions despite the fact that, as we have claimed, they also remain uncertain of them. Schizophrenics, we maintained, disbelieve in the reality of their delusions because these delusions confict with their other experiences. At the same time, they believe in the reality of the delusions because they demand attention and because they possess a high positive value. This combat between doubt and conviction could be resolved if schizophrenics could only relinquish their delusional worlds and return solely to the consensually validated world of other people. But they cannot relinquish their delusional experiences because they remains inescapably preoccupied with them. As a result, they try to overcome any disbelief in them by convincing themselves that they are absolutely real. This striving for certainty will fail, however, because other, conflicting items will also unavoidably assert themselves. Yet this conflict does not lead to living with doubt but rather to opposing it even more forcefully. The schizophrenic is *determined* to believe in what he or she disbelieves. The certainty and incorrigibility of the schizophrenic's belief in his or her delusions is not then simply a pure and unalloyed absolute certainty. It is a certainty motivated by the need to combat doubt. It is a certainty which would not have to aspire to absoluteness if it did not need to grow extreme in order to overpower disbelief.

4. Illustrations of the Patient's Double Orientation to Reality

We shall now describe two examples of this "will to believe." In each instance a schizophrenic patient performs an action designed to elicit confirmation of his delusional belief. The confirmation, however, will consist precisely in the absence of disconfirmation. Because the other person, when given the chance, does not deny the truth of the schizophrenic's delusion, the patient can take this as proof that his delusion is true. But because the patient suspects that his delusion is untrue and desires to believe in its truth, he craftily performs this action in such a way as to circumvent the falsifying evidence that he fears could easily emerge. If the risky action succeeds, the schizophrenic's disbelief in his delusion will be weakened, and his belief in it strengthened.

Example (A). As the doctor walks into his room, the patient says "Hello, Dr. White"—(mumbles quietly under his breath) "You hate me, don't you?"—(immediately in a normal voice) "How are you?" Suppose that the doctor hears only the friendly greeting and does not detect the mumbled question because the patient voices it too indistinctly and quietly. The doctor as a result responds in the customary fashion, "I'm fine, Mr. Clark. How are you getting along this morning?"

Because the doctor fails to deny that she hates him, Mr. Clark can assume that the doctor has just admitted that she does hate him, that she assents to his question. In this way the patient confirms his delusional belief that Dr. White hates him. Yet Mr. Clark, in posing this question to Dr. White, has purposefully mumbled it quietly and indistinctly precisely so that the doctor was very unlikely to hear it. Mr. Clark mumbled the question in this fashion because he suspected that Dr. White would deny its truth if she only heard it. At one level the patient believed that Dr. White did not hate him and that the doctor would accordingly deny the accusation should she hear it. Mr. Clark thus mumbled his question in order to avoid receiving disconfirming evidence of his delusional belief that Dr. White hates him. But because Dr. White, when given the opportunity, does not deny what Mr. Clark says, the patient can take this as evidence that his belief is true. Mr. Clark is striving to strengthen his delusional belief although he also suspects that it is untrue. Or perhaps we should say that he is striving to strengthen his delusional belief *because* he suspects that it is untrue. This shows not only that Mr. Clark both believes and disbelieves that the doctor hates him. It also discloses that the patient needs and seeks confirmation of his belief precisely because he also disbelieves it, and his disbelief shapes the way he seeks confirmation of his belief: he craftily avoids having his disbelief verified.

The patient is walking a tightrope between belief and disbelief. His need to have his delusional beliefs confirmed leads him to perform actions that place him in danger of having them disconfirmed. At some level he is aware of this danger because he too suspects that his beliefs are false. He thus performs these dangerous actions in a manner that is as safe as possible for his delusional beliefs: he only *half* performs them: he *mumbles* the dangerous question. This half performance reduces the risk because it protects the patient from falsifying evidence while it does generate results that the patient can view as verifying evidence.

It is like a scientist who sets up a purposefully flawed experiment to test a cherished hypothesis. The scientist wants to perform an experimental test of her beloved hypothesis. But why should she? If she deeply cherishes her confidence in the hypothesis, why should she engage in an experiment which may just prove the hypothesis false? She would do so only if she were in desperate need of confirmation of the hypothesis. She desperately needs confirmation because of a gnawing doubt that it is false. But because her need of confirmation is so desperate, she purposefully designs a flawed experiment. She constructs a faulty experiment so that it will be unlikely to deliver the falsifying evidence that she fears a sound experiment would produce. Moreover, she so designs the experiment that it will produce evidence which is so ambiguous that it can with some maneuvering be viewed as supporting the hypothesis. It is the perfect experiment! It is flawed in just such a way as to circumvent readily available falsifying evidence and to produce evidence so ambiguous as to appear verifying.

Let us explicate another example (B). In a British hospital a schizophrenic patient catches sight of his doctor walking toward him down the hospital corridor. The patient (1) bends down and touches the floor midway between his two feet with perfectly straight arms. He then stands erect and (2) holds his right forearm and hand in a perfectly vertical position in the center of his torso. He makes a final movement which consists in (3) spreading out his right hand and fingers with the open palm facing the oncoming doctor. The physician does not know what to make of these unusual movements and merely greets the patient in a customarily cordial manner. The patient interprets this greeting as a signal by the doctor that, yes, she is, as the patient knew, an undercover agent for the British Secret Service, MI5. Movement (1), bending down and touching one's toes with straight arms, has been the patient's way of signaling through the shape of his arms, shoulders, neck, and head an "M." Movement (2), the perfectly vertical forearm and hand in the middle of the torso, has signalled an "I." And finally posture (3), the spread hand and fingers, has represented a "5."

The doctor, when she addresses the patient, does not deny that she is a covert agent for MI5. At the same time she does not explicitly admit it either. People who *are not* covert agents deny that they are such agents when asked. People who *are* undercover agents do not admit that they are when asked. The doctor, in the patient's mind, clearly recognized the signal. However, the doctor could not explicitly concede that she was such an agent; to do so would "blow her cover." Therefore, she simply does not deny it. This absence of denial is the only admission that any agent could give in the circumstances. The patient, consequently, has gained firm confirmation of his delusional belief that the doctor is a secret agent for MI5.

Now the physician does not deny that she an is agent because in fact she has been unable to interpret the patient's communication. And the patient believed that the doctor would in all likelihood fail to interpret his communication. That is precisely why the patient chose to communicate with the doctor with such idiosyncratic symbolism. At some level of awareness the patient believed that the doctor was not an MI5 agent, but he did not want the doctor to say so. If the doctor had said that she was not, this would have disconfirmed the patient's delusional belief. Fearing this disconfirmation, the patient chose an idiosyncratic code he suspected the doctor could never comprehend.

At another level of awareness, however, the patient can still assume that the doctor did accurately decode the coded message. Assuming this successful communication, the patient can view the absense of a response by the doctor as a clear admission that he is an agent. The patient's delusional belief thereby receives confirmation.

5. Other Kinds of Psychotic Experience: the Delusions of Delirious Patients

In another kind of delusion the double orientation to reality is absent, and as a result the patient is unequivocally certain of the actual existence of the delusional realities. These are the delusions of delirious patients.

The psychotic experiences of delirious patients can completely envelop every aspect of their consciousness, leaving no room for an awareness of another world. Imagine a patient, a bus driver in a chronic delirium. Although he is in fact confined to a hospital bed, he feels that he is struggling desperately to manage a speeding, run away bus. In this psychotic episode he is experientially asborded in the bus, its felt speed and irregular directions, the terrified screams of the passengers, the sights and sounds of cars whizzing passed with their horns blowing, etc. The doctor can see the patient's hands turn red and his muscles tighten as he grips and quickly moves the hallucinated steering wheel. She observes the fear and determination in the man's eyes, his tightly clenched teeth, and his sweating brow. The patient loudly blurts, "Look out!" as he stomps on the hallucinated brake peddle and feverishly jerks the hallucinated steering wheel to one side. For this patient, the bus, the steering wheel, his passengers, and the other cars on the highway are unequivocally real and they are the only realities. He harbors no doubt whatsoever in their concrete and actual existence, and he is conscious of them alone. He has no awareness of the hospital or hospital room that he presently inhabits. He remains unaware of the nurses and doctors who observe him and administer to him. He lives exclusively in the world of his runaway bus, with fear and determination to save the lives of his passengers, and absolutely certain of the immediate reality of this speeding bus and its terrified, screaming passengers.

Schizophrenic patients, particularly in the acute phase, can undergo psychotic episodes in which they too have no distance from the delusional phenomena that envelop and consume them because these phenomena are for them the only reality. This is frequently produced by the intense emotional arousal of the novel, frightening experiences. Usually, however, schizophrenics evince a greater experiential distance from their delusional world. This distance exists, we think, because schizophrenics are oriented to two realities at once, and they both believe and disbelieve in each of these realities. Schizophrenics inhabit two worlds simultaneously, and this doubling and even splitting of consciousness usually prevents them from being wholly enveloped by either.

6. The Use of Psychotherapy for the Treatment of Schizophrenic Delusions

While we shall now insist on a role for psychotherapy in the treatment of schizophrenia, we wish to stress the importance of viewing this role within the standard context of comprehensive therapeutic management of the patient. Appropriate medication and programs of rehabilitation as well as psychotherapy are crucial for effective treatment. We shall here presuppose rather than explicitly discuss the necessity of this larger, more inclusive management program.

The double orientation to reality of the schizophrenic patient provides an opening for psychotherapy to supplement other treatment procedures. Because the patient already doubts the reality of his delusional world and believes in the existence of the consensually validated world, the psychiatrist can intervene to increase the doubt in the delusional world and also strengthen the belief in the shared world. Doing so will require, however, that the clinician sympathetically acknowledge the schizophrenic's firm belief in the delusional world and doubt of the shared world.

It will prove difficult for the schizophrenic to reduce his allegiance to his delusional world for the two reasons we cited above. (1) The delusional world continues to present itself directly to the schizophrenic's consciousness; and moreover, it forcefully solicits and preoccupies his consciousness. In these ways the delusional world demonstrates its reality to the patient. (2) A strong positive value may attach to the meaningfulness of this delusional reality; the schizophrenic has a deep personal commitment to this world. If the schizophrenic admits its unreality, he may have to face numerous unpleasant facts about himself, including his foolishness for having been taken in so thoroughly and so long by a "mere delusion." It is painful to sacrifice that world to which one has so strongly committed oneself and that has thus far instilled one's life with meaning, purpose, and direction. Because one's life has been lived "for the sake" of this world, to lose such a world seems tantamount to losing one's life. This is especially true for chronic schizophrenics, whose life apart from delusional experiences is so often encumbered by failure, loneliness, emptiness and error.

We would like to argue that because it will prove difficult for the patient to withdraw his commitment to the delusional world, it is crucial for the psychotherapist to develop a fully *phenomenological understanding* of the patient's experience. By the phrase "phenomenological understanding of the patient's experience" we mean an understanding of the patient's mental processes precisely and fully as the patient lives through them. A phenomenological understanding of the patient's mental life is an understanding "from the inside," i.e., from the patient's own experiential point of view.

But the psychotherapist must also view the patient's experience "from the outside." The doctor must understand why the patient's life "is not working." This means comprehending what the persistent conflict is between the patient's own experiences and the environment in which the patient is seeking to function. Viewing the patient's life from both the "inside" and the "outside," the therapist can come to perceive how the patient needs to change his beliefs and actions so that he will succeed more effectively in achieving some of his own most important goals. These goals consist in such common human aims as maintaining intimate ties with other people and feeling valued in one's chosen pursuits. Such goals can be realized only in the shared world of other people. Consequently, the schizophrenic must learn to gear into this world successfully.

A full phenomenological understanding of the patient's mental life will lead the psychotherapist to attempt to comprehend the patient as the patient understands himself. And the patient must appreciate these efforts to understand (and not misunderstand) if the patient is to begin to trust the therapist. Only then can the patient find it possible to begin to comply, however tentatively, with the therapist's view that he should withdraw from his commitment to his delusional system.

The patient sees the positive value of his life as dependent upon the truth of his delusional system. To concede the falsity or the irrelevance of that system is to admit that one's life has had no value. The therapist must see and communicate to the patient the fact that the patient's life has a positive value that lies deeper than the literal truth of his delusional system. Consequently, even if the delusional system is relinquished as false or irrelevant, the positive value of the patient's life will continue to be seen and recognized by the therapist. The moral support of the psychotherapist is crucial because it is necessary for another person to perceive the enduring positive value of the patient precisely when the patient fears that he is losing his positive value. The other person, whose view the patient trusts, must view the patient as "right" precisely when the patient admits that he was "wrong." Without this positive conception of himself derived from another person, the patient would feel that only despair would result from devaluing the delusional system.

The patient's delusional system is hardly ever entirely false. The system is usually rooted in some essential truth concerning the patient's life. This truth, however, has undergone a convoluted and distorting elaboration. The patient who insists that he is Christ may in fact find satisfaction in selflessly serving others and in cultivating a heightened spirituality. The conviction that he is Christ may be an expression of his conviction that he, *more than anyone else he can possibly imagine,* is *devoutly* and *fervently* attempting to serve others and to seek true spirituality. Others are spiritual and selfless to some degree. He, however, attempts to be spiritual and selfless to the highest degree; to be *absolutely* spiritual and selfless. On account of his selflessness, he suffers immensely. But he is willing and even determined to do so. This absolute spirituality and exceptional selflessness must signify that he really is Christ. Furthermore, in his fanatical and relentless pursuit of his one, all-consuming goal, he ignores or denies dysconfirming evidence—his flaws, his weaknesses, the genuine historical record of his life.

Psychotherapy in such a case aims at undermining the patient's firm conviction that he is Christ. If this conviction is ever to be relinquished, the patient must still be able to retain the truth about himself that underlies the delusional distortion of it. Therapy thus consists in helping the patient realize that his belief in his delusional system motivates him to do things that conflict with even his own goals and wishes. The patient who believes that he is Christ and who accordingly seeks to lead a truly spiritual existence cannot lead that life if he tries to persuade others that he is Christ. He must orient himself more to what he also already believes to be true: namely, that these others do not and will not believe that he is Christ and will therefore interfere with his strivings for spirituality. The therapist must help the patient see that he should not try to convince the others. For him to concede that he should not try to convince them is for him to relinquish one hoped-for source of confirmation of his divine being. Since he in his own disbelief needs this confirmation, he will not at first want to relinquish this possible source of it. But if he can come to recognize that confirmation will never be forthcoming from this source in any event, then he can recognize that only disconfirmation can be given by others when he seeks confirmation from them.

The patient will not withdraw his commitment to his delusional system if someone tries to disprove it directly. On the contrary, such direct attack will only fuel the patient's determination to defend and embrace his delusional beliefs. The therapist's attempt to undermine the schizophrenic's confidence in this system must appeal to the doubt in it that already haunts the patient, and the therapist must undermine this system *indirectly*, by planting additional "seeds of doubt." The therapist can in a very sympathetic and empathetic way follow the patient into the labyrinth of the delusional world and then, having patiently and sympathetically travelled the full distance, indicate that this labyrinth by itself turns into a dead-end that leads nowhere. Moreover, it can become evident that the delusions themselves block genuine conversation with the therapist. Such blockage, produced by the patient's delusions, threaten the very relationship and trust that has been established between the therapist and patient. The patient can then begin to appreciate that these delusions are obstacles and hindrances that cut him off from a highly valued, ongoing communication with others.

While sowing these seeds of doubt, the therapist can also help the patient find ways of engaging in the consensually validated world that will successfully fulfill the patient's own goals. In this regard psychotherapy must be supplemented with rehabilitation efforts that necessarily occur outside of the therapist's office. Occupational, recreational or art therapy, as well as therapeutic programs in half-way houses, day hospitals, and the like all may play a part here. Such programs can provide a path for experimentation and creativity and for a movement toward a personal redefinition of self and of self's relationship to the world. This kind of rehabilitation can prove far more fruitful that anything else the therapist can do.

If this success grows and the patient comes to find a more and more fulfilling mode of living with others in the shared world, still undergirded by the patient's own genuine truths and values, the reality of this world will become more convincing, massive, and solid. As the reality of the common world becomes more persuasive and solid, this world will displace the delusional world. For a long time, perhaps even for the rest of his life, the patient will probably not relinquish all commitment to the delusional world. Yet the patient's preoccupation with this world, undermined both by growing doubt and by successful involvement in the consensually validated world, will wane. The delusional world persists, but now weakly and on only the fringes of the patient's consciousness: the patient is focused on events in the shared world and grows increasingly committed to them. From being absorbed by extraordinary occurrences in the delusional world, the patient has become focused on more ordinary events in the consensually validated world. From assigning primacy to the reality of the delusional system, the patient now remains aware of this system, but in a way that retains only its "essential truth."

7. Conclusion

We have described the belief and disbelief that permeates the schizophrenic's mental life. Schizophrenics both believe and disbelieve in the consensually validated world; and they both believe and disbelieve in their delusional worlds. Because such patients doubt the reality of their delusional systems, they strive to overcome this doubt and replace it with a firm certainty. This anxious striving for certainty—a certainty not experienced but only devoutly sought—frequently expresses itself as absolute certainty in order to convince both oneself and others. Such expressions of absolute conviction in one's delusional world have misled some astute observers into claiming that certainty and incorrigibility of belief characterize schizophrenic delusions. We have contended that if researchers would look below the surface of these expressions of certainty, unquestionably sincere when uttered, they would find a deeper uncertainty that the schizophrenic simply cannot endure. Consequently, schizophrenics will seek from others confirmation of their delusional beliefs. Such searches for confirmation are frequently disguised and indirect because the patient knows that direct and unambiguous requests for verification will only produce falsification.

Finally, it is important to recognize this co-occurrence of certainty and uncertainty because it opens the way for psychotherapy as an effective component of comprehensive treatment. The therapist can exploit the doubt that the patient already feels towards the delusions: treatment can aim at increasing and extending this doubt until the delusions play only a marginal and minimal role in the patient's experience. In addition, the therapist can reinforce the orientation towards the consensually validated world that the patient already has. The patient's weak commitment to an intersubjectively shared world can be strengthened through psychotherapy and through the patient's own practical success in this world.

Summary

The customary view that *certainty* and *incorrigibility* characterize the beliefs that schizophrenics hold toward their delusions is challenged. Such patients sometimes display a double orientation to reality, as first described by Jaspers: Schizophrenics are oriented toward both, their delusional world, and the "real", i.e., the consensually validated, world. In this double orientation they are certain and dubious of both worlds. Because these patients remain uncertain of their delusions, they desperately strive to eliminate their doubt and replace it with certainty. This striving to achieve as-yet-unattained certainty manifests itself in the words and behavior of schizophrenics, which may in turn be mistaken for expressions of absolute certainty. The strive for certainty is motivated by the secondary elaboration of delusions as follows: Delusion formation can be understood as a process leading from primary delusions to secondary delusional elaboration, which aims at providing an *integrated view* of the primary delusions and the consensually validated world. As such an elaboration is destined to fail because the two worlds cannot be integrated, and as the patient continues to experience inconsistency and incoherence, repeated invalidation of delusions, and hence, uncertainty about them must result. However, such doubt remains unbearable, and the patient strives with greater determination for certainty. This hypothesis of an interweaving of certainty and uncertainty has psychotherapeutic implications. Without directly confronting the patient, psychotherapy can undermine his preoccupation with his delusions and can strengthen his belief in the consensually validated world. In this way the intersubjectively shared world can come to play a more massive, prominent, and rewarding role in the patient's life, and the delusions can grow marginal and irrelevant.

References

American Psychiatric Association: Diagnostic and Statistical Manual of Mental Disorders, Third Edition, Revised. Washington, DC, American Psychiatric Association, 1987

Hamilton M (ed): Fish's Schizophrenia. Bristol, Wright, 1984

Jaspers K: General Psychopathology. Chicago, University of Chicago Press, 1963

Kräupl Taylor F: Psychopathology: Its Causes and Symptoms. London, Butterworths, 1966

Kräupl Taylor F: Descriptive and Developmental Phenomena. In: Shepherd M, Zangwell OL (eds): Handbook of Psychiatry 1: General Psychopathology, pp. 59-94. Cambridge, Cambridge University Press, 1983

Slater E, Roth M: Clinical Psychiatry, Third Edition. Baltimore, Williams and Wilkins Company, 1969

Wiggins OP, Schwartz MA, Northoff G: Towards a Husserlian Phenomenology of the Initial Stages of Schizophrenia. In: Spitzer M, Maher BA (eds): Philosophy and Psychopathology, pp. 21-34, New York, Springer, 1990

M. Spitzer, F.A. Uehlein
M.A. Schwartz, C. Mundt
(eds.): Phenomenology
Language & Schizophrenia.
Springer-Verlag, New York, 1992

Rationality and Delusional Disorders

Grant Gillett

1. Introduction

An abiding theoretical problem for psychiatry and philosophy is that, on most accounts of rationality, a severely deluded patient may qualify as quite rational. For instance, a paranoid psychotic patient may seem very plausible to a person not versed in psychiatry and even where he does not seem rational, his mistakes are often so minor that they fail to account for the evident thought disorder. Consider Mrs. A, who was examined by a forensic psychiatrist after she had killed her infant. She justified this action in the following way.

1. When we die our souls are judged.
2. They are judged on the basis of our actions and decisions.
3. My baby has neither made decisions nor performed actions.
4. Therefore she did not have a soul.
5. Therefore it did not matter that I killed her.

This chain of reasoning occurred within the context of other features of a psychotic disorder but is itself clearly insane despite the fact that the irrationality is hard to discern. I will try to explain the difficulty in accounting for psychotic irrationality in a way that also explains the fact that delusions typically have highly personal content.

2. Rationality

Theories of rationality usually rest on the need for adequate foundations for knowledge (based either in axioms or observations), a reasonable attitude to evidence, the logical structure of reasoning, or the cultural propriety of an individual's belief and value system.

Foundational theories of rationality come in rationalist or empiricist forms. There are problems with both. Rationalist theories build a structure of knowledge from a base of axioms. Axiomatic foundations for epistemology form a series of (innate) truths which cannot be questioned e.g. 'sensory experience reveals objects to us', or 'all souls are judged according to their actions'. When one comes to examine the justification for holding such axioms to be true, either no answer can be given or their givenness is related to social norms. We shall return to the latter view below. Empiricist theories claim that knowledge is based on sensory experiences. Their problem is that all beliefs are under–determined by their empirical base. It is quite possible, for instance, that the chair I see before me is a fake constructed by a mischievous German psychiatrist. That would explain my sensory data even though it may not be sustainable on investigation. Thus it is my interpretation or belief–forming processes that are rational or irrational and not just the relation (or lack of it) between those beliefs and sensory experiences. This implies that the processes of inference or derivation of mental content must be brought into focus and here the empiricists have little to offer apart from the laws of logical inference (both deductive and inductive). But it is obvious that Mrs. A's beliefs about her baby are as logically deduced as many vaguely religious convictions which do not qualify as being psychotic.

Therefore, in order to deliver a substantive account of irrationality, any epistemological theory needs to specify the norms which govern belief formation. For instance, why should it be wrong for John B to form the belief that his mother is a witch when the evidence he cites includes facts like, she wears black dresses, she goes out after sunset, I saw a black cat rubbing itself on her legs, she makes my tea so that I can't see what she puts into it, and so on. We are in no doubt that he is wrong, but why?

A different answer to this question ties rationality to cultural norms. So, for an animist, it is rational to believe that when you eat an animal you imbibe some of the spirit of that animal and animal spirits can dwell in people or even take possession of them. On the cultural endorsement view, a belief is irrational or delusional if it is not endorsed by one's social group. But this fails to explain the difference between psychotics and thinkers like Wilberforce or Copernicus who revolutionized the thinking of their day. We admire rather than treat such outstanding or innovative thinkers but their existence can only be accommodated in an account of rationality and irrationality which 'makes conceptual room' for individuals to "transcend the herd" (Nietzsche) in rationally commendable ways.

I will develop an interpersonal or intersubjective view in which rationality and truth are linked to rule–governed techniques of articulating one's activity with the world. On this view, beliefs, rationality, and values combine to form an interconnected cognitive repertoire which is holistic, instrumental, explains behavior, aims at truth, and arises in discourse.

The resulting conception of rationality copes well with many different areas of thought. It also enables an analysis of factual, evaluative, and religious delusions and explains why they tend overwhelmingly to have personal content. The common delusions—of persecution, grandiosity, control, thought broadcast, thought insertion, reference, Capgras' syndrome, autoscopy, de Clerambault's syndrome and Cotard's Syndrome—are commonly *personal* in the sense that they relate to the subject himself, significant others with whom he has relationships, or his own status as a personal agent in the world. They are also transcultural and therefore do not solely constitute aberrations of culturally determined beliefs (Rust 1990). My (phenomenological/genetic) account of the defects of rationality shown in psychosis will explain these facts about insight and delusion. It will also suggest why Fulford focuses on "reasons for action" (which involve both conative/evaluative and cognitive/factual content) as central in understanding psychotic disorders (Fulford 1989).

3. Insight and Delusion

As soon as we consider delusional content and the nature of insight we are struck by the inadequacy of a conception of rationality according to which a subject is rational if she forms beliefs by using valid inferential processes based on factual evidence. Insight is not purely factual but involves a "correct attitude to a morbid change in oneself" (Lewis 1934). This involves a recognition that one is suffering an illness, the realization that the illness is mental and the ability to relabel certain events as being pathological (cf. David 1990) none of which are easily located in the standard models of rationality. Delusions are also problematic in that, far from being mere false beliefs held in an irrational or incorrigible way they can involve "extreme value judgments... so extreme as to defy credibility" (DSM–III–R), true beliefs, or beliefs which are impossible to assess as being either true or false (such as those of Mrs. A; cf. Spitzer 1990a). Other aspects of the phenomenology of insight and delusion also highlight characteristic features of human thought.

First, insight is a matter of degree (cf. David 1990, p. 800) and concerns an "amount of realization about one's own condition" (Lewis 1934, p. 332). Patients come to see the truth about themselves as an increasing realization that they have been mentally deranged and that many of their supposed experiences were fanciful. This usually happens as the patient reestablishes himself in relationships with others i.e. as the famous 'glass wall' begins to break down. Such differences of degree are widespread in cognitive activity, we believe some things with great certainty and others we are not so sure about, we understand some things fully and others a little, we can be very systematic or more impressionistic in our knowledge and habits of belief formation, and so on.

Second, there is the phenomenon of pseudo–insight, where the patient produces utterances that seem to capture what is wrong with her but that are not integrated into her general thought and self–reflexive abilities; "the patient merely regurgitates overheard explanations arising out of different theoretical perspectives" (David 1990, p. 801). This is particularly interesting in that the lack of integration of these superficially true beliefs is a failure of self–understanding. If we accept Socrates' dictum 'Know Thyself' as a desideratum for human conduct, then the patient with pseudo–insight would fail to evince the wisdom or virtue (Aristotle) that would be part of the proper understanding of the propositional knowledge involved in the dictum. This, of course, is a defect of her person as a reasoning acting being and not just a defect in declarative knowledge.

Third, delusions are not completely insulated from real life because some patients are influenced by evidence that counts against their delusions (Jones et al. 1987). They do, however, often find some pseudo-rational explanation for conflicts between their beliefs and presented evidence. What is more, the superficial acceptance of evidence and consequent adjustment of belief structure at one level preserves the underlying interpersonal or reactive attitudes that one discerns at the center of their psychiatric disorder. Thus, even though they are not totally insulated from normal evidential–inferential confirmation, there is reason to think that the beliefs of a psychotic, because of the perceived inter–personal dynamics which support them, are not susceptible to the reality testing that a normal subject would impose.

A related manifestation of psychotic cognition is the ability of deluded patients to believe in impossible things such as "existing in the past as well as the present... having inside one's body something larger than oneself (e.g. a nuclear power station): being in two places at one time" (David 1990, p. 804). Such patients may even give reasons for their beliefs but, in so doing, they obey none of the canons of commonsense scrutiny of beliefs and inference. Again we see a coming apart from standard account in that the normal person obeys informal constraints which embed a common-sense, physics, metaphysics and psychology and make certain kinds of mistaken belief inconceivable (even though they are logically possible). This unwritten code of *reasonableness* is not followed by the psychotic.

These features of psychotic irrationality do not easily fit into the justified–factual–belief model and tend to highlight the *personal*, or, in Fulford's terms, "evaluative" dimension of the disordered mental content. I will make free use of Fulford's insistence that evaluation and action are key notions in understanding mental illness and also of Lewis' observation that insight is involved with "looking inwards rather than looking outwards" in looking for a better account of rationality.

4. The Nature of Rationality

I believe that the difficulty of conceptualizing psychotic rationality indicates a deeper disquiet in our understanding of thought and reason. In the psychological sciences, we have inherited a tradition which regards reason and sound belief as emerging from a series of information processing steps based on evidence plainly available to the thinker (this Empiricist Representational view of the mind is descended directly from Locke, Berkeley and Hume; cf. Gillett 1992). The empiricists have emphasized the evidence which produces certain beliefs and tried not to think too hard about the source of the warrant for the favoured transitions between propositional attitudes such as belief (or indeed the warrant for taking the evidence this way rather than that). The rationalists have stressed the axioms and self–evident transitions underpinning valid trains of thought and stressed the intellect's role in imposing a definite order on the chaotic realm of unstructured experience. On their view, sensory information can only awaken the categories which structure thought so that it yields true knowledge. Both traditions tend towards *internalism*—the idea that thought can be specified without regard to what is outer—and *individualism*—a focus on the individual thinker. In both traditions the rules governing transitions in thought and the use of concepts (which are the building blocks of propositions) are neglected. Even Kant, who did most to merge the strongest claims of rationalism and empiricism, discussed the cognitive world as a product of rational individuals and neglected the evident intersubjectivity of concepts and mental ascriptions.[1] This oversight leaves thought as an essentially inner set of goings on which explains a thinker's behavior. Because the norms or rules operating in thought are not investigated, the stage is set for aberrations in thought content to be regarded as surd or attributable only to a physiological, causal or meaningless derangement of the subject.

The fact that the common mental aberrations found in delusional disorders all have personal and interpersonal content should lead us to explore the role of intersubjectivity in the justification of belief, and the development of what we might call 'epistemic virtue' (after Blackburn). Epistemic virtue or the ability to distinguish between right and wrong beliefs becomes a fundamental aspect of human thought life and places real constraints on the thinker's contribution to experience whether their thinking involves factual or evaluative aspects of that experience.

My argument will pick up several threads left hanging by others.

5. The Subject in Social Context: A Hypothesis

Spitzer (1990a), following Jaspers, mentions the centrality of I–thoughts in psychotic thought disorders and suggests that there might be some level of validity not well captured by a concentration on truth and falsity but available to phenomenological analysis of psychosis. He regards the subject as an active synthesizer of knowledge who achieves objectivity rather than receiving objective impressions and ideas. Hundert (1990), in a similar Kantian vein, focuses on the cognitive work done by a subject in categorizing experience (he wisely avoids an in–depth discussion of the categories of judgment). Hundert's subject brings concepts to experience as a cognitive individual "by the rediscovery and reinvention of these concepts" (Hundert 1990, p. 62). He is inspired by Piaget (whom I have criticized elsewhere, cf. Gillett 1987), and therefore sees the subject as an active thinker who organizes her world. I have no quarrel with this as part of the truth but the analysis needs a Wittgensteinian flavor. This can be

---

1 Strawson (1966) pinpoints this with characteristic lucidity, elegance and economy in *The Bounds of Sense*.

done through the concept of empathy of interpersonal feeling–which is explored by Margulies (1990).

The roots of such a project are consonant with Spitzer's discovery of the idea of a "sensus communis" in Kant's Anthropology (cf. Spitzer 1990b). Kant remarks that the insane subject loses sight of a touchstone of ordinary experience namely "that we relate our understanding to the understanding of others, and do not merely isolate ourselves within our own opinions". This is surely where answers must be found if we are to understand everyday rationality and thereby the phenomena of insight and delusion in psychosis.

We can begin an Wittgensteinian analysis of rationality and delusion by recalling the problem of 'inner awareness' or self–reflective thought. This is often more difficult for a patient than thinking about others or the outside word: "insight into another's illness may be preserved despite the loss of personal insight" (David 1990, p. 800). However, to a traditional epistemologist this seems very odd; the Cartesian view is that knowledge of the contents of one's own mind is clear, immediate, and incorrigible. Therefore, how can self–reflexive thought be more flawed than other types of thought under certain conditions? I will argue that self–referring thought and judgment are vulnerable to deep disruptions of cognition because thought is essentially based on what happens in inter-personal/inter–subjective transactions which focus on self as a person–in-relation. The possibility is that the subject whose phenomenological world is in disarray feels "ontologically" threatened (R.D. Laing 1965) as a subject of experience and thus the level of the personal becomes the focus of disturbing or irrational thought content. The ontological threat, we could say, arises from the fact that it is the core *being* of the patient as a person–in–relation that is perceived as endangered when psychosis disturbs one's cognitive equilibrium.

6. The Norms Governing Thought

It is at least plausible that it is because we do not understand the normal controls on thought that we scratch about for appropriate conceptualiza-tions of the phenomena we encounter when it goes out of control. When we consider the normative constraints or demands for justification which operate within thought we usually begin with an epistemology that concentrates on the bare dyad of thinker and world. If this starting point were deficient, then the resulting picture of rationality would yield no insight into psychotic irrationality.

Wittgenstein suggests that the ability to make warranted judgments and come to justified beliefs is developed and maintained in human forms of life. On this view, thinkers grasp the rules governing the use of a concept (both in its application and cognitive manipulation) by imitating their fellow human beings and responding to the corrections of others. One makes certain judgments—such as "that is red", "that dog is running" and so on—to the best of one's lights, in the same way as others. One then adjusts one's responses according to their responses. Thus, cognizing experience would be based on a colloquy of skills developed in inter-personal situations—"those situations where language is taught and learnt" (Quinton 1955)—and not on a set of individual (rediscovered or reinvented) cognitive operations. An analysis of this kind does not base concept use and transitions in thought either on the law–like causal impingement of environmental regularities or on an innate system of axioms and formal operations occurring in mental structures.

On the favoured view, the mind is fluid, dynamic and open to inter-personal effects, its operations governed by informal norms. The relations between persons qua persons who think and act in a context of inter-action, are crucial in the internalization of these norms. The norms are pervasive, governing judgments about the contents of an experience, techniques of belief formation and the conduct of mental life in general. Thus mental life is seen to rest on techniques or skills which are informally conveyed from one person to another and difficult to define or specify. There is therefore no surveyable set of operations based on independently available inputs or axioms which go to make up right thinking. Human beings latch on the thinking (and the warranted use of the concepts in which it is conducted) by participating in situations and relationships where linguistic terms or signs mark certain ways of responding to the world.

For any individual, the techniques are not a matter of his own choice; they obey prescriptive norms and in grasping them he must appreciate that there is a right and wrong way of using a given concept. And he learns these techniques of concept–use in forms of life where normative con-straints determining the meaning and content of concepts are imparted by other thinkers who train him to follow the requisite rules. Absent such participation, he will never develop the techniques of data extraction and selective response involved in using a concept because they are learnt by *doing* not by contemplating or formulating theories. Thus my very being as a thinking, experiencing subject is constituted inter–personally and a threat which splits me off from others is a fundamental threat to my person.

This approach offers a plausible account of the role of self–reflexive thought in rationality. A thinker learns to mould her own use of concepts according to the reactions of others to her own judgments. And, just as she imitates their responses to objects of mutual attention, so she can learn to mimic their responses toward her. Thus, in the process of mastering concepts, she masters the ability to judge of herself whether or not she is correct in making a range of judgments about the content of experience. These self–reflexive judgments about one's own judgments are, I have suggested, internalized on the basis of interactions with other thinkers. Lewis observes "with every mental activity—or act—there is an observing or registering of its apprehended quality apart from the material upon which the function in question is being exercized" (Lewis 1934, p. 19).

On the present view, regarding self as an object for self is an internalization of the fact that others regard self as an object of thought as they train one to use concepts. The fact that they do so within inter-personal relationships is significant. It colors thought (even where that is factual) with an affective or (in Fulford's terms) "evaluative" quality. Thus, in mastering right thinking, one is being formed as a person and one's personality is taking shape. Techniques of self-thought are, therefore, more difficult than straightforward judgments about external states of affairs and replete with conative/evaluative nuances and implications. It is small wonder that thinking rightly about oneself is difficult, prone to disruption, and that irrationality classically strikes here first.

This approach to thought and belief implies that human thought and action are essentially relational skills which correlate responses with contexts in which the activity of other persons has illuminated the world. But this does not collapse phenomenological analysis into a variety of unconstrained relativism which removes the distinction between delusion and exceptional beliefs. Rational, insightful thinking (which may include social, credal or political deviance) is distinguished from insanity by the ability to take a normative attitude toward one's own judgments. When one exhibits a grasp of the rules which govern thinking and can correct oneself according to the perspectives of others, one shows insight and rationality. When these normative procedures of self-correction and adaptation of one's dispositions to think or act thus and so are defective then one lacks insight and tends to think and act irrationally.

The broad checks on one's thought arise from the ways in which thought is linked to effective action in the world and the resulting coherence between thoughts. Both individuals and groups can be defective in either way but if an individual's thoughts are consistent with a conceptual structure imparted by his primary cognitive group or a role he takes in the discourses of that group then one need not invoke aberrations in that individual to account for the flaws in his thought. On the other hand, when a set of ill-judged thoughts involving aberrant attitudes particularly toward oneself are held for reasons which seem to go far beyond what *sensus communis* would endorse then psycho-pathology is the obvious explanation.

It is difficult to define rationality and insight because it is difficult to say what constitutes 'getting it right' in the hurly-burly of everyday human activity where the norms on right thinking are part of the framework of interpersonal life. This framework rests on recognitional skills that are holistic and participatory, operating in human 'forms of life'. It is well known in philosophical semantics that such skills make it virtually impossible to spell out in cogent terms just what is involved in grasping even the simplest concepts or making the most ordinary judgments. So difficult is this that even Kant was obliged to fall back on "mother wit" as an indispensable element in the use of concepts (or 'rules of the understanding'). Raitonality, or right thinking, rests on this bedrock.

It should be evident that the skills which constitute insight and rational belief formation are susceptible to both biological and inter-personal forces. Thus a distorted interpersonal milieu will upset and derange the secure practice of those skills of mental ascription and self ascription that underpin belief formation and, especially, self–reflexive knowledge. A biological lesion which unhinges or dedifferentiates asso-ciations and orderly patterns of inference and judgment will also cause derangement. But it is likely that the elements of right thinking are so closely tied to adaptive action that the system will be moderately robust, at least in terms of its basic epistemic functions, in the face of the former type of impairment and that the greater aberrations of thought and action will require the collusion of biological derangement. However, the contrast between functional and purely biological causes of thought disorder, leaves us with the task of explaining the systematicity, persistence, coherence and deeply personal content of the former.

On the present view, the elements of thought life—concepts—are ways of responding to things around one which are repeatable and communicable and gained from one's formative interactions with other thinkers. Their approvals and disapprovals map the structure of right thinking for the apprentice cognizer and agent. Therefore, there is a holism about human mental life in that the relational aspects of our being, heavily imbued with conative and moral overtones, are formative in the epistemic aspects of our being. Thus the elements of my mental life are formed in a process centred on me and grounded on my nature as a person.

In this way, one's mental life, including a cognitive map of the world and a repertoire of cognitive techniques for using that map to understand and negotiate situations, are constructs of the integrating subject who is a person in relation to others. Mental content is therefore based on doing things and relating to others rather than receiving and connecting data from a purely objective world and the construction of mental life does not proceed via purely formal or causal, truth–preserving operations. The mental life of the insane stands out as strange and unfamiliar as an orange shirt at Wimbledon because they do not fit the informal norms governing what people normally do and their attitudes (and shifts of attitudes) toward each other.

This analysis illuminates psychotic irrationality particularly as it is revealed through insight and delusion.

7. The Phenomena of Psychosis

Insight is best seen, as Lewis suggests, in terms of "a rough notion of the patient's sanity of judgment, or commonsense attitude towards his illness" so that the patient cannot "look at his data and judge them as we, the dispassionate, presumably healthy outsiders do" (Lewis 1934, p. 19; notice the resonance with Kant's *sensus communis*). This is not just a set of beliefs which happen to be true or a mechanism which happens to work but a set of cognitive skills which are refined through relationships with others so that one is not "thinking only along one's own lines without caring for dialogue and intersubjective feedback" (Spitzer 1990a, p. 392). The resulting defect undermines right thinking about oneself which is an ability comprising self–reflective techniques of judgment and concept–use. Insight therefore involves the awareness of what Fulford calls "illness" (Fulford 1989, p. 216), a realization that there is a mismatch in one's adaptation to the world. The realization that one lacks the normal warrants for one's contentful mental acts is, as I have tried to show, linked to actions and relationships in a way hinted at but not described by Fulford. The interpersonal, intersubjective or relationship–based nature of attitudes toward one's own ideas implies that evaluation, prescription, and shared norms are intrinsic to such activity. And because the integrating effect of such self–reflexive activity constitutes me as an experiencing, intentional, subject of thought and action, these skills and anything which disrupts them, play a key role in my psyche. Thus one might expect a deterioration in mental function which deranged or dis–integrated cognitive content but did not blunt conscious activity would give rise to phenomenology which focussed on the self as threatened or subject to unusual influences and would deny the psychotic the shared, rational perspective implicit in insight.

Delusions, on this account, would not just include false beliefs and immoderate evaluative attitudes but would rather express a deep disquiet in the mind intimately connected to the integrity self–as–subject–and–agent. The characteristic malfunction in delusional thought is the tendency to take a 'Cartesian attitude' toward judgments in which one would normally follow established epistemic or evaluative procedures (Spitzer 1990a, pp. 389ff). Common delusions such as those of reference, control, or broadcast thought, in fact, resemble common suspicions or fleeting fancies held by normal people. But in the normal subject these are not supported by a disordered phenomenology which lends (pseudo–)validity to them and they are constantly subject to the normative scrutiny of the internalized perspective of the other. Commonsense dismisses these fancies as absurd but the insane patient who is split off from the normal processes of establishing cognitive credentials or warrants and who is plagued with experiential content that is difficult to accommodate uses her 'rational faculty' to attempt to impose some organization on what is otherwise dis–integrated and threatening. This systematizing activity then becomes the principal manifestation (to self) of self–as–subject and imbued with "ontological" significance leading to desperation and irrational commitment (because otherwise self is threatened with non–being).

It is understandable that many delusory systems revolve around a failure or major disruption of one's integrity as a human agent. If, as Jean Paul Sartre suggests, we exist primarily as subjects who become what we are through what we do, the relevance of action and intention to delusions is immediately obvious. This discussion recalls the relation between delusional thought and the mental attitudes toward the 'I' or "active subject of experience" (Wiggins et al. 1990). The subject "intends itself" through processes of active constituation as a being in the world among others. Spitzer borrows from Jaspers the categories of "activity, unity, identity and the me–not–me distinction" (Spitzer 1990a, p. 50). The successful use of these categories of self in everyday experience rests on highly integrated cognitive mechanisms of identifying and relating oneself to objects and situations, organizing that activity by using concepts, and so on. I would posit that it is the interpersonal validation of these techniques that goes astray when a person becomes psychotic. This introduces a Cartesian, isolated within one's own experiences, or 'split–off from others' quality to psychotic thought in which the patient finds herself adrift in a strange and disorganized world in which other people are also seen as alien to one, vaguely threatening and can only be understood in terms of a bizarre construction of events.

I have argued that belief formation is an active set of techniques based on rule–governed use of concepts. Shared norms give validation, and self–reflective balance to the data gathering, classification, review of experience, inference, and modification of behavior involved in mental life. The psychiatrically disordered patient has, in greater or lesser measure, a defect of the requisite cognitive skills as a result of some combination of meaningful and biological influences. The picture of rationality and mental activity that emerges enables us to understand the central place of I–functions and personal thoughts in psychotic mental content. Any subjective validity for this content is found in the disruption that has split the schizophrenic not only from the *sensus communis* but also from *vita communis*. This split threatens the psychotic in the bedrock of his life as a human thinker because that being is primarily relational.

8. Conclusion

Our shift of focus has illuminated the complex bio–psycho–social phenomenon that is mental disorder in a way that allows us to accommodate brain aberrations and relationship aberrations as effective causes of psychiatric disorder. This implies that to understand psychiatric phenomenology we must make use of both causal and meaningful explanations. The former focus on brain mechanisms, physiological disorders of neutral function, psychological determinants of temperament and behavior, and social influences. The latter need not disregard these effects but tends to emphasize the meaningful connexions that pervade mental life. We can see the interaction of both effects in paranoid schizophrenic disorders especially where the patient has systematized and organized his aberrant experience. The understanding of rationality and delusion, indeed of mental life and content, that emerges from this preliminary account is both dynamic (in a broad sense) and person–centred. It emphasizes, lest we ever forget it, that the basis of rationality is personal integrity and the basis of personal integrity is relational. What is more, it explains why the lady who killed her baby is irrational in a deep and disturbing way. Normal human beings feel a sensitivity to the vulnerability and needs of infants, are moved by the appeals they make, and tend to include them as fledgling participants in moral and interpersonal discourse. If rationality involves competence within this discourse and an awareness of the informal norms and meaningful realities that pervade it, then Mrs. A is irrational. She has acted without regard for a deep and intuitive feature of our *sensus communis*. It is the peculiar combination of this defect with a superficial competence in reasoning that distinguishes her from the run-of-the-mill child-abusing borderline personality disorder patient and puts her psychotic irrationality in quite a different class.

Summary

Psychotic irrationality is difficult to define or explain on the basis of traditional models of rationality. Rationality and concept use are, however, grounded in the rule-governed use of concepts to categorize experience. This activity is mastered in the interpersonal milieu of language-use and human relationships. This milieu pivotally involves the person as subject and agent. Therefore it is understandable that psychotic irrationality should be associated with deep disruptions of self-knowledge and personal thoughts.

References

David AS: Insight and psychosis. British Journal of Psychiatry 156: 198–808, 1990
Fulford KWM: Moral theory and medical practice. Cambridge University Press, 1989
Gillett G: Concepts, structures and meanings. Inquiry 30: 101–12, 1987
Gillett G: Representation, meaning and thought. Oxford, Clarendon, 1992
Hundert E: Are psychotic illnesses category disorders? In: Spitzer M, Maher BA (eds): Philosophy and Psychopathology, pp. 59–70, New York, Springer, 1990
Jones B, Garety RA, Helmsley DR: Measuring delusional experiences: a method and its application. British Journal of Clinical Psychology 26: 256–7, 1987
Laing RD: The divided self. Harmondsworth, Penguin, 1965
Lewis A: The psychopathology of insight. British Journal of Medical Psychology 14: 332–348, 1934
Margulies A: When the self becomes alien to itself: psychopathology and the self-recursive loop. In: Spitzer M, Maher BA (eds): Philosophy and Psychopathology, pp. 146–155, New York, Springer, 1990
Quinton A: The problem of perception. Mind 64: 28–51, 1955
Rust J: Delusions, irrationality and cognitive science. Philosophical Psychology 3: 123–138, 1990
Spitzer M: On defining delusions. Comprehensive Psychiatry 31: 377–97, 1990a
Spitzer M: Kant on Schizophrenia. In: Spitzer M, Maher BA (eds): Philosophy and Psychopathology, pp. 44–58, New York, Springer, 1990b
Strawson PF: The Bounds of Sense. London, Methuen, 1966
Wiggins OP, Schwartz MA, Northoff G: Toward a Husserlian phenomenology of the initial stages of Schizophrenia In: Spitzer M, Maher BA (eds): Philosophy and Psychopathology, pp. 21–34, New York, Springer, 1990

M. Spitzer, F.A. Uehlein
M.A. Schwartz, C. Mundt
(eds.): Phenomenology
Language & Schizophrenia.
Springer-Verlag, New York, 1992

The Role of Affect in Delusion Formation

Manfred Spitzer

1. Introduction

Patients with acute delusions of persecutory type almost always experience anxiety. Delusions of grandeur mostly occur in a manic state in which, by definition, an elevated mood is present. Depression leads to certain types of delusions, such as nihilistic and hypochondric delusions, as well as delusions of sin, guilt, and poverty. A peculiar kind of love seems to be the root of DeClerambault's syndrome, the delusion of being loved by another person, and delusions of jealousy seem to be motivated by some mixture of love and distrust. In short: There seems to be a relationship between emotions and delusions. What kind of relationship is this? Do disturbed emotions lead to the development of delusions or do delusions lead to disturbed emotions? What evidence can be derived from the literature in support of the theories which have been proposed about such relationships?

In this paper I will reconsider views about emotions and delusions. I will not offer a "final" comprehensive theory, but rather attempt to illuminate what Austin might have called a "mixed bag" of problems (cf. Fulford 1990). My intention is to stimulate further empirical research and conceptual thought.

2. Affect—a Plethora of Approaches

As affect is the term most often used in psychiatry, I employ it here to denote the topic at issue. However, the terms *emotion, mood,* and *feeling* might as well be used here. What do we mean by "affect"? We all have some opinion about what affect is, but if we attempt to spell this out, we immediately encounter problems. For example, if our concepts were clear, we would be able to tell how many affects there are. But we can't! When we reflect upon this question we begin to wonder how to identify and distinguish affects, and by what criteria. Is fear, for example, a different affect when compared to dread and anxiety? If the answer is "yes", how can we find out all the many affects that there seem to be, and how can we be sure that some of our terms denoting affects are not mere synonyms? And what about joy, happiness, cheerfulness, gladness, pleasure, and delight? If the answer is "no", then we must ask why there are so many different words to denote the same thing. We may prefer the answer "yes and no", that is to say, we may want to introduce clusters of nearly similar, but not identical, affects. However, how do we determine which terms belong to a given cluster, and how do we find out how many clusters of "really different" affects there are? It seems as though the answer we might be most inclined to give—"yes and no"—merely iterates, rather than answers, the question we had in mind when starting this discussion.

Related to the question of the sorting out of the various affects is the question of what an affect is—a feeling, a sensation, a cognition, a pattern of behavior or a mere tendency to behave, a state or a trait of the mind or of the body?

Several solutions to these problems have been proposed. If we begin with an analysis of language, the number of different emotions seems quite large. As William James already noted:

"The varieties of emotion are innumerable... The mere description of objects, circumstances, and varieties of the different species of emotion may go to any length. Their internal shadings merge endlessly into each other, and have been partly commemorated by language, as, for example, by such synonyms as hatred, antipathy, animosity, resentment, dislike, aversion, malice, spite, revenge, abhorrence, etc., etc." (James 1892/1984, p. 325).

On the other hand, by means of semantic analysis, all of the terms we use to denote emotions can be described by a system of only three dimensions: evaluation (pleasant vs. unpleasant), potency (much vs. little), and activity (active vs. passive; cf. Miller & Glucksberg 1988, pp. 440-441). Such an analysis, however, does not necessarily lead to types. Research on the organizational structure of various semantic fields, such as, for example, color, kinship, pronouns, prepositions, evaluative terms, and emotions, showed clearly that some of these semantic fields, like color and kinship terms, can be represented by dimensions, whereas others, like prepositions, are better represented by a hierarchy. Emotion-terms, however, defy any clear-cut characterization (see Miller & Glucksberg 1988).

From the biological viewpoint, different levels of arousal can be distinguished, leaving only one dimension onto which all emotions are to be placed. From his work with patterns on the electroencephalogram (EEG), Machleit et al. (1989) proposed that the number of basic emotions is five: Intention, anxiety, aggression/pain, sadness, and happiness.

Darwin (1872/1965) distinguished several elementary emotions, such as happiness, anxiety, hatred, surprise, etc., relying on facial expressions as criteria for his distinctions. Such facial expressions seem to be universal across cultures, as empirical studies have shown (Ekman 1973). Scoring systems for emotional facial expressions have been proposed containing six basic emotions, happiness, sadness, anger, surprise, fear, and disgust. Measures of autonomous nervous system activity such as heart rate, finger temperature, and skin conductance can be used in addition to facial expressions to measure the emotional experiences of people. However, as Oster et al. note, there is no single "via regia" to the emotions of another person:

"In sum, there is no single, infallible 'touchstone' measure that we can use to verify the emotion experienced by the sender. The best strategy ... is to use multiple, converging lines of evidence" (Oster et al. 1990, p. 120).

From this rather incomplete list of attempts to come to terms with what seems to be among the nearest to us—our feelings—it is clear that there is neither a genuine method of studying affect nor a final answer to the basic questions that we can ask. Therefore, in the following section, a brief historical outline of the concept of emotion/affect/feeling is given in order to specify the roots to which we cannot help but turn when we want to clarify our own ideas (cf. Ritter 1973, pp. 89–99). This will establish various aspects of the concept which in one way or another still contribute to its meaning.

3. Affect—A Brief Historical Background

In pre-Socratic thinking, affect was considered something that a person suffers from passively, and hence was labeled ethically negative. *Passivity* and *negative value* have prevailed as features of the concept of affect ever since. Affect was related to the *physical existence of the body* by Plato, and, since Aristotle, affects have been investigated psychologically. Aristotle regarded affect as playing a major role in motivational processes, and viewed the problem as one of the right level of affect.

Stoic philosophers, in contrast, emphasized that the goal of human life is to totally get rid of affects. Interestingly, false judgments of reason were regarded as the cause of affects (and not, as we tend to assume at present, vice versa). For example, the affect of greed for money was thought to be caused by the assumption that money is of positive value—a assumption which surely was wrong in the view of the stoics. According to the stoics, all affects are inseparable from reason.

"Affect is reason, but bad and unrestrained reason, resulting from bad and incorrect judgment which is compounded by fierceness and vehemence" (Chrysipp, quoted from Ritter 1973, p. 90, my translation).

Passivity and relatedness to the body are the main features of the concept in the Middle Ages; Thomas Aquinas (quoted from Ritter 1973, p. 92) defined affects as "acts of sensual striving, insofar as they are linked to bodily changes." The second part of the definition is a result of the feature of passivity and suffering, as the soul—without the body—cannot be subjected to purely passive suffering experiences. To these features, the notion of *affect in contrast to reason* was added.

In the 18th century, affects and madness were strongly linked by Spinoza, who carefully investigated the nature of affects in his book on ethics. Spinoza stated that when a person is possessed by only one affect for a prolonged period, this affect can become so strong that the person may become mad, and, for example, see things that are not present.

During the 17th and 18th century, the distinction between affects and passions was established. This distinction was based mainly on time: *Affects as short bursts* were distinguished from passions, i.e., longer lasting movements of the soul, such as love and hatred.

To sum up, during its long history, the notion of affect has acquired a number of features: passivity, negative value, relatedness to the body, opposition to reason, relation to madness, and short duration. These features, especially opposition to reason and passivity, play an important role in arguments about affects as a possible cause of delusions. Before we return to this (cf section 6), the main issues as they have emerged in psychiatry will first be introduced.

4. Pro Affect: Hagen, Specht, and Bleuler

The role of affect in the formation of delusions has been intensively debated in German academic psychiatry since it came into existence in the middle of the last century (for an overview, cf. Lewis 1970). Two opposite views have gained strong influence, the major proponents being Hagen, Specht, and Bleuler on the one side, and Jaspers, Gruhle, and Schneider on the other.

The view that emotions play a major role in the formation of delusions was first expressed by Hagen (1870), who stated that delusions "grow rapidly in the breast-warmth of affects and passions" (p. 59). In 1889, even Kraepelin noticed that the roots of delusions are in the intellectual processing of ideas, "which, however, may be influenced [...] by feelings and affects" (p. 109).

In his famous monograph *On Pathological Affect in Chronic Paranoia—a Contribution to the Theory of the Development of Delusions*, Specht (1901) gave one of the most detailed account of the role of affect in delusion formation. He started out with the assumption that emotions influence thought in normal life. As an example, Specht mentioned visual illusions caused by strong affects such as fear and anxiety. Specht also viewed the development of delusions as ensuing from perceptual disturbances of the kind just mentioned, and therefore as ultimately caused by affective disturbances.

In addition, Specht paid special attention to the incorrigibility of delusions, and linked this feature to their affective nature. His argument is one of analogy: Strong emotions cannot be influenced by reason, and the same is true for delusions. Therefore, patients adhere to delusions because they suffer from a disturbance of their emotions, which were thought to be "overcharged". We will see below that this line of analog reasoning, although not logically valid, must have been, and still seems to be, appealing to quite a few clinicians.

The eminent psychiatrist Eugen Bleuler also saw a disturbance of emotions as a possible cause of delusions. Like Specht, Bleuler (1906, 1911/1950, 1916) drew parallels to normal life. In his famous monograph on schizophrenia, Bleuler wrote on the formation of delusions in schizophrenic patients:

"To a certain degree, the affects inhibit in everyone contradictory associations and facilitate those that serve their purpose. Thus even the healthy person is often deceived when he is under affective influences. [...] When we are angry at someone, we see only his faults, or at least magnify them; when we want something very badly, we minimize the obstacles that are in our way; when we are afraid we magnify the obstacles. When someone considers the external world as hostile for some reason, he will find causes for suspicion everywhere. In healthy persons whose affectivity is persistent and comparatively very strong in relation to their powers of thinking, dogmatism and incapacity to engage in reasonable discussion lead to error and can without transition pass over into paranoia" (Bleuler 1911/1950, pp. 384–385).

In fact, Bleuler thought that this process explained the formation of all the various kinds of schizophrenic delusions, as can be seen from the following quote:

"In every case, these autistic worlds develop under the dominance of one or several of the most important human drives: love, power, and wealth are the desired goals; fear or lack of, or inadequate, sexual activity, of personal inferiority, and of persecution is linked to these drives. This concept of the genesis of the schizophrenic basic delusion completely explains the innumerable observations which have been made in this field" (Bleuler 1911/1950, p. 385).

Bleuler then goes on to criticize other theories of delusion formation, which explain the phenomenon in terms of faulty logical deductions, altered body sensations, altered perception, or the affect of mistrust, which for him is not an affect at all (cf. Bleuler 1906, pp. 75, 83).

With respect to delusions in affective disorders, Bleuler said strikingly little about affects as—rather obviously—the primary cause. In his textbook on psychiatry, which first appeared in 1916, we only find a short passage about the development of delusions of poverty in depression:

"Delusions develop as a result of affects, in such a manner that all that is appropriate to the affect is primed, and all that is opposed is inhibited, and does not occur at all in this connection, or occurs with insufficient logical weight. Hence, the melancholic will, when thinking of his wealth, constantly see his debts and bad odds, and he will not see his assets, as he either regards these as worthless or insecure, or will not be able to relate these assets to the idea of his debts, i.e., will not be able to use them to annihilate the idea of being in debt. In such a manner, he arrives at the delusion of poverty" (Bleuler 1916, pp. 65–66, transl. by the author).

Our discussion of Bleuler's view of affect and delusions would not be complete unless we also mention his concept of weakened associations (between concepts as well as between brain structures[1]) in schizophrenia. According to Bleuler, affect has a weakening influence on the logical connections (viz., associations) between ideas, and once logic is weakened, the flow of thought can be subject to other influences. Among these influences are, again, the affects: "once logical connections are weakened, the influence of affects is strengthened" (Bleuler 1911, p. 814, transl. by the author). Bleuler's view can therefore be summarized as follows: affect influences formal thought, and, ultimately, through this process, can cause delusions.

To many clinicians, the ideas of Hagen, Specht and Bleuler have been convincing. Only recently, Zigler and Glick (1988) have proposed that paranoid schizophrenia really is "camouflaged depression". Weinschenk (1955) claimed that disturbed affects can distort perception and even lead to hallucinations. These experiences ultimately result in delusional explanations, which the patient makes up. Weinschenk's view is not very far from a more recent approach pursued by Maher (1974), in which delusions result from anomalous experiences which patients want to explain for themselves. However, in Weinschenk's view, affective disturbances are responsible for the anomalous experiences, whereas in Maher's view, the anomalous experiences can be due to a wide variety of reasons or causes.

5. Contra Affect: Jaspers, Gruhle, and Schneider

While Friedrich Wilhelm Hagen, Gustav Specht and Eugen Bleuler favored the affective genesis of delusions, Karl Jaspers, Hans–Walter Gruhle and Kurt Schneider proposed an opposite view. According to these authors, *real* delusions (delusions proper, primary delusions), by definition, are *not* caused by any other mental phenomena, but spring into existence without any "reason" whatsoever. How did this view originate? How was it motivated, and what are its consequences?

When Jaspers wrote his famous *General Psychopathology* in 1913, psychiatry had its set of problems and its set of already worked out solutions. In other words, the concepts developed by Jaspers, and the way in which he structured his concepts to cut through vaguely defined areas of disordered mental life, were influenced by the general framework of psychiatric reasoning of his time. In particular, the distinction introduced by Jaspers between primary and secondary delusions, which is crucial to our discussion, cannot be understood without taking into account some facts about the state of psychiatry at the turn of the century.

Most importantly, the spirochete Treponema pallidum had just been discovered as the cause of one of the most enigmatic disorders, the veneral disease syphilis, which often leads to a variety of psychiatric symptoms,

---

1 The concept of association has been used to denote relations between concepts as well as neurones (cf. "association fibers").

including hallucinations and delusions. However, in other cases, seemingly similar symptoms could be explained in terms of a patient's personal history. Hence, symptoms could either historically and understandably *develop*, or they could be part of a disease *process*. In the first case, no disease was present, while in the second case, the symptoms were caused by a disease. Therefore, the question arose whether the distinction between these diagnostic alternatives could be determined on purely psychopathological grounds, i.e., without any reference to somatic pathology. With respect to the endogeneous psychoses, which Kraepelin just had described and distinguished on the basis of their course, it must have seemed quite likely that pathogenic agents would sooner or later be found, just as the spirochete had already been discovered. However, until such causes were discovered, the diagnosis of these disease processes had to be based on psychopathology. For this reason, the distinction between—to take the most prominent historical example which is at the same the subject of our discussion—the understandable *development* of delusions, and the non-understandable coming into existence of delusions by some supposedly present disease *process*, was of great importance. Furthermore, some of the disorders which Kraepelin just had described, the affective disorders, were known to have a good prognosis. As these may exhibit delusions as one of their symptoms, the distinction between delusions as a part of an affective disorder and delusions apart from these disorders was seen as being of great clinical importance.

Accordingly, Jaspers distinguished "primary delusions" from delusions secondary to other mental changes. He had already developed a similar idea in one of his early writings,[2] and merely pushed this further in his *General Psychopathology*.

"We can ... distinguish two large groups of delusion according to their origin: one group emerges understandably from preceding affects, from shattering, mortifying, guilt–provoking, or other such experiences, from false–perception or from the experience of derealisation in states of altered consciousness etc. The other group is for us psychologically irreducible... We give the term 'delusion-like ideas' to the first group; the latter we term 'delusions proper'." (Jaspers 1963, p. 96).

As we can see, if the development of delusions can be understood in terms of the patient's history or in terms of any other mental events present in the patient at the time of the genesis of the delusions, then these delusions are *secondary*. In contrast, *primary* delusions spring into existence without any "good reason", their genesis cannot be understood.

"Primary delusions. If we try to get some closer understanding of these primary experiences of delusion, we soon find we cannot really appreciate these quite alien modes of experience. They remain largely incomprehensible, unreal and beyond our understanding" (Jaspers 1963, p. 98).

---

2 Cf. Jaspers (1913), *Kausale und verständliche Zusammenhänge zwischen Schicksal und Psychose bei der Dementia Praecox* (*Causal and understandable relations between fate and psychosis in dementia praecox*).

It is these primary delusions, of course, which were thought, at the time of Jaspers, to indicate a disease–process (i.e., the progressively deteriorating dementia praecox in a Kraepelinian sense). Therefore, delusions which turn out to be understandable in terms of any other psychological event (the most prominent being affect!) are in fact not true delusions and instead are called delusion–like ideas by Jaspers.

"The term delusion should properly only be given to those delusions which go back to primary pathological experiences as their source, and which demand for their explanation a change in the personality. As such, they constitute a group of primary symptoms. The term delusion–like ideas is reserved by us for those so–called 'delusions' that emerge comprehensibly from other psychic events and which can be traced back psychologically to certain affects, drives, desires and fears. We have no need here to invoke some personality change but on the contrary can fully understand the phenomenon on the basis of the permanent constitution of the personality (Anlage) or of some transient emotional state. Among these delusion-like ideas we put ... the 'delusions' of mania and depression ('delusions' of sin, destitution, nihilistic 'delusions', etc.) ..." (Jaspers 1963, pp. 106–107).[3]

Note that according to Jaspers, delusions due to affective changes are in fact not real delusions but are only delusion–like. Although in a footnote Jaspers added the disclaimer that "depressive delusions can only be attributed to affect comprehensibly if we presuppose in severe melancholia a temporary change in the psychic life as a whole" (Jaspers 1963, p. 107), the opinion stated in the main text is straightforward: By definition, real delusions are not caused by affective changes.

According to Gruhle, primary delusions are a major symptom of schizophrenia[4] and have to be distinguished from secondary delusions which are due to the prevailing affect. On several occasions, he stated that primary delusions cannot be understood in psychological terms. In his view, primary delusions have an organic cause.

"Real delusion is not functionally related to any previous experience of the patient; it does not spring from a particular feature of character, and is neither related to habitual mistrust and suspicion, nor to jealousy, insecurity, anxiety, etc. In contrast to recent researchers, who are partly oriented toward Freud, I am convinced that schizophrenic delusion is neither the result of a flight into psychosis, nor the result of internal conflicts, nor due to complexes or the like, although previous experiences emerge when it come to the *content* of the delusions. We are not primarily interested in the question of the specific content of the delusion (he is, for example, persecuted by a married couple), not even the question of why somebody is persecuted at all, but rather, *why somebody has a delusion at all. I think, true delusion is a primary symptom of schizophrenia, a non–derivable, non–understandable, organic symptom*" (Gruhle 1932, p. 178, my translation).

In Kurt Schneider's rigid system of psychopathology, psychoses by definition were conceived of as diseases, and a sharp line was drawn

---

3 The single quotes around the word delusion are not in the original German book but have been introduced by the translators.
4 Gruhle admits, though, that primary delusions also occur in some alcohol–induced psychoses as well as psychoses of patients with epilepsy (cf. Gruhle 1932).

between those mental disorders which are "merely" reactive and those which were thought to be due to a disease process.

"[It is] important ... that we should differentiate clearly between psychotic event [on the one hand] and psychopathic development or psychic reaction [on the other hand]" (Schneider 1959, p. 108).

As his system was conceptually similar to that of Jaspers, Schneider's views on delusions were also similar: True delusions are not understandable, occur without any psychologic reason, and indicate severe pathology, such as schizophrenia or a form of organic mental disorder.

Schneider emphasized delusional perceptions as a particularly important symptom of schizophrenia (a first rank symptom) as compared to delusional ideas (a symptom of the second rank). Therefore, we would expect that the view that affectively motivated delusions are not real delusions would be transferred to the problem of delusional perceptions. In other words, we would expect Schneider to claim that affectively motivated delusional perceptions are not real delusional perceptions at all. This is exactly what we find in his writings on this subject:

"Delusional perception (Wahnwahrnehmung) refers to the abnormal significance attached to a real percept without any cause that is understandable in rational or emotional terms... Delusional perception is not the same as investing an experience with abnormal significance for some reason. We need not concern ourselves here with misinterpretations or errors of reasoning for which there is an understandable, rational cause. But when the cause is understandable in emotional terms—that is to say, when misinterpretations take place against a prevailing emotional background, or mood, particularly one of anxiety or mistrust—they are of some interest. The content of such delusion–like reactions is very much in keeping with this affective background and can be understood in terms of it. The presence of delusional perceptions, however, excludes a reactive experience, and always indicates a true psychosis which, in practical terms, is a schizophrenic illness" (Schneider 1949/1974, p. 33)

In other words, according to Schneider, a delusional perception, by definition, is not motivated, caused, or due to a disturbance of affect or emotion.

6. Discussion and Conclusions for Further Research

From the different views so far presented, it is obvious that the problem of the relationship between affect and delusions has *empirical as well as conceptual* aspects. It is an empirical question, for example, how often delusions occur in affective versus other (e.g., schizophrenic) disorders. However, this question is confounded by a conceptual question: Do we call a particular illness "affective" even though severe delusions are present, or do we call it "delusional" even though strong affects are present.[5]

---

5 It may be argued that this is a mere question of names and not, as stated, a conceptual one. However, it should become clear in this discussion that the problem is in fact a conceptul one and not one of mere names, since the whole question of delusion proper, secondary delusion, delusional perception, and delusion-like reaction pivot on this conceptual issue.

If we assume that currently used diagnostic systems are robust, reliable and valid instruments which to at least some degree "carve nature at the joints" (as Plato put it), then we can ask empirical questions about the frequency of delusions in various disorders. From the answer that delusions occur more frequently in schizophrenia—a disorder mainly of cognition—than in mania and depression—the two main affective disorders—, we might conclude that affect plays a minor role in delusion formation. However, this epidemiological argument is opposed by the fact that affective disturbances are common in schizophrenia, especially at the beginning, i.e., when delusions begin to form. Proponents of the "affect-genesis-theory" have always emphasized this latter finding. However, such a view begs the question, as its proponents tend to assume the presence of a disturbed mood, whenever delusions are formed. That is to say, they turn the inference upside down: There are delusions, hence, there must have been a disordered affect.

Such a view is sometimes accompanied by an argument by analogy which deserves consideration here, since it is based heavily upon features of affect which were mentioned above. It is argued that, by definition, delusions are incorrigible to reason, i.e., they are as *opposed to reason as is affect*. When I am in love, I know that I am in love and nobody will "talk me out" of it. Just as in the case of the deluded patient, I will not listen to "reasonable arguments". Moreover, many patients experience their delusional experiences passively, *just as we often are the passive subjects of affects*. Additionally, it has been claimed that delusions must have a *somatic basis* because they represent a way of thinking quite removed from ordinary, healthy thought. Since affect is also conceived of as embedded within somatic functioning, a third analogy emerges. Finally, as we have seen above, affect has come to be viewed as a phenomenon of rather *short duration*, precisely what is necessary to explain the origin of delusions at the beginning of a psychosis.

As we can see, the main thrust of the argument that affect is involved in delusion formation comes from analogy: In several respects, affect has the very same characteristics as delusions. Hence, the argument goes, affect must be involved in delusion formation.

The concepts of delusional mood and of the mood congruence of delusions provide two further examples of the ways in which our views on affect and delusions are interrelated.

6.1 Delusional Mood

Delusional mood (delusional atmosphere, Wahnstimmung) is defined as a state of anxiety and suspicion which often precedes the formation of delusional ideas, especially in schizophrenic patients. Proponents of the affective–genesis–theory portray the delusional mood as a classic example of affect involvement in delusion formation. In a delusional mood, according to Hagen, patients feel "as if they have lost grip on things, they feel gross uncertainty which drives them instinctively to look for some fixed point to which they can cling. The achievement of this brings strength and comfort, and it is brought only by forming an idea, as happens with healthy people in analogous circumstances. Whenever we find ourselves depressed, fearful or at a loss, the sudden clear consciousness of something, whether false or true, immediately has a soothing effect. As judgment gains clarity, the feelings loosed by the situation will (ceteris paribus) dwindle in their force. Conversely, no dread is worse than the danger of unknown" (Hagen 1870, translation quoted from Jaspers 1963, p. 98).

This idea that delusions are directly derived from the affects of the delusional mood was a subject of debate in psychiatry. Whereas Jaspers merely found it "doubtful whether the foregoing analysis will hold in all cases" (1963, p. 98), a clear dismissal of this position was advocated by Kurt Schneider.

"We stated that delusional perception does not derive from any particular emotional state, but this does not contradict the fact that delusional perception is often preceded by a delusional atmosphere brought on by the morbid process itself, an experience of oddness or sometimes, though more rarely, of exaltation. Furthermore, in these vague delusional moods, perceptions gain a sense of something 'significant' yet not defined. The delusional atmosphere is, however, very vague and can offer no content pointing to the delusional perception that follows later, nor can we understand the specific content of the delusional perception in terms of it. The most we can say is that these perceptions are characteristically embedded in this atmosphere but are not derived from it" (Schneider 1959, p. 109, transl. slightly changed by the author).

Schneider' view is quite clear: Neither the coming into being of delusions nor their specific content can be meaningfully related to delusional mood.

When we reconsider the two contrasting views on the role of affect in delusion formation, the issue of the affective genesis of delusions in the special case of delusional mood narrows down to the following kind of question: Can, for example, persecutory delusions be derived from suspicion (pro–affect view) or is it more accurate to state that they merely occur in such states, but are not determined by them in any way (contra–affect view).[6] Disagreement obviously concerns the derivability of the content of the delusion as well as its form, that is to say, its mere existence as a delusion. Although data do not yet exist to solve this problem, psychiatrists have reasoned from both perspectives. Some think that affect always plays a role in delusion formation, while others hold the opposite view. As Arthur (1964, p. 110) pointed out in a review article, "many leading psychiatrists deny that delusional persons show any excessive affect or that it was present before the delusions appeared." We seem to be left with a decision to make, and, to go back to our example, to either take suspicion and persecution as related or to not do so.

---

6 It should be noted here that within this context the question of whether or not suspicion should be called an affect has been debated. If suspicion were an affect, then persecution could understandably be derived from it, and hence, delusions of persecution could be said to have an affective cause.

It may be possible to further elucidate this issue by undertaking careful case studies. Such studies must not be confounded by conceptual flaws and unspoken biases.[7] In other words, conceptual clarification is a necessary part of empirical research of this sort.

6.2 Mood Congruence

The distinction between delusions that spring into existence without any good reason and delusions that can be derived from the prevailing affect (i.e., Jaspers' distinction between primary and secondary delusions) has been given a new and less precise name: Since DSM-III, we refer to mood–congruent delusions and mood–incongruent delusions .[8] Mood–congruent psychotic features are defined as follows:

"Delusions or hallucinations whose content is entirely consistent with either a depressed or a manic mood. If the mood is depressed, the content of the delusions or hallucinations would involve themes of either personal inadequacy, death, nihilism, or deserved punishment. If the mood is manic, the content of the delusions or hallucinations would involve themes of inflated worth, power, knowledge, or identity or special relationship to a deity or famous person" (DSM–III–R, pp. 401–402).

It is quite obvious that this definition is derived from the view of delusions held by Jaspers, Gruhle and Schneider. Another example of the dependence of the DSM-III-R upon the views of these authors can be seen in the discussions in DSM-III-R of delusions of persecution without any reference of their possible congruence with the delusional mood. In fact, the term "delusional mood" is not mentioned in the entire DSM–III–R nor is it included in the official glossary of the American Psychiatric Association (cf. Stone 1988).

By handling mood congruence in this way, the DSM–III–R does not solve the problem at issue. Definitions (of what is mood congruent and what is not mood congruent) are given instead of analyses of mental states and their complex relationships. Moreover, such analyses are blocked because the terms in which they have historically been cast (such as delusional mood and genetic understanding; see Spitzer & Uehlein, Wiggins et al., this volume) are not included in the official vocabulary of psychiatry. In other words, the DSM-III arbitrarily takes the contra-affect view to be the correct one, and, in doing so, completely obscures the fact that the problem has not yet been solved. As we already have mentioned, most psychiatrists are biased toward one of the two views, and one way of not overcoming such biases is to fail to be aware of them. The issue of mood congruence further conceals the problem of the possible role of affect in the formation of delusions.

---

7 In Husserl's terms, the case studies have to undergo the process of eidetic variation (cf. Uehlein, this volume).
8 As I have argued elsewhere, the notion of congruence does not match with the process of actually making decisions about the degree of understandability of particular delusions in terms of particular affects (cf. Spitzer, in press)

6.3 The Conceptual and the Empirical: Final Comments

A final answer to the question of the role of affect in delusion formation is far beyond the aim of this paper. However, the first thing one must do in order to solve a problem is to spell it out clearly and to exemplify it. Having done so, for the case of affect and delusion formation, it is easy to see that this problem has conceptual as well as empirical aspects. In other words: The question of the role of affect in delusion formation must be addressed through a number of related questions, such as: Is there a necessary relation between delusions and affect or an empirical one? What is affect? Upon what features do we want to do empirical research?[9]

It is important to permit such difficult questions to remain within the domain of psychiatric inquiry. They must not be abolished by authority, i.e., by mere definition, and by the abolition of related terms.

States such as delusional mood, for example, should not be excluded from clinical practice and research merely because they are somewhat difficult to operationalize. On the contrary, such states are important fields upon which research must be carried out in order to produce empirical data relevant to our question.

Only a careful dialogue with the patient can yield such relevant data. Such data will be almost completely subjective, since they will be based upon reports of experienced affect as well as subjectively important propositional attitudes. As van Praag recently pointed out, delusional mood

"is not readily observable, not spontaneously and concisely verbalized, and not unmistakably acknowledged when a straightforward question is posed. A standardized structured interview is unsuitable to trace this undisputably pathological experience. To this end, one needs unrestricted access to the realm of the subjective" (van Praag, 1992, p. 268).

In this sense, we need to keep, or even to reconquer, subjective experience as a legitimate research domain for psychiatry. After all, it provides us with data which cannot ever be replaced by data from other sources. Introspective data are vital to our understanding of basic symptoms in psychopathology.

Summary

After the concept of affect is analyzed from a systematic and historical perspective, views about the role of affect on the formation of delusions are presented. Hagen, Specht and Bleuler favored the idea that affective changes, even if we do not notice them, are among the main causes of delusions. In contrast, Jaspers, Gruhle and Schneider proposed the opposite view, i.e., that real (primary, proper) delusions are not caused by

---

9 A recent article on *Fear and anger in delusional (paranoid) disorder* by Kennedy et al. (1992) may serve as an example of the kind of empirical research, which has to be done in order to clarify the issue.

affects. The state of the delusional mood and the issue of mood congruence are discussed. These issues exemplify the ways in which the two views contrast and are still influential. Furthermore, they reveal the incapacity of present psychiatric approaches which fail to handle investigate the role of affect in delusion formation in a scientifically sound way. The necessary conditions for any answer to this question lie in a clearer view of the conceptual and empirical aspects of the problem.

References

Arthur AZ: Theories and explanations of delusions: a review. American Journal of Psychiatry 121: 105–115, 1964

Bleuler E: Dementia Praecox or the Group of Schizophrenias (1911), transl. by Ziskin J, Lewis ND; New York, International Universities Press, 1950

Darwin C: The expression of the emotions in man and animals. Chicago, university of Chicago press (orig. publ. in 1872), 1965

Ekman P: Cross–cultural studies of facial expression. In: Ekman P (ed): Darwin and facial expression: A century of research in review, pp. 169–222. New York, Academic press, 1973

Fulford KWM: Philosophy and medicine: the Oxford connection. British Journal of Psychiatry 157: 111-115, 1990

Gruhle H–W: Allgemeine Symptomatologie. In: Bumke O (ed): Handbuch der Geisteskrankheiten, vol. 9: Die Schizophrenie, pp. 135–292, Berlin, Springer, 1932

Hagen FW: Studien auf dem Gebiete der ärztlichen Seelenheilkunde. Erlangen, Eduard, Eduard Besold, 1870

James W: Psychology: Briefer Course (first published in 1892). Cambridge, Mass., Harvard University Press, 1984

Jaspers K: Kausale und verständliche Zusammenhänge zwischen Schicksal und Psychose bei der Dementia Praecox. Zeitschrift für Neurologie 14, pp. 158–263, 1913. [parts of this paper have been translated by J. Hoening, reprinted in Hirsch, S.R., Shepherd, M. (Eds.): Themes and Variations in European Psychiatry. An Anthology, pp. 81–93. Charlottesville, University Press of Virginia, 1974

Jaspers K: General Psychopathology (transl. by Hoenig J, Hamilton MW) Manchester University Press, The University of Chicago Press, 1963

Kennedy HG, Kemp LI, Dyer DE: Fear and anger in delusional (paranoid disorder: The association with violence. British Journal of Psychiatry 160: 488–492, 1992

Lewis A: Paranoia and paranoid: a historical perspective. Psychological Medicine 1: 2–12, 1970

Machleit W, Gutjahr L, Mügge A: Grundgefühle. Phänomenologie, Psychodynamik, EEG–Spektralanalytik. Berlin, Heidelberg, New York, London, Paris, Tokyo, Hong Kong, 1989

Maher BA: Delusional thinking and perceptual disorder. Journal of Individual Psychology 30: 98-113, 1974

Miller GA, Glucksberg S: Psycholinguistic aspects pragmatics and semantics. In: Atkinson RC, Herrnstein RJ, Lindzey G, Luce RD (eds): Steven's Handbook of Experimental Psychology (ch. 6), pp. 417-472. New York, Wiley, 1988

Oster H, Daily L, Goldenthal P: Processing facial affect. In: Young AW, Ellis HD (eds): Handbook of research in face processing, pp. 107–161. Amsterdam, New York, Oxford, Tokyo, North Holland, 1989

Overall JE, Gorham DR: Brief Psychiatric Rating Scale. In: Guy W: ECDEU Assessment Manual for Psychopharmacology, Rev. ed., Rockville, Maryland, pp. 157–169, 1976

Ritter J (ed): Historisches Wörterbuch der Philosophie, Vol. I, pp. 89-99. Darmstadt, Wissenschaftliche Buchgesellschaft Darmstadt, 1971

Schneider K: Clinical Psychopathology (transl. by Hamilton MW, Anderson EW). New York, London, Grune & Stratton, 1959

Schneider K: The concept of delusion (1949). In: Hirsch SR, Shepherd M (eds): Themes and Variations in European Psychiatry. An Anthology, pp. 33–39. Charlottesville, University Press of Virginia, 1974

Specht G: Über den pathologischen Affekt in der chronischen Paranoia—Ein Beitrag zur Lehre von der Wahnentwicklung, Festschrift, Erlangen, 1901

Spitzer M, Uehlein FA: Phenomenology and Psychiatry. This volume

Spitzer M: The basis of psychiatric diagnosis. In: Sadler JZ, Schwartz MA, Wiggins OP (eds): Philosophical perspectives on psychiatric diagnostic classification. Baltimore, The Johns Hopkins University Press (in press)

Stone EM: American Psychiatric Glossary, 6th ed. Washington, DC, American Psychiatric Press, 1988

Van Praag HM: Reconquest of the Subjective. Against the Waning of Psychiatric Diagnosing. British Journal of Psychiatry 160: 266–271, 1992

Weinschenk C: Über die Wirksamkeit der pathologischen Affektivität bei der Wahnentstehung der endogenen Psychose. Schweizer Archiv f. Neurologie, Neurochirurgie und Psychiatrie 95: 91-119, 1965

Wiggins OP, Schwartz MA, Spitzer M: Phenomenological/descriptive psychiatry: The methods of Edmund Husserl and Karl Jaspers. This volume

Zigler E, Glick M: Is paranoid schizophrenia really camouflaged depression? American Psychologist 43: 284-290, 1988

M. Spitzer, F.A. Uehlein
M.A. Schwartz, C. Mundt
(eds.): Phenomenology
Language & Schizophrenia.
Springer-Verlag, New York, 1992

The Brain's Capacity to Form Delusions as an Evolutionary Strategy for Survival

Edward M. Hundert

> *I made some studies, and reality is the leading
> cause of stress amongst those in touch with it.*
> Jane Wagner (1986, p. 18) in Lilly
> Tomlin's one-woman play, *The Search for
> Signs of Intelligent Life in the Universe.*

1. Introduction

Delusions have long been considered a hallmark of mental illness. When individuals begin to believe that they are Jesus here to save the world or the devil here to destroy it, they are quickly labelled "psychotic" and thought to be in need of some form of psychiatric treatment. Throughout history, such individuals have been stigmatized and ostracized from the community because their souls have been taken over by evil demons, their mental structures have deteriorated, their brains have malfunctioned, or whatever other paradigm is employed to account for the "pathology" that delusions are assumed to represent.

Our modern biological paradigm looks to a "broken brain" to account for the locus of delusions; it is a simple matter so conceptualize such psychopathological symptomatology in terms of neurobiological malfunction. Modern researchers are now actively studying delusional patients using every new brain scan as it becomes available. The absence of any definitive results thus far is taken as a reminder of the complexity of the human brain and not as cause for pessimism over whether "the lesion" will ever be found. After all, a broken brain must be broken *somewhere*, whether at the anatomical, physiological, or molecular genetic level. It is only a matter of time, so they say, until the malfunction that causes delusions is discovered.

This human brain that forms the center of our biological paradigm is itself an effect as well as a cause, however. The brain evolved over millions of years through the process of natural selection and it has come to hold a special place in that evolutionary process. We might in fact say that, along with the organs of reproduction, the brain is the organ most responsible for our continuing evolution, since it solves the many unexpected problems that would prevent our survival through reproductive age. In this "decade of the brain" (as dubbed by the U.S. National Institutes of Health), we become more amazed with every new discovery at the brain's miraculous plasticity and myriad mechanisms for surviving fortune's slings and arrows. It is largely the brain's responsibility to adapt to an often hostile world so that the species can survive another generation.

If the brain evolved to maximize our chances for survival through its many subtle adaptive mechanisms, we may well ask whether one such mechanism is the brain's capacity to form delusions. A biological view of psychopathology does not limit us to the hypothesis that delusions represent a form of brain *pathology* to be discovered by MRI, PET, or EEG. An alternative biological hypothesis focuses on a brain that has developed complex ways to keep its body alive (its evolutionary mission) and one of these ways may well be the alteration of an individual's contact with reality in a manner that immediately labels them as a "delusional patient" in need of "treatment" for this "condition".

This alternative hypothesis can be looked at in clinical, philosophical, or evolutionary terms, but before taking up each of these, a brief case study will clarify matters for the discussion that follows.

2. A Case Study: Timothy G.

One of my patients whom I will call Timothy G. is a 32 year old, single, white, unemployed male whose psychiatric illness began at approximately the age of 20. Until that time he had done very well, and his high school yearbook describes him as a quite popular, fun-loving person. During his second year of college, however, his social functioning began to deteriorate and he became increasingly isolated and depressed. He also had marked insomnia, as well as paranoia, and it was his harassing of several local women that led to his first hospitalization.

Between the ages of 20 and 22, the patient had numerous short hospitalizations for the treatment of severe depression following several nearly-fatal suicide attempts. These sometimes dramatic attempts to take his life included stabbing himself in the abdomen (causing liver damage), trying to ignite himself with gasoline, jumping off a bridge into an icy river, cutting his wrists, and taking several overdoses, the last of which left him unconscious for two days. At about the time of this last serious suicide attempt, the patient began to feel that he had "blasphemed the Holy Spirit". By about the age of 23, Tim developed a fixed delusional system which has been present in stronger and weaker forms for nearly 10 years. His delusional system involves the belief that he is Adolf Hitler reincarnated to do penance for his war crimes. He claims to have experienced being buried for five years in Hitler's grave and then coming back to earth so that he can suffer through his many suicide attempts and multiple hospitalizations. When things are going relatively well for him, he continues to state that he is doing penance, although he describes this in a more non-specific way. When he is stressed in any way, however, his full belief about being the reincarnation of Hitler returns with many elaborate details.

To complicate matters, the patient was diagnosed at about the age of twelve with multiple sclerosis when he had an episode of double vision. MRI scans show multiple white matter lesions throughout his brain, especially in the frontal lobes and in the temporo-occipital regions adjacent to the occipital horns. He does not have all the classic features of multiple sclerosis, particularly since his neurological symptoms of early onset have not progressed at all in the last ten years, and one hypothesis has been raised that a severe bicycle accident leading to loss of consciousness at age ten could be responsible for the lesions seen on brain scans and causing some of his symptoms.

Tim's family history is significant only for one maternal great-aunt and one maternal uncle who suffered from recurrent depressions. He has had a rocky course over the years, living in halfway houses and frequently being rehospitalized when he becomes more paranoid, impulsive, and depressed. He has not attempted to hurt himself in nearly ten years.

3. Clinical and Evolutionary Perspectives

Tim presents an interesting case for our discussion because he has identifiable brain pathology and a rather classic delusional system. Many delusions take this form where patients think themselves evil or sinful or somehow contaminating the world and those around them. It is tempting so assume that the brain pathology which lights up so clearly on his MRI scan is the direct cause of his fixed belief that he is the reincarnation of Adolf Hitler.

But the course of his illness speaks of another story. It is a story in which, perhaps because of his neurological condition, perhaps because of an inherited familial depressive disorder, or perhaps because of some other unknown reason, the patient became suicidally depressed in his early twenties and "reality" as he knew it left him with only one option: suicide. It was the isolation of his meaningless suffering that drove him to impressive lengths to take his life, and it is almost miraculous that he is alive today.

Meaning was returned to his life, however. This meaning arises from his delusion because, like so many psychotic patients, his "symptomatology" is an organizing feature of his continued existence. To end his life would be to end the world's only hope for bringing justice to the perpetrator of the Nazi holocaust. Since the time his brain figured this out, his continued survival has not been in jeopardy.

By referring to Tim as a "psychotic patient", I include delusions under the general label of *psychosis* and this requires some explanation. Melges (1982, p. 134) summarizes the usual definition: "The term psychosis refers to defective reality testing. Simply stated, defective reality testing means that the person has difficulty in telling the real from the unreal." Tim's delusion is psychotic if we take it that he is not really the reincarnation of Adolf Hitler and he is unable to tell the real from the unreal in that simple sense.

What we are considering here, however, is the possibility that continued contact with the "real" would *lead to the end of Tim's life.* We may then wonder whether it was the lesions on his MRI scan that led to his delusion, or whether it was the *healthier* part of his brain that came to the rescue to keep him alive by giving him a reason not to end his life.

This view of delusions as a secondary or reparative effort of the brain in the face of some other breakdown in human experience was popularized by Minkowski over 50 years ago. His famous patient had the fixed elusion that he was about to be executed the next day. After a monumental effort to get with this patient's experience, Minkowski (1933, p. 187) concludes that:

> "... the delusion is not completely a product of the imagination. It becomes grafted onto a phenomenon which is a part of our life and comes into play when the life-synthesis begins to weaken. The particular form of the delusion, the idea of execution, is in fact only the attempt of that part of the mind which remains intact to establish a logical connection between the various sections of a crumbling edifice."

The model of a "primary breakdown" with "secondary symptoms" is actually quite familiar from other schools of psychiatric thought, as Havens (1973, p. 140) reminds us. The psychoanalytic model appeals to primary ego deficits giving rise to secondary symptoms whose content may vary. The cognitive-behavioral model likewise appeals to primary deficits in the patient's mental set which give rise to secondary "depressiogenic cognitions" whose content may also vary. We see this most strikingly in a biological model where a primary breakdown such as drug-induced visual hallucinations give rise to secondary symptoms whose contents are almost completely ignored for diagnostic purposes. (What it is that hallucinating patients think they are seeing does not make any difference to the diagnosis assigned by DSM-III-R.) Elsewhere (Hundert 1989, 1990, 1991), I have discussed some of the implications of this perspective for how we might reconsider such classification schemes, and Spitzer (1990a) has recently reviewed the definitional problem of delusions in some detail.

From an evolutionary perspective, it should be clear why the brain would choose a delusion over death. The actual mental experience of the individual is not, after all, a matter for natural selection, except as it leads to some maladaptive behavior or change in the physical characteristics that are needed for reproduction and survival until reproductive age. As Maher (1990, p. 75) puts it, "Natural selection operates upon physical structure and/or upon action, and not upon thinking itself". The brain evolved for nothing if not survival. When the "real world" leaves an individual with no option other than suicide (or perhaps murder) we should naturally expect a healthy brain to let go of that real world. Semrad (1973, p. 5) once said that "psychosis is... the sacrifice of reality to preserve life". It is sobering to wonder how many suicides we precipitate when we miss this point that a "delusion" can be a reparative effort of the healthier part of the patient's brain (the part that does *not* light up on Tim's MRI scan) when our well-intentioned therapies finally convince these unfortunate people that it is not true that they are being punished for a past life and thereby deprive them of the meaning their brains have created for themselves.

But if we begin talk of what is "true" and "not true", we move beyond the clinical and evolutionary perspectives to a question of philosophy that is now thrown into relief by this adaptive view of delusions.

4. Whose Reality is It Anyway?

The well known problem of simply defining psychosis as Melges did above in terms of an inability to tell the "real" from the "unreal" is the complete absence of consensus as to what counts as *real*. Certainly many cultures would take Tim's belief in reincarnation at face value and the only question might be whether he is indeed Hitler in particular. When we attempt to frame a view of the brain's capacity to form delusions as an evolutionary strategy for survival, we must remember that it is not just the individual but the species that survives through evolution. What is "adaptive" is what is adaptive for the collective whole. This has major implications for any view of what can count as "real".

It is within this context of the species rather than the individual that we can understand the brain's capacity to form delusions as an evolutionary strategy without stepping into the philosophical quagmire of whether a single "truth" exists. Miller (1983, p. 138) was not entirely accurate when he wrote that "philosophers have not known what to make of madness"—although he was certainly correct in his conclusion "that there is a big opportunity here for new orientations". In *The Bounds of Sense*, Strawson (1966, p. 151) notes that "another name for the *objective* is the *public*", thus connecting the objectivity of truth with its collective accessibility. Another philosopher, Kant (1798, p. 117), understood delusions in just this way when he wrote: "The only general characteristic of insanity is the loss of a sense for ideas that are common to all (sensus communis), and its replacement with a sense for ideas peculiar to ourselves (sensus privatus)...". Spitzer (1990b) has written an interesting analysis of Kant's views on schizophrenia in just these terms.

What makes it so difficult to address the collective rather than the individual level is that human experience reveals the remarkable possibility of being either real *or* unreal. *Both* are "real" parts of human experience, and it would be quite improper to suggest that Tim is wrong about his *experience*, even as we separate the question of whether he is right or wrong in his belief system. Contact with reality is for each of us a fluid function, which is why Klein (1958, 1959) urges us to speak not of "stages" of reality testing as so many developmental theories do, but to speak rather of "positions" of reality testing. Just as a boxer may move forward to a new position, but then under attack may return to an earlier, more defensive position when appropriate, so we all have varying degrees of contact with reality depending upon the stresses on our system. It is easy to see how this capacity is adaptive in the evolutionary sense, since without it we would likely suffer the same fate as the boxer who is unable to move back to an earlier defensive position when needed.

From another perspective, it is tempting to wonder whether most of us are "deluded" most of the time! It has been suggested that in our usual good humor, we are not in maximum contact with reality, since we happily carry on with assumptions that our boss thinks we are doing a great job, our families love us, and so forth. As Tim reminds us, *severe* depression can lead to even grosser reality distortions. But it may well be that *mild* depression maximizes reality contact as we realistically assess both the positive and negative elements of our condition. This irony provides the humor in the comment made by Lily Tomlin's character of the bag lady Trudy that opens this essay. In fact, she describes how adopting this *position* "saved her life", and we can see the evolutionary survival value of a brain with the capacity to remain fluid and move into positions of more and less reality contact as is adaptive to the situation.

Empirical studies of the dramatic differences in the lived realities across individuals reveal a startling lack of consensus as to the "real". The psychologist William James (1890) was driven to abandon all reference to any distinction between "the real" and "the unreal", and spoke instead of "the realities", the subuniverses of the world of "scientific reality" and the world of what he called "idols of the tribe" (shared myths, illusions, and fantasies). The anthropologist Castañeda (1969, 1971) was likewise compelled by his studies of different cultures to recognize that there exist separate realities completely alien to the thinking of the modern scientific mind. Given such a multiplicity of "real worlds" we can see why, in the political arena, thinkers such as Thomas Szasz (1962) might argue for the abandonment of any distinction between the real and the delusional, and attempt to recognize psychosis as simply another way of "being in the world", with mental illness no longer a meaningful concept. We need not, however, abandon all we know about psychopathology in the light of the existence of multiple realities. We need only recognize with Strawson that the "objective" does not refer to some single unified truth, but rather to that which is available to the public: to the collective whole—the group whose survival is maintained by subtle evolutionary strategies that include the brain's capacity to form delusions.

But now we recognize that there is as much a political as a philosophical matter to be understood when we consider the adaptive value of delusions.

5.   The Politics of Reality and Survival

I would therefore like to conclude this discussion by broadening it to consider the political side of the problem of reality and survival. While I have thus far emphasized the adaptive survival value of delusions for the individual, social history offers a continuous series of examples of the awful price paid by those who have perceived a reality different from the "agrees-upon real world". Although different tribes, communities, nations, or cultures have held sharply different world-views between them, a large group within each has always managed to condemn, persecute, or even kill those who perceive reality differently. From Galileo to the Salem witches so Soviet dissidents in this century, the threat posed by those who might raise questions of the consensual view is a powerful reminder of how shared beliefs cement a culture together. The risk of death by burning at the stake or exile to Siberia raises a serious question as to the ultimate survival value of the brain's capacity to form delusions in our political world.

In his provocative paper, *Do We Need 'A' Reality?* Carl Rogers (1980) reminds us how many realities we each experience even instantaneously. I look up to see the heavens moving around me and am at once the focal point of the revolving universe and a small insignificant part of it. I am both standing firmly on the earth beneath me and moving at breathless speed through space. The pen I hold is both solid and composed in its matter more by space than by atoms. Even without the empirical work of a James or a Castañeda, such introspection itself delivers a final crushing blow to our comfortable belief that "we all know what the real world is".

The operative term here is *comfortable* because our growing appreciation of differences in world-view (catalyzed by mass communication across nations and cultures) creates what Rogers (p. 102) calls "a most burdensome dilemma, one never before experienced in history." If the comfort of a shared world-view has indeed been part of the cement that holds cultures together, the imminent loss of this comfortable myth challenges us to find a new way to share our world together.

We have seen how the brain's capacity to form delusions may have evolved as part of a strategy for collective survival. But that collective survival may now depend upon an even greater adaptive ability to live in a world *less dependent* upon a shared view of reality. Only once in this century have large masses of people pretended to enjoy the comfortable luxury of complete agreement as to the nature of social and cultural reality. This was the agreement brought about by Adolf Hitler's Nazi Germany that nearly marked the destruction of western culture. It may be a wonderful twist of fate if our collective ability to survive as a species through an increased acceptance of differences in realities draws upon a capacity of the brain that originally evolved for the purpose of giving rise to life-saving loses of contact with those very realities.

There is thus a distinct irony to Tim's delusional belief that he is the reincarnation of Hitler, since he reminds us that we walk a fine line between two dangerous extremes. The first is the persecution of an individual who perceives reality differently from the collective whole. (We may wonder whether Tim would still have been hospitalized and labelled psychotic if his *beliefs* were the same but he had not harassed others or attempted suicide). The second is the threat to civilization as we know it if our brain's adaptive capacity is not up to the even greater task of caring for our fellow humans no longer because we are comfortable that they are the same as us, but because we prize and treasure them for their differences from us.

Perhaps Tim's "penance" is a beacon of hope that our human brain—the brain that has adapted so survive in part through its ability to move fluidly through realities as needed—will provide us with the capacity to survive together in a new era that no longer requires the comfort of a simplistic view of one shared reality. Evolution works in wondrous ways. Who knows; the brain's evolved capacity to form delusions may turn out to provide the basis for a new strategy that will ensure our collective survival even in the modern world.

Summary

It is all too easy to view delusions and other psychopathological symptoms as evidence of some brain process or structure that has malfunctioned and given rise to "psychotic" experience. In this essay, the brain's capacity to form delusions has been discussed not as pathology, but as an adaptive strategy that evolution has provided for our continuing survival. It is nearly always possible to ask of a psychotic symptom whether it represents primary brain pathology or a reparative effort of the healthier part of the individuals's mental apparatus to find a way to continue living in a crumbling world. This essay reviews some of the clinical, evolutionary, philosophical, and political implications of this view of delusions, and challenges us all to become more comfortable with the varieties of human experience.

References

Castañeda C: The Teachings of Don Juan; A Yaqui Way of Knowledge. New York, Ballantine Books, 1969

Castañeda C: A Separate Reality; Further Conversations with Don Juan. New York, Pocket Books Division of Simon and Schuster, 1971

Havens L: Approaches to the Mind; Movement of Psychiatric Schools from Sects Toward Science (1973). Cambridge, Repr. by Harvard University Press, 1987

Hundert EM: Philosophy, Psychiatry and Neuroscience; Three Approaches to the Mind. Oxford, Oxford University Press, 1989

Hundert EM: Are psychiatric illnesses category disorders? In: Spitzer, M, Maher BA (eds), Philosophy and Psychopathology, pp. 59-70. New York, Springer, 1990

Hundert EM: Thoughts and feelings and things: A new psychiatric epistemology. Theoretical Medicine, 12: 7-23, 1991

James W: The Principles of Psychology. New York, Holt, 1890

Kant I: Anthropology (1798), transl. by Dowdell VL, rev. and ed. by Rudnick HH, Carbondale and Edwardville, Southern Illinois University Press, 1978

Klein M: On the development of mental functioning (1958). Repr. in Envy and Gratitude and Other Works by Melanie Klein 1946-1963, pp. 236-46. London, Hogarth Press, 1975

354   E. Hundert

Klein M: Our adult world and its roots in infancy (1959). Repr. in Envy and Gratitude and Other Works y Melanie Klein 1946-1963, pp. 247-63. London, Hogarth Press, 1975

Maher BA: The irrelevance of rationality to adaptive behavior. In: Spitzer M, Maher BA (eds), Philosophy and Psychopathology, pp. 73-85. New York, Springer, 1990

Melges FT: Time and the Inner Future: A Temporal Approach to Psychiatric Disorders. New York, John Wiley & Sons, 1982

Miller JW: In Defense of the Psychological. New York, Norton, 1983

Minkowski E: Lived Time; Phenomenological and Psychopathological Studies (1933), trans. by Metzel N. Evanston, Northwestern University Press, 1970

Rogers C: Do we need "a" reality? In: A Way of Being, pp. 96-108. Boston, Houghton-Mifflin, 1980

Semrad E: The clinical approach to the psychoses: heuristic formulation of regressive states. Unpublished transcript of the Academic Conference Presentation of September 14, 1973, McLean Hospital, Belmont, MA, 1973

Spitzer M: On defining delusions. Comprehensive Psychiatry, 31: 377-97, 1990a

Spitzer M: Kant on Schizophrenia. In: Spitzer M, Maher BA (eds), Philosophy and Psychopathology, pp. 44-58. New York, Springer, 1990b

Strawson PF: The Bounds of Sense. London, Methuen & Co., 1966

Szasz TS: The Myth of Mental Illness (1962). London, Repr. by Granada, 1972

Wagner J: The Search for Signs of Intelligent Life in the Universe. New York, Harper & Row, 1986

M. Spitzer, F.A. Uehlein
M.A. Schwartz, C. Mundt
(eds.): Phenomenology
Language & Schizophrenia.
Springer-Verlag, New York, 1992

Thought Insertion and Insight: Disease and Illness Paradigms of Psychotic Disorder

K. William M. Fulford

1. Introduction

Present day psychiatry displays contradictory attitudes to the concept of insight. The conventional line is that the distinction between psychotic and non-psychotic disorders, as marked traditionally by loss of insight, has outlived its usefulness (Gelder et al. 1983). Insight is considered too obscure a notion, too opaque to clear, descriptive definition, for the notion of psychosis to be incorporated into modern classifications of mental illness (World Health Organization, 1978). Yet the term psychosis continues to be widely employed in academic journals as well as in everyday clinical work. Indeed, the intentions of their authors notwithstanding, the concept of psychotic disorder remains firmly embedded even in our official classifications. DSM-III (American Psychiatric Association, 1980) and ICD-10 (World Health Organization, 1991), for example, both contain a category for psychotic disorders "not elsewhere classified".

This contradiction is both practically important and philosophically interesting. In psychiatry there is a tendency to believe that clear definition is a sine qua non for a concept to be clinically useful. According to this view the continued use of the concept of psychosis, in the face of evident difficulties of definition, is no more than a linguistic bad habit. But in philosophy it is recognized that the use of a concept can sometimes come first. After all, we learn our concepts mainly by using them rather than by reference to definitions. And many of our most useful concepts are indeed highly resistant to explicit definition—the concept of time for instance. The continued use of psychosis thus suggests, philosophically, that difficulties of definition or not, the concept has an important role to play in clinical psychiatry. Indeed following Wittgenstein (1958), we should expect the use which is made of the concept of psychosis to be a better guide to its meaning than received definitions.

It is this broadly Wittgenstinian line that will be followed in this paper. The everyday clinical use of the concept of psychosis will be shown to exhibit certain features. These features reflect the meaning of the particular kind of loss of insight by which psychotic disorder is marked out from non-psychotic. The conventional approach to defining insight will be found to be inconsistent with these features and an alternative will be proposed. This switch of approaches, or paradigms, will amount to a change of perspectives, from that of the doctor to that of the patient. The conventional approach seeks, in effect, to assimilate loss of insight to medical models of disease. Certain kinds of loss of insight can indeed be analyzed in this way. But it is in terms rather of the patient's experience of illness that specifically psychotic loss of insight is to be understood.

2. Insight in Clinical Use

Insight is a complex notion incorporating a wide variety of meanings, non-medical as well as medical. In the Shorter Oxford English Dictionary it is defined as "seeing into a thing or a subject", "perception", "discernment", "understanding", and so on. In medicine, similarly, insight may include awareness of symptoms, appreciation of their seriousness, cooperation with treatment, understanding of causes, and recognition of psychological processes, both intrapersonal and interpersonal (David 1990).

These diverse senses of insight are clearly too wide and too non-specific to capture the psychotic/non-psychotic distinction. As we will find in the next section, the non-specificity of the notion of insight has been an important factor in its rejection as a nosological entity. Here, though, as noted a moment ago, we will be arguing the other way. Instead of pursuing the relevant sense of insight directly in terms of received definitions, we will be approaching it indirectly, as revealed by the actual use which is made of the psychotic/non-psychotic distinction. In this respect we have already noted the persistence of the distinction in journals, textbooks and classifications. Careful examination of these and similar materials can provide important information (Fulford 1990). More behavioral techniques are possible, however, and the results of a small pilot study along these lines are described here. I should emphasize in advance that studies of this kind are not intended to be "scientific" investigations of diagnostic practice. They are simply techniques for helping to make more visible the diagnostic concepts implicit in everyday clinical practice.

The study in question involved the use of a case-vignette questionnaire. This was developed originally in the context of work on the conceptual basis of compulsory psychiatric treatment. For each of a series of 14 cases (illustrated in Figure 1) respondents were asked to say whether they would treat the patient against his or her express wishes. The results were scored 2 for yes, 1 for possibly, 0 for no. The questionnaire was prepared in a one-page format designed to be completed in less than five minutes. This time limit, and the instructions to the respondents, made it clear that they should react as they would be likely to react in the heat and disorder of everyday practice. It was not a test of discursive ethical reasoning but an attempt to reflect ordinary clinical decision-making with all its inherent uncertainties.

Figure 1: Examples of the case vignettes used in the questionnaire study

Case 1. Miss A.N. Age 21. Student. Four year history of intermittent anorexia. Currently seriously underweight, exercising and using laxatives; amenorrhoeic. Refusing admission on the grounds that she is "too fat".

Case 3. Mr S.D. Aged 48. Bank manager. Presents in casualty with biological symptoms of depression and nihilistic delusions. Asking for something to "help him sleep". He refuses to stay in hospital when he is told that he may be suffering from depression.

Case 4. Miss H.M. Aged 25. Novice nun. Brought by superiors for urgent outpatient appointment as they are unable to contain her bizarre and sexually disinhibited behavior. Shows pressure of speech, grandiose delusions and auditory hallucinations. Refusing to stay.

Case 8. Mrs R.C. Aged 47. Housewife. Refusing investigation of breast lump discovered on routine screening. Understands that she does not have to accept treatment if the lesion is found to be malignant. Normal mental state.

Case 9. Mr S. Aged 18. Student. Emergency psychiatric admission from his College. Showed thought insertion (Mike Yarwood "using his brain"). Complaining that people were talking about him. Refusing medication and planning to leave hospital.

Case 13. Mr P.P. Aged 23. Unemployed man. Seen in casualty by the duty psychiatrist. Brought in by girlfriend because he is angry and threatening to kill a rival. Has been drinking. History of criminal assault. No other symptoms. Refusing to stay.

For all this the results were unequivocal. These are summarized in Figure 2. As will be seen, out of a wide variety of both mental and physical conditions, case 9 (schizophrenia) and case 4 (hypomania) scored nearly 100 %. Thus almost all respondents would have treated both these patients against their wishes. In addition, case 3 (depression) scored 50% and case 1 (anorexia nervosa) 25%. The remaining cases all scored zero or close to zero. Given the uncertainties of compulsory treatment, and the limitations of the case-vignette approach, this indicates a remarkable degree of consistency of practice. To some extent this was to be expected since all the respondents were doctors and all were attached to the same clinical department (the Department of Psychiatry in the University of Oxford). However, although the study is still on-going, the results are thus far proving highly robust. The findings to date across different professional groups working in different clinical situations confirm that (1) almost

358   K.W.M. Fulford

everyone would treat cases 4 and 9 against their wishes, (2) there are sharp differences of view about cases 1 and 3, and (3) almost all respondents considered the remaining cases to be unsuitable for involuntary treatment.

Figure 2: Sumary of responses to case vignette questionaire (N = 22)

Cases	respondents opting for involuntary treatment (%)	Mental Health Act 1983	severe mental disorder life threat-ening	Butler criteria
1 Anorexia	25	+	?	?
2 Obsessional disorder	10	+		
3 Depression	50	+	+	+
4 Hypomania	100	+		+
5 Optic Atrophy	1			
6 Acromegaly	0			
7 Hysteria	3	+		
8 Breast lump	0			
9 Schizophrenia	100	+		+
10 Osteoporosis	0			
11 Agoraphobia	0	+		
12 Marital problems	1			
13 Personlity disorder	1	?	+	
14 Bronchial carcinoma	1			

So what lies beyond these responses? It is natural, particularly among psychiatrists, to point to the relevant mental health legislation. In most of the United Kingdom involuntary treatment is governed by the Mental Health Act 1983. However, as Figure 2 shows, the criteria for involuntary treatment in the Act are too comprehensive to explain the responses in the questionnaire. The criteria, essentially, are that the patient should be both mentally ill and a danger to themselves or others. But a direct application of these criteria would include some patients who were excluded by respondents and vice versa. The degree of seriousness, although not directly referred to in the Act, could of course be relevant. But this imme-diately begs the question, in what sense "serious"? The most natural sense is "immediately life-threatening". But as Figure 2 also shows, defined in this way, seriousness picks out a quite different subgroup of patients from those identified by respondents.

We can get closer to the relevant sense of serious by going back to some of the groundwork for the 1983 Act. In the 1970's the British Government set up a Royal Commission to consider the treatment of mentally ill offenders in law (Butler 1975). Among a wide range of issues, the Committee gave detailed consideration to which groups of mentally disordered offenders should be regarded as not responsible for their actions. The principle behind this, that insanity is an excuse in law, has a long history, but its application has always been problematic (Walker 1985). The Butler Committee argued that only seriously disordered offenders were not responsible, and that the relevant sense of "serious" corresponded broadly with the medical concept of psychotic disorder. This concept was however considered too imprecise to serve as a legal test. Hence they suggested that "serious" should be defined by the presence of one or more specific symptoms from such areas of (traditionally) psychotic psychopathology. These were to include, in addition to impairments of cognitive functioning, hallucinations, delusions and certain forms of thought disorder, including thought insertion.

The "Butler" criteria of seriousness were not incorporated into the Mental Health Act, 1983, which as noted earlier, is rather widely drawn. However, as shown in the right-hand column of Figure 2, the Butler criteria correspond closely with the patients selected by respondents in our questionnaire study. Patients 9 (schizophrenia) and 4 (hypomania), selected by nearly 100% of respondents, each had symptoms in two of the "psychotic" areas defined by the Butler Committee, while patient 3 (depression), selected by 50%, had one. Apart from patient 1 (anorexia), the remaining patients had no symptoms referable to the Butler criteria. Patient 1 is particularly interesting in Butler terms. Anorexia has traditionally not been classified as a psychotic disorder. Yet the lack of insight often shown by patients with this condition may be psychotic in quality. In particular their beliefs, about their need for food, their body size, and so forth, may be delusional in all but name. By the Butler criteria, therefore, at least some anorexic patients should be considered seriously ill, and this is reflected in the 25% of respondents who considered that patient 1 should be treated on an involuntary basis.

The correspondence between the intuitive selection of patients in our questionnaire study and the Butler criteria thus provides direct evidence that the psychotic/non-psychotic distinction is alive and well. Much could be said about the artificiality of a questionnaire study. Yet it is surely the more remarkable that even under these artificial conditions the psychotic/non-psychotic distinction should emerge so decisively. Moreover this result has a good deal of face-validity. There is surprisingly little direct evidence about which patients are treated involuntarily in practice. But such as there is, points directly to the importance of the concept of psychosis in this respect. It is largely psychotic patients, traditionally defined, who are treated under the Mental Health act. It is also largely psychotic patients who are considered not responsible in law (Grubin 1991).

But our questionnaire study takes us an important step further than this. For it helps to make explicit the characteristics of the particular kind of loss of insight by which psychotic disorders are marked out from non-psychotic. Thus psychotic loss of insight, as reflected in the selection of patients considered suitable for involuntary treatment, is (1) a feature of mental rather than physical disorders, (2) associated specifically with mental illness rather than other mental disorders (such as personality disorder—case 13), (3) instantiated by a range of specific symptoms—delusions, hallucinations and certain forms of thought disorder, and (4) a mark of mental illnesses which are serious, in the sense, specifically, that they have serious ethical and medicolegal implications. Set out in this way, these characteristics of psychotic loss of insight may seem trivially self-evident. They are characteristics, nonetheless, which conventional accounts of the meaning of insight fail to reproduce. It is to these accounts that we turn next.

3. Definitions of Insight—The Disease Paradigm

The conventional rejection of the psychotic/non-psychotic distinction can be traced in part to a paper by Aubrey Lewis published in 1934. Emphasizing the wide variety of senses of insight, Aubrey Lewis proposed a provisional definition for the use of the term in medical contexts as "a correct attitude to a morbid change in oneself". After carefully elaborating this definition (as discussed below) he then applied it to a range of clinical cases. This showed that insight, so defined, could be lacking in a number of conditions—physical as well as mental—not traditionally regarded as psychotic, while on the other hand it could be present in some cases of psychotic disorder. He thus concluded that the psychotic/non-psychotic distinction is false in principle and had outlived whatever usefulness it may once have had. This conclusion could have been (could still be) right. In our attempts to order and make sense of the world we often adopt distinctions which turn out to be spurious. We tend to see shapes in the clouds, as Kendell has noted, writing of psychiatric classification (1975). Some distinctions, indeed, have been readily enough abandoned in the face of empirical or conceptual considerations; the distinction between endogenous and reactive depression, for example. But as we have seen the psychotic/non-psychotic distinction has not been abandoned. Fifty years on from Aubrey Lewis, and despite attempts to exclude it from our classifications, it remains in active use. Which suggests that it is clinically useful. And this in turn suggests that it is not the concept of insight which we should abandon but the Aubrey Lewis definition.

There are various ways in which one might search for a different definition. One approach is to look more closely at Aubrey Lewis' definition in order to see whether it can be fine-tuned to meet the requirements of clinical usage. This shows that his definition implies, indeed depends on, a conventional disease model of mental illness. That is to say, the "morbid change" to which Aubrey Lewis takes insight to involve a "correct attitude", means morbid as understood from the doctor's perspective; it involves essentially factual or descriptive considerations; and these relate the patient's condition to disease entities defined (ultimately) in terms of disturbances of functioning. Thus, in Aubrey Lewis' words, insight is all to do with "knowledge", with "data of change", with viewing symptoms "objectively", and, presaging a later paper on the nature of health (1955), "with the integration of ... part function ..." Moreover, a "correct" attitude to a morbid change in oneself, turns out to be no less than an attitude which approximates to "that of the physician". Unpacking Aubrey Lewis' definition in this way, however, suggests that rather more than fine-tuning would be needed to adapt it to clinical usage. For the disease model itself is in many respects inconsistent with the clinical features of insight outlined a moment ago. The disease model is derived from physical medicine (Fulford 1991), whereas psychotic loss of insight is a feature (feature 1 above) of mental disorders. Similarly, the disease model is derived from physical disease, whereas psychotic loss of insight is a feature (feature 2 above) of mental illness. It might seem that the disease model should fare better with individual psychotic symptoms (feature 3 above): hallucinations, in particular, have been successfully analyzed in terms of impaired functioning (Horowitz 1975). However delusions, which in clinical phenomenology are integral to psychotic hallucinations (Jaspers 1913), have consistently evaded satisfactory analysis in these terms (Maher & Ross 1984). Hence even in respect of its instantiation in particular symptoms, the disease model fits at best uncomfortably with the phenomenology of psychotic loss of insight. While as to its ethical and legal significance (feature 4 above) it is wholly off-target. As Boorse, a proponent of the disease mode, has pointed out, accounts of irrationality in terms of impaired functioning may actually be inconsistent with the status of psychotic disorder as the central case of mental illness as an excuse in law (Boorse 1975). And the whole orientation of this approach, as a science-based approach, is at best tangential to ethical considerations.

None of this amounts to final proof that a disease-model is incapable of providing a satisfactory analysis of the meaning of psychosis. But it does suggest that a change of tack may be worthwhile. Instead of fine-tuning the Aubrey Lewis approach, that is, we could try tackling the meaning of insight from a different perspective altogether. This leads naturally to an approach from the perspective of the patient's experience of illness rather than the doctor's knowledge of disease.

4. The Meaning of Insight—an Illness Paradigm

Consistently with the disease-orientation of most doctors, the experience of illness has until recently been largely neglected by the medical profession. It has been at the focus of interest of other professions concerned with health care, however. The "lived experience" of illness is at the heart of nursing theory for example (Mckee 1991), and the characteristics of this experience have been described in detail in sociological theories of deviance (Parsons 1951). Philosophers, too, have made a contribution, with detailed analyses of the meaning of illness, and of its logical relationships with other concepts, including that of disease (Boorse 1975, Fulford 1989, ch.3).

Work of this kind has brought out the extent to which the experience of illness differs from medical models of disease. For a start, illness is overtly value-laden (Sedgwick 1973)—it is as a negatively evaluated experience that illness prompts us to seek medical help, for example. It is also, though, a particular kind of negatively evaluated experience—it is illness, not, say, wickedness or foolishness, which prompts us to seek (specifically) medical help. Just how this particular kind of negatively evaluated experience is to be analyzed is a large question. The disease model suggests that illness is to be understood merely as a condition caused by an underlying disturbance of functioning (Boorse 1975). But authors writing from the perspective of illness theory have emphasized the primary importance of incapacity, of the experience of being unable to do things which one can ordinarily do. In the sociological tradition, this is integral to Talcott Parsons' (1951) now classical work on the varieties of deviance; and it comes through clearly in Lockyer's (1981) more empirical studies. It is to be found in a different guise in the emphasis on empowerment in theories of care (Alderson 1990). Among philosophical theories, it is central to my own work (1989) and an important theme in a number of Scandinavian studies of the medical concepts (Nordenfelt 1987).

It is the notion of incapacity, or failure of action, which is the key to understanding psychotic loss of insight in terms of the experience of illness. There is a sense in which this takes us into all the complexities of the philosophy of action. These, indeed, and other areas of philosophy, are highly relevant to a full understanding of the experience of illness, and this in turn is necessary to a complete account of insight (Fulford 1989, ch.7). Without going into all this, however, there is an element of the experience of illness as incapacity which, as we will see, is highly illuminating to the concept of insight.

Thus incapacity (my arm becoming paralyzed, say) is distinguished experientially as something wrong with me, both from things that are done or happen to me (my arm being prevented from moving, perhaps by someone holding it still) and also from things that I do (my arm not moving because I am not moving it). This two-way distinction can be shown to be a very general feature of the experience of illness (Fulford 1989, ch.7-10). Hence lack of insight could be understood in terms of this same two-way distinction. Lack of insight, that is to say, an "incorrect attitude" in Aubrey Lewis' terms, could mean misconstruing something wrong with me either as something that is being done or is happening to me, or as something that I am doing. As we will see, there is more to it than just this. But the power of an illness-theory rather than disease-theory approach is shown by the fact that, alone and unanalyzed, this idea takes us a long way towards an account of the particular kind of loss of insight by which psychotic disorders are characterized. This will now be illustrated by considering the differential diagnoses of a number of specific psychotic symptoms.

4.1 Thought Insertion

Thought insertion is an important psychotic symptom. In the absence of cognitive impairment it is one of the defining characteristics of schizophrenia (Gelder et al. 1983). Yet it has been almost entirely neglected in accounts of the nature of psychosis. This is perhaps surprising given that it is such an odd symptom. Most symptoms are understandable as extensions, in intensity and/or duration, of normal experiences. But thought insertion is qualitatively different from normal thinking. It is the experience of having someone else's thoughts in your head. There are thoughts there which you are thinking and yet which you experience as the thoughts of some other person. Mellor (1970) gives an example of this: "The thoughts of Eamonn Andrews come into my mind. There are no other thoughts there, only his." Similarly, in Leff and Isaacs (1990) we find "I'm picking up thoughts from other people. Its like being a receiving station."

The sheer oddity of thought insertion means that it has to be carefully differentiated from other superficially similar experiences, normal as well as pathological. It must be distinguished, first, from one's thoughts being merely influenced by others. Thinking is something we do. It is in a sense most intimately our own. But as with other things that we do, we may be to a greater or lesser extent influenced in what we think by other people. This is a normal experience. It is also one to which psychotic patients may give unusual twists. Hypomanic patients, for example, may claim that their thoughts are inspired by God. Depressives may believe that their thoughts are under the influence of the Devil. Schizophrenic patients may believe that they are being influenced telepathically. But in all these cases the person concerned retains the experience of thinking their own thoughts. Their thoughts may be deeply influenced by some other agency. But there is not the experience, as in thought insertion, of the thoughts themselves being those of that other agent.

Thought insertion has also to be distinguished from all the various ways in which one's thoughts may be to a greater or lesser extent out of control. Much of our thinking, like most of the things we do, is more or less automatic. Yet it remains our own. Creative thinking, notably, though invariably dependent on hard preparatory work, is often actually blocked by deliberate goal-directed thought. Solutions arrive in our minds apparently spontaneously when our attention is directed elsewhere. But we have no inclination to disclaim responsibility for such solutions. Then again, we may sometimes be unable to get a particular thought out of our mind. This may be because it is, say, emotionally charged, as in grief. But it may also be apparently senseless, for example when a tune gets "stuck in one's head". Obsessional symptoms are like this but in an extreme form. Obsessional thoughts, moreover, especially if they are violent or sexual in nature, are sometimes described by the patient as not their own. Even here though, there is no suggestion that they are the thoughts of some other agency (Sims 1988). What is meant is simply that such thoughts are wholly out of character.

Table 1: A differential illness-diagnosis of thought disorder

Phenomenon	Construal					
	by patient			by others		
Thoughts in patients mind	done by	wrong with	done to	done by	wrong with	done to
Normal thoughts	+			+		
Thoughts influenced by others	+			+		
Obsessional thoughts		+				+
Thought insertion			+			+

Returning now to the experience of illness it will be apparent that the phenomena just described can be distributed across the two-way distinction by which this experience is defined. This indeed generates a differential diagnostic table—what I have called elsewhere a differential illness-diagnostic table (Fulford 1989, ch.10)—of the kind illustrated in Table 1. The left-hand column of the table lists the four varieties of thought just described: normal thinking, thoughts influenced by others, obsessional thoughts and thought insertion. The remainder of the table shows how these are construed by the patient and by others in terms of the two-way distinction—the done by/wrong with/done to distinction—by which the experience of illness is characterized. What is shown by this is that with thought insertion, and only with thought insertion, there is a mis-match between the way the experience is construed by the patient and the way it is construed by others. Normal thinking is construed by the patient and by others as something he or she does. One's thoughts being influenced by others is construed by the patient and by others as something (in part) done to them. Obsessional thoughts are construed by the patient and by others as something wrong with him or her. But thought insertion is construed by the patient as something that is being done to him or her, while everyone else construes it as a symptom, as something wrong.

Table 2: A more extensive differential illness-diagnosis of thought disorder

Phenomenon	Construal					
	by patient			by others		
	done by	wrong with	done to	done by	wrong with	done to
Normal thoughts	++			++		
Thoughts influenced by others	++ -		+ -	++ -		+ -
Obsessional thoughts		++			++	
Thought insertion (full)			++		++	
Thought insertion (partial)	+ -	+	+ -		++	
Flight of ideas	++				++	
Flight of ideas (partial insight)	++ -	+ -			++	

A more extensive differential illness-diagnosis of thought insertion is shown in Table 2. This has essentially the same structure as Table 1: varieties of thought in the left-hand column distributed across the done by/wrong with/done to distinction, as construed first by the patient and then by others. In this table, however, locations are indicated by two +s instead of one, allowing the representation of intermediate or partial cases. Thus partial thought insertion is the experience of thoughts inserted into one's mind but from one's own subconscious. Hence this incomplete alienation of thought appears in the table partly as a "done to" and partly as a "done by" experience for the patient. There may however be a degree of insight into this symptom, represented in the table as a shift in the patient's construal of their experience to the "wrong with" column. Flight of ideas provides a second example of this shift. Flight of ideas is a symptom of hypomania in which the patient's thoughts race from subject to subject, linked by meaning, pun, rhyme, or other association, but in a wild progression. The hypomanic patient characteristically lacks insight in that he or she experiences this as something they are doing (i.e thinking), and doing in a particularly inspired way. But as the condition begins to resolve the patient may gain partial insight, acknowledging at least the possibility that their speeding thoughts may be abnormal.

4.2 Hallucinations and Delusions

Thought insertion, although interesting in its own right, may be considered something of a rarity. The above analysis can readily be extended, however, to the perhaps more familiar psychotic symptoms of hallucination and delusion. Thus hallucinations are standardly defined broadly as perceptions occurring in the absence of a stimulus. Their differential diagnosis can be set out diagrammatically in a table (Table 3) similar to that illustrated above for thought insertion. As Table 3 shows, however, there is the added complication that perception is normally something that is in part passive (being induced by the environment and hence a "done to"experience) as well as being in part active (and hence a "done by" experience). Hallucinations have thus to be differentiated both from illusions, which as distortions of a stimulus are "done to" experiences (we are "tricked by the light", for example), and from imagery, which, however vivid, remains under voluntary control (Gelder et al. 1983) and hence is a "done by" experience.

As Table 3 also shows, however, there is more to a true or psychotic hallucination than merely a perception in the absence of a stimulus. In the first place true hallucinations are persistent. The tired doctor who hears the phone ring as she drops off to sleep is not psychotic. She readily accepts the switchboard operator's explanation that she "must have imagined it". Secondly, true hallucinations involve a persistent belief in the reality of the perceived object. Hallucinations can be highly persistent and yet recognized for what they are. This indeed may be especially so with chronic or recurrent psychotic disorders. The more acutely ill patient, however, not only believes in their hallucinations but clings to them even in the face of apparently disconfirmatory evidence. A patient who is shown that there is no one in the room in which they heard people talking about them, will claim that the people concerned have climbed out of the window, or that their voices were projected electronically, or even that they are invisible.

Table 3: A differential illness-diagnosis of hallucinations

Phenomenon	Construal					
Perception	by patient			by others		
	done by	wrong with	done to	done by	wrong with	done to
Normal	+		+	+		+
Illusion			++			++
Imagery	++			++		
Hallucination (brief)	++	+		++	+	
	−	−		−	−	
Pseudohallucination (partial)	+	+		+	+	
Hallucination (true)	+		+		++	

All of this is fully consistent with an illness-theory analysis of psychotic loss of insight. Persistence is a well recognized feature of all illness experience, physical as well as mental. Moreover the patient who recognizes their hallucinations for what they are is said to show "partial insight"; and hallucinations of this kind are described standardly as one form of "pseudohallucination" (Hare 1973). But the introduction of belief suggests that it is delusion which underpins the true psychotic hallucination. This is a contentious suggestion. It has been argued that delusions can be explained as attempts to account for anomalous perceptual experiences (Maher and Ross 1984). The more traditional view, however, makes delusions the central psychotic symptom (Jaspers 1913). This is reflected in our standard terminology; the elaboration of beliefs in support of hallucinations is called "delusional elaboration" (Wing et al. 1974); and thought insertion is sometimes actually classified as a delusion (Sims 1988). The traditional view, furthermore, has a degree of face-validity. After all, the most natural explanation of anomalous perceptual experiences is not "invisible people" and so forth, but, where these experiences are persistent, that there is "something wrong". This indeed is the explanation which the epileptic with "forced thoughts", an experience not unlike thought insertion, more or less readily accepts (Lishman, personal communication).

There is an important sense then, in which delusions are at the heart of the phenomenology of psychotic loss of insight. And with delusions we move from the experience of illness as such, to the analysis of this experience in terms of incapacity. This leads us, as anticipated, into the deep waters of the philosophy of action. I have discussed this in detail elsewhere (Fulford 1989, ch.10). But the steps in the argument are essentially these. Delusions can be distributed according to their content across the two-way distinction by which illness is defined: delusions of persecution, for example, are "done to" experiences; delusions of guilt are "done by" experiences; and even delusions concerned with matters apparently remote from the patient are "done to" or "done by" experiences to the extent that they are imbued with personal significance (Wing et al. 1974). But, as with other psychotic symptoms, not all delusions (i.e false beliefs) are psychotic. Indeed it is not the content but the form of a belief which is crucial to its status as a psychotic symptom. This has been evident clinically for some time from the occurrence, as in the so-called Othello syndrome (Shepherd 1961), of beliefs which though concordant with fact are nonetheless delusional (i.e psychotic). It is also evident logically from the occurrence of the otherwise paradoxical delusion of mental illness (Fulford, 1989 ch.10).

Just how the form of a delusional belief is to be analyzed is a matter of considerable controversy (Hemsley and Garety 1986). But delusions have turned out to be highly resistant to analysis in conventional disease-theory terms. Delusions are in some sense irrational beliefs and hence might be expected to be analyzable in terms of impaired cognitive functioning. But while ancillary symptoms (such as impaired memory in dementia) may be analyzed in these terms, the best efforts of the cognitive psychologists have thus far failed to identify an impairment of cognitive functioning which is characteristic of delusions. Illness-theory, on the other hand, drawing on the philosophy of action, suggests that the irrationality of delusional thinking should be understood in terms not of defective cognitive functioning but rather of impaired reasons for action. This provides an analysis of delusions which is consistent with the full range of their remarkable phenomenology, including not only rarities like true beliefs and the delusion of mental illness, but also the commonplace if poorly recognized delusional value judgments. It also explains the central place of delusions in relation to other psychotic symptoms. And it can be shown to assimilate delusion to "lack of intent", and thus to go part way towards an explanation of the particular ethical and legal significance of psychotic disorders (Fulford 1989, ch. 10).

5. Conclusions

The main purpose of this article has been to illustrate the way in which switching from a disease to an illness paradigm can help to illuminate the concept of psychotic loss of insight implicit in everyday clinical work in psychiatry. The relevant features of the concept were first made explicit by the use of a case-vignette questionnaire. Theories of the meaning of insight developed within a disease paradigm were then shown to be inconsistent with these features. An illness paradigm on the other hand has now provided an account which in principle covers each of them: such an account is neutral with regard to mental and physical disorders, the two-way distinction by which illness is defined being a feature of both; it is, by definition, concerned with mental illness rather than disease; it is compatible with and indeed explains a wide variety of the particular symptoms with which psychotic lack of insight is associated; and it explains the particular ethical and legal significance of loss of insight of this kind.

The two paradigms, however, illness and disease, should not be thought to be incompatible. On the contrary, like the perspectives they represent, that of patient and doctor respectively, they are mutually complementary. The disease paradigm has become prominent in medical thinking essentially because of the success of medical science. It is therefore far from redundant. This is true not least in relation to insight. There are many kinds of loss of insight which are better analyzed in terms of the disease paradigm: failure to "see" a symptom, to recognize its cause, and so forth, as noted earlier. Severe cognitive defects, for instance, as in confusional states and dementias, often involve a lack of insight in the sense of simply not being aware that anything is wrong. Much the same is true, though in a different way, with the remarkable denial of disability shown by some patients with parietal lobe lesions (Lishman 1987). All such defects of insight are in principle straightforwardly analyzable as impairments of cognitive functioning.

This of course is not to undermine our analysis of psychotic loss of insight in terms of an illness paradigm. On the contrary it emphasizes the specificity of such an account. The point is rather that if the disease paradigm is not redundant it is also not sufficient. In itself it provides us with what I have called elsewhere only a half-field or hemianopic view of medicine (Fulford 1989, ch.12). And the value of philosophical analysis in this area is that it can help to increase the conceptual resources of medicine by making the other half-field visible, by giving us a more complete or whole-field view of the subject. As we have seen, this is important theoretically. But it is also important practically. The questionnaire study described at the start of this chapter illustrates the degree of consensus that is possible in psychiatry in relation even to such contentious issues as involuntary psychiatric treatment. But it also shows that even within a single clinical department there can be important areas of disagreement (cases 1 and 3, to be specific). A full-field view of medicine may not in itself resolve such disagreements but it could help to provide a better understanding of what they consist in.[1]

1 Acknowledgements: Tables 1 and 3 are adapted from my Moral Theory and Medical Practice and are reproduced here by kind permission of Cambridge University Press. I am grateful to Dr. Anthony David for his helpful comments.

Summary

Despite its continued active use in clinical research and practice, the notion of psychotic disorder, marked by loss of insight, has been widely considered too obscure in meaning for it to be retained in modern psychopathologies. The difficulties of definition of psychotic loss of insight are shown to be due to the adoption of a disease paradigm of mental disorder, one based on medical knowledge of disease processes. In terms of an illness paradigm on the other hand, derived from certain general features of the patient's actual experience of illness, psychotic loss of insight is found to be relatively transparent in meaning. This is illustrated by an analysis of the differential diagnoses of certain key psychotic symptoms—thought insertion, hallucination and delusion. It is emphasized, however, that disease and illness paradigms of mental disorder are nonetheless complementary parts of the conceptual structure of medicine.

References

Alderson P: Choosing for children: parents' consent to surgery. Oxford, Oxford University Press, 1990

American Psychiatric Association: Diagnostic and statistical manual of mental disorders (third edition). Washington, DC, American Psychiatric Association, 1980

Boorse C: On the distinction between disease and illness. Philosophy and Public Affairs 5: 61-84, 1975

Butler Rt Hon, the Lord: Chairman, Report of the Committee on Mentally Abnormal Offenders, Cmnd., 6244. London, Her Majestey's Stationery Office, 1975

David AS: Insight and psychosis. British Journal of Psychiatry 156: 798-808, 1990

Fulford KWM: Moral theory and medical practice. Cambridge University Press, 1989

Fulford KWM: Philosophy and medicine: the Oxford connection. British Journal of Psychiatry 157: 111-115, 1990

Fulford KWM: The concept of disease. In: Bloch S, Chodoff P (Eds): Psychiatric ethics (second edition), ch. 6, pp. 77–99. Oxford University Press, 1991

Gelder MG, Gath D, Mayou R: Oxford textbook of psychiatry. Oxford University Press, 1983

Grubin DH: Unfit to plead in England and Wales, 1967-88, a survey. British Journal of Psychiatry 158: 540-548, 1991

Hare EH: A short note on pseudo-hallucinations. British Journal of Psychiatry, 122: 469-76, 1973

Hemsley DR, Garety PA: The formation and maintenance of delusions: a Bayesian analysis. British Journal of Psychiatry 149: 51-6, 1986

Horowitz MJ: A cognitive model of hallucinations. American Journal of Psychiatry 132: 789-795, 1975

Jaspers K: General psychopathology (first published in 1913). Transl. by Hoenig J & Hamilton MW. Manchester University Press, 1963

Kendell RE: The role of diagnosis in psychiatry. Oxford, Blackwell Scientific Publications, 1975

Leff JP, Isaacs AP: Psychiatric Examination in Clinical Practice. Third edition. Oxford, Blackwell Scientific Publications, 1990

Lewis AJ: The psychopathology of insight. British Journal of Medical Psychology 14: 332-48, 1934

Lewis AJ: Health as a social concept. British Journal of Sociology 4: 109-24, 1955

Lishman AW: Organic psychiatry. Second edition. Oxford: Blackwell Scientific Publications, 1987

Lockyer D: Symptoms and illness: the cognitive organization of disorder. London and New York, Tavistock Publications, 1981

Maher B, Ross JS: Delusions. In: Adams HE, Suther P (eds): Comprehensive handbook of psychology, ch. 14, pp. 383–409. New York, Plenum Press, 1984

Mckee C: Breaking the mould: a humanistic approach to nursing practice. In: McMahon R, Pearson A (Eds): Nursing as Therapy, ch. 8, pp. 170–191. Suffolk, Chapman and Hall, 1991

Mellor CS: First rank symptoms of schizophrenia. British Journal of Psychiatry 117: 15-23, 1970

Nordenfelt L: On the nature of health; an action-theoretic approach. Dordrecht, Holland, Reidel, 1987

Parsons T: The social system. Glencoe, Illinois, Free Press, 1951

Sedgwick P: Illness—mental and otherwise. The Hastings Center Studies I, 3: pp. 19-40 Institute of Society, Ethics and the Life Sciences, Hastings-on-Hudson, New York, 1973

Shepherd M: Morbid jealousy: Some clinical and social aspects of a psychiatric syndrome. Journal of Mental Science 107: 687-704, 1961

Sims A: Symptoms in the mind; an introduction to descriptive psychopathology. London, Bailliere Tindall, 1988

Walker N: Psychiatric explanations as excuses. In: Roth M, Bluglass R (eds): Psychiatry, human rights and law, ch. 9, pp. 96–113. Cambridge University Press, 1985

Wing JK, Cooper JE, Sartorius N: Measurement and classification of psychiatric symptoms. Cambridge University Press, 1974

Wittgenstein L: Philosophical investigations (2nd ed). Transl. by Anscombe GEM Oxford, Basil Blackwell, 1958

World Health Organization: Mental disorders: glossary and guide to their classification in accordance with the ninth revision of the International classification of diseases. Geneva, WHO, 1978

World Health Organization: Mental disorders: glossary and guide to their classification in accordance with the tenth revision of the International classification of diseases—draft. Geneva, WHO, 1991

M. Spitzer, F.A. Uehlein
M.A. Schwartz, C. Mundt
(eds.): Phenomenology
Language & Schizophrenia.
Springer-Verlag, New York, 1992

Subjectivity, Error Correction Capacity, and the Pathogenesis of Delusions of Reference

Hinderk M. Emrich

1. Introduction

One of the major goals in recent developments in understanding the constitutional factors leading to schizophrenic disorders is the unification of different aspects of psychotic psychopathology within one single neuropsychological principle. The present paper aims at a discussion of this aspect of schizophrenia research within the perspective of the concepts of censorship-impairment, error-correction dysfunction and the systems theory approach of "comparator-systems", in relation to the psychopathology of delusions of reference.

2. Comparator-Systems

Within the recent past, out of neuropsychological considerations regarding the pathogenesis of anxiety and fear, the concept of "comparator-systems" (Gray & Rawlins 1986) has emerged, leading to a deeper understanding of many of the phenomena of psychopathology and behavior. Furthermore, utilizing the perspectives of the theory of dynamic processes and self-organization, systems theory has provided an instrument to describe the relations between "endo-systems" and "exo-systems" (cf. Wassenaar et al. 1992), thereby leading to a better formalization of the description of subjective phenomena. In this essay, these concepts will undergird a systemic explanation of the pathogenesis of delusions of reference in psychotic disorders.

The essence of "hippocampal comparator systems" is that they are memory-driven, i.e. that they are able to relate actual events to representations of the past, representations of stored regularities, which are called "world models". In pure sensualism or so-called "naïve realism", perception is assumed to be a unidimensional unidirectional process in which the objective reality is simply imaged by the combination of sensory inputs with data processing, in the sense of using a camera and microphone and a data-handling computer. This, however, is an oversimplification. Before sensory data processing is possible, a primary conceptualization (a hypotheses-generating process) has to be realized which belongs to a world-model in the sense of the "betting of proposals" regarding possible "reality-fictions" (cf. Gregory 1973).

Such a conceptualizing world-model also plays a central role within the concept of hippocampal comparator-systems. According to Gray and Rawlins (1986) the comparator generates plans and predictions on the basis of stored regularities, and the exo-system, the structure of "the world" has an influence on this through actual sensory data. In the instance of greater discrepancies between predictions and actual data, a signal arises in the sense of "alarm" which is interpreted by cognition and emotional systems as fear and anxiety. Antianxiety drugs are assumed to exert their tranquilizing effects by the impairment of a behavioral inhibition system which is activated by the above–mentioned comparator–triggered "alarm", thereby leading to a greater degree of "buffering" of behavior against discrepancies between prediction and actual events. Comparator-systems are not only capable of explaining the psychopharmacological effects of antianxiety drugs, they also are suitable in understanding the actions of psychedelic compounds.

Recently, Devane et al. (1989) have demonstrated the existence of specific cannabinoid-receptors in hippocampal and related systems. Thus, neuropsychological effects exerted by cannabinoids, such as tetrahydro-cannabinol (THC), may be interpreted as effects on such world-models-containing hippocampal comparator-systems. This can be demonstrated e.g. by the use of the 3-dimensional depth inversion illusion (Emrich 1989). When the directions of the disparities of retinal images are exchanged artificially, hollow objects have to be perceived as convex ones and vice versa; however, due to internal censorship in the instance of semantically meaningful objects incorporated into the world-model of the comparator-system, this inverted 3-dimensional depth is not perceived: the censorship-induced reorganization of the sensory data represents an illusionary perception of the outer world. Under the influence of THC this illusion is strongly impaired (Emrich et al. 1991).

An additional feature of comparator-systems, which is of greatly philosophical importance, is that they are "intentional", i.e. they can handle "meaning". How intentionality is realized neurobiologically is not known; only "quasi-intentionality" is—to some extent—understood. In this instance, intentionality is only a projection into a self-organizing or a cybernetic system which is programmed to fulfill a "goal"; however, the interpretation of goal-directedness is a perspective from the exo-point of view and not an intrinsic feature of the system. It may, however, turn out that this view about "quasi-intentionality" contains some truth: Whatever we know about intentionality, whatever we can argue about an intentional system, we derive from an "exo"–point of view insofar as we—also in the instance of observing ourselves—are "exo"–observers, and the real "machinery" which brings about our intentions is hidden from us. In biological systems "quasi-intentionality" is explored and explained using theories of synergetics, i.e., the theories of (dissipative) dynamical systems under the aspect of "self–organization" (cf. Becker 1991); here aspects of "neural darwinism" (Edelman 1987), i.e. considerations about evolutionary dynamics, are discussed. It should be mentioned, however, that intentionality from an intrinsic point of view represents self-transcendence of a system and that, obviously, this self-transcendence has to do with coupling between the endo– and exo–parts of the system–totality.

3. Subjectivity

The problems of subjectivity are basically related to the phenomena of "meaning", "representation", and the relation between "wholeness" and the having of a "point of view". Basic questions investigate how the relationship between external reality (S) (in an exo-world, an exo-system) and internal reality ($\sum$) (in the endo-system) is constituted.

According to the quantum-physicist Atmanspacher this problem may be formalized in the following way:

> "Consider a situation where I observe how another observer perceives an event. From my point of view the corresponding interaction belongs purely to S. The observer himself, however, will state that an interaction between S and $\sum$ has taken place, namely a process of representation. ... An interactive understanding of events in S provides an additional complication. It destroys the unidirectional character of the representation - the interactive interpretation implies that any representation S → $\sum$ is a "presentation" $\sum$ → S at the same time" (Atmanspacher 1992)

The question of generating "objectivity" and the problem of raising a "scientific" description of *internal* and *external* reality of the situation may be formulated within the terminology of Thomas Nagel as the task of construing the "view from nowhere", i.e. the "god-eye's view", of totality-reconstruction. How is one subjective perspective related to this asymptotic view of the construction of wholeness, of objectivity, and a perspectiveless view of the total? To some extent, the endo-system must construe a view-independent, view-invariant model of the exo-system, the "world". In this remote, to some extent "absolute" reconstruction of the situation of the system the "ego", the representation of the "endo-system", itself is only partially or not at all occurring.

This has an interesting implication: subjectivity is not at all present in this absolute, perspectiveless system, i.e., a system which is not able to care of an exo-system, since subjectivity is the relation of the "self" to the "not-self" or the perspective *on* the self and *of* the self in relation to (or so to say, in "comparison" to) the outer world.

Thus, subjectivity generally contains the philosophical aspect of mediating something which is hermetically closed like a windowless

Leibnizian monad with an "open" system or at least—in the sense of Maturana (1982)—a system which can be "perturbated" by an outer reality; and the perspectives of the endo-system in regard to these "perturbations" are the "subjective" ones.

However, the construction of an "objective" and to some extent invariant outer reality is a very remote and sophisticated higher development of a system. Questions occur, such as how disturbances of this high development may take place and which consequences for the system may result.

4.   Error-correction and Delusions of Reference

Fundamentally, error-correction capability may be regarded as an ability of a system to correct, to eliminate, to reformulate, to work-over, and to reorganize intentional representations. If it is true that the representation of outer reality has to construe a great degree of subject-invariance, it follows that the ego, the subjective point of view, has to be withdrawn and be eliminated from the world construction of outer reality (which is construed from perturbation-data within the endo-system). This internal reconstruction of perturbation-data results, for example, in the subjective impression that to see and have vision does not mean to perceive light beams but rather to become aware of objects in the neighborhood, i.e. to be closely related to objects. When we close our eyes we do not believe the object is disappearing but know that it is continuously present only we do not observe it presently. This is due to the partial subject-invariance and partial subject-independency of our world construction, i.e., of our internally presented intentional world-model.

However, if this ability to create a quasi subject-unrelated objective exo-world is impaired by an insufficiency of the "correction-system" (which normally reformulates the data from the subjective point of view in a way that "objectivity" results), different types of "world-experience-disturbances" have to be anticipated.

From a constructivistic point of view one may argue that delusions represent not or only partially communicable reality-constructions, which often manifest themselves especially in abnormal assumptions about causal relationships i.e., delusions represent interpersonally not agreeable world models. Thus, two types of delusions have to be anticipated: Those which arise due to primary distortions of the reality-construing neurobiological machinery, and secondly, those which depend on disturbed value-balances in self-esteem. (However, since valuating functions may also depend upon neuropsychological/neurobiological factors, primary delusions of self-esteem may also be possible.) The delusions discussed here are of the first type. The disturbance I would like to discuss in this way is the impairment of the ability to *eliminate* the subject. It may be regarded as a form of a "regression" (in a non-analytical understanding). The reformulation of the world-relation of the subject is disturbed in a way that leads to the experience that everything is related to me in a positive or a negative manner, i.e.

it may be a relation of prosecution or a relation of abnormal grandiosity of myself.

Relating this to the above mentioned effects of psychedelic compounds one may state that psychedelics obviously create a world-relation in which the objectifying abilities of the endo-system are impaired, leading to an increase in the subjectivity of the point of view of the subject. A similar kind of regression may take place in psychosis during the generation of delusions of reference. Finally, it should be mentioned that similar hypotheses can be expressed regarding the psychopathology of schizophrenic disturbances of the structure of the ego, namely splitting phenomena as well as disturbances of the ego/environment-borders.

Summary

Delusions of references appear to be due to disturbances of the ability of the system to eliminate the subjective point of view in apperception of "the world". In subjectivity, active processes of self-relation take place in the sense that object-constitution to some extent eliminates the subjective point of view and construes the "view from nowhere". Consequently, subjectivity means the establishment of a very refined artificial fictional world that always is corrected for naïve intentional data which would represent a non–relative point of view. Therefore, to reach and stabilize subjectivity means to continuously correct a naïve ego-related world. To be psychotic, however, means to regressively fall back from this refined and corrected artificial world and to thereby acquire the delusion: everything and everybody relates to me. From a systems-theory perspective, this means being in a disturbed state involving impairment of data correction by the endo-system.

References

Atmanspacher H: Categoreal and acategoral representation of knowledge. Cognitive Systems, (in press) 1992

Becker J: Evolutionary systems as prototypes for self-organization. Paper presented at a workshop on "The Paradigm of Self-Organization II" in Wildbad Kreuth, September 4-6, 1991

Devane WA, Dysarz FA, Johnson MR, Melvin LS, Howlett AC: Determination and characterization of a cannabinoid receptor in rat brain. Molec Pharmacol 34: 605-613, 1988

Edelman GM: Neural darwinism: the theory of neuronal group selection. New York, Basic Books, 1987

Emrich HM: A three-component-system-hypothesis of psychosis. Impairment of binocular depth inversion as an indicator of a functional dysequilibrium. Brit J Psychiatry 155 (suppl 5): 37-39, 1989

Emrich HM, Weber MM, Wendl A, Zihl J, von Meyer L, Hanisch W: Reduced binocular depth inversion as an indicator of cannabis-induced censorship-impairment. Pharmacol Biochem Behav 40 (in press), 1991

Gray JA, Rawlins JNP: Comparator and buffer memory: an attempt to integrate two models of hippocampal functions. In: Isaacson RL, Pribram KH (eds) The hippocampus, vol. 4. New York, Plenum Press, pp 159-201, 1986

Gregory RL: The confounded eye. In: Gregory RL, Gombrich EH (eds): Illusion in nature and art, pp 49-96. Oxford, Freeman, 1973

Maturana HR: Erkennen: Die Organisation und Verkörperung von Wirklichkeit. Braunschweig, Vieweg, 1982

Wassenaar JS, Hesselink HF, Pesso A: The representation of interactions and the neurobiology of subjectivity; applications in psychotherapy. In: Dalenoort GJ (ed): Self-Organization (in press) 1992

Name Index

Coleridge ST 75, 76, 79,
85
Conley RR 251
Conrad K 222
Cornblatt BA 241
Cramer P 177, 178
Crider A 228
Crockett D 274, 286
Cromwell R 264
Cromwell RL 298
Crow TJ 155, 240, 241,
251, 267, 270
Cutting J 126, 132, 222,
224, 274

Danziger K 117
Darwin C 332
David AS 321, 322,
324, 356
Dawson DFL 211
Dawson E 291, 297,
298
de Man P 141
Deese J 160, 203
Degkwitz R 123
DeJong R 262
DeLisi LE 274
Derrida J 78
Descartes R 135
Devane WA, 373
Dilthey W 39, 40, 50,
64, 151
Dixon WJ 247
Dreyfus H 128, 141
Driesch H 118
Edelman GM 374
Edwards W 232
Einhorn HJ 234
Ekman P 332
Emrich HM 14, 373
Endicott J 241
Eriksen BA 229
Eriksen CW 229
Ewald G 147
Exner S 161, 162

Falkai P 235
Faust D 123
Fischer 1925
Fischoff B 232
Fish B 266
Fish FJ 155
Fisher M 186
Flaum M 241
Fliess W 162

Flor-Henry P 274, 285
Francis WN 184
Fraser WI 201
Freeman T 262
Frege, G 50
Freud S 130, 161, 162
Friedreich N 17
Frith CD 224, 231, 292
Frommer J 11, 28, 211,
214, 215
Fulford KWM 14, 321,
322, 326, 328, KWM
331, 356, 361, 362,
364, 368, 369
Fünfgeld M 12
Funke G 82
Fürstner C 17, 22

Gabrial TM 127
Gadamer H-G 49, 104
Gainotti G 274
Galton F 162, 163, 193
Garety RA 232, 233,
368
Garrett M 203
Gaupp R 17, 22
Gelade G 291
Gelder MG 355, 363,
366
George L 235
Gill MM 162
Gillett G 13, 322, 323
Gilmore GC 241
Glick M 336
Glucksberg S 182, 183,
332
Goetz KL 241
Goffmann E 242
Goldberg G 198, 207
Goldberg SC 251
Goldstein K 28
Golinkoff M 284
Gorham DR 37
Gosset 1965
Gould LN 208
Gray JA 221, 236, 372
Green M 241, 250
Gregory RL 373
Griesinger W 18, 119,
147, 153, 211
Grinnell F 104
Gross G 246
Grubin DH 360
Gruhle H-W 13, 21, 22,
24, 27, 151, 153,

156, 240, 334, 336,
338, 342, 344
Gudden BA v 16
Gur RE 274, 284
Gurwitsch A

Haeckel E 120, 122
Häfner H 22-24
Hagen FW 13, 334-336,
340, 341, 343
Hahn R 169
Hall G 228
Halliday M 212
Hamilton M 247, 308
Hamilton W 50
Hanson NR
Hare EH 367
Harrow M 217, 228
Harrow M 230, 242
Hartley D 160
Harvey PD 250
Hasan R 212
Havens L 349
Hebb DO 180
Heelan PA 105
Hegel GFW 13, 79, 82
Heidegger M 9, 21, 49,
126-141
Heimer L 270
Hellwig P 212, 213
Helwig J 247
Hemingway EM 213
Hempel CG 109
Hemsley DR 11, 221-
224, 228, 231, 233-
235, 243, 368
Henrich D 217, 218
Heraucourt W 58
Herbart JF 149
Hess R 12, 292, 295,
299, 300
Hiller W 276
Hirsh SR 242
Hobson JA 162
Hoche AE 17, 22
Hoening J 50
Hoff P 8, 119, 149, 164
Hoffman RE 10, 148,
199, 201, 203-206,
209, 213, 215
Hogarth RM 234
Hogarty GE 242
Hölderlin F 9, 27, 129
Holm-Hadulla R 28
Holsboer F 285

Subject Index

grammatical analysis 200
grammatical deviances 201
Grundverhältnisstörung 218

habit 82
habitual attitudes 99
hallucinations 5, 43, 44, 97, 98, 106-
113, 129-131, 208, 300, 366, 367
and will 208
and language production processes
208, 209
Heidelberg 16-18, 21, 28, 29, 151
Psychiatric Hospital 8, 21, 22
School 28
hemispheric dysfunction 274
hermeneutics 65, 103, 105-113
horizonedness (Horizont) 79, 89
in phenomenology 83-86
humanities 39
Huntington's disease 260, 269
hybrid conceptions 92
hypotonia of consciousness 154

ICD-10 4, 123, 148, 355
idealism
relevance to psychopathology 217
idiographic vs. nomothetic 39
Illenau 16, 17
illness vs. disease paradigm of mental
disorder 360-363
immediate impression 79
incoherence 11, 147-158, 211-213
incorrigibility of delusions 305-317
indirect semantic associations 172,
189-190
information overload 230, 293, 298
information processing 42
inner speech 208, 209
insight 110, 321, 322, 327, 355-369
clinical use 356-360
definition 360-364
loss of 14
intentional acts 42, 72-74
intentional arc, span of 152
intentionality 42, 51, 54, 72, 73, 82
interpersonal relations
impaired in schizophjrenia 6, 13
interpersonal view
on schizophrenia 13
interpretation 60
interstimulus intervall (ISI) 186
intersubjectivity 13, 56
intrusions of associations
in schizophrenia 187

intuition 50-53, 55, 57, 58, 63
of essences 52, 55

knowledge, certainty of 54

language 6
deviances in schizophrenia 201
levels of analysis 7
mediating symptoms 7
language disturbances
monograph by Berze & Gruhle 27
language plans
in schizophrenia 11
language production 199
in schizophrenia 199
latent inhibition 224-228, 236
laterality 12, 274-287
lebendige Anschauung 50
left hemishpere dysfunction
in schizophrenia 230
lexical decision 184
required time 181
lexical ties 212
life-world (Lebenswelt) 70-72, 98
limited capacity channel 290, 295
linguistic philosophy 355
living intuition
as source of knowledge 50, 51

mannerisms 258, 259
mediated associations 172, 189-190
memory traces 183
Mental Health Act 358-360
mental lexicon 184
mental phenomena, constitution of 38
mind, representational view 322
mood 331
motor phenomena in schizophrenia
258-271
and formal thought disorder 259
motor synchrony deficit 265

Naturalism
in Kraepelin 122
negative schizophrenia 11
negative symptoms 155, 230, 241-244
and cognitive deficits 241
and neuropsychological dysfunction
241
hypotheses of occurrence 243, 244
in neurotic patients 249, 251
primary vs. secondary 243
social factors 242
neologisms 201